SELF AND EMOTIONAL LIFE

INSURRECTIONS:
CRITICAL STUDIES IN RELIGION,
POLITICS, AND CULTURE

INSURRECTIONS: CRITICAL STUDIES
IN RELIGION, POLITICS, AND CULTURE

SLAVOJ ŽIŽEK, CLAYTON CROCKETT, CRESTON DAVIS,
JEFFREY W. ROBBINS, EDITORS

The intersection of religion, politics, and culture is one of the most discussed areas in theory today. It also has the deepest and most wide-ranging impact on the world. Insurrections: Critical Studies in Religion, Politics, and Culture will bring the tools of philosophy and critical theory to the political implications of the religious turn. The series will address a range of religious traditions and political viewpoints in the United States, Europe, and other parts of the world. Without advocating any specific religious or theological stance, the series aims nonetheless to be faithful to the radical emancipatory potential of religion.

SELF

AND EMOTIONAL LIFE

PHILOSOPHY,
PSYCHOANALYSIS, AND
NEUROSCIENCE

ADRIAN JOHNSTON | CATHERINE MALABOU

COLUMBIA UNIVERSITY PRESS   NEW YORK

COLUMBIA UNIVERSITY PRESS
Publishers Since 1893
New York   Chichester, West Sussex
cup.columbia.edu
Copyright © 2013 Columbia University Press
All rights reserved

Library of Congress Cataloging-in-Publication Data

Johnston, Adrian, 1974–
Self and emotional life : philosophy, psychoanalysis, and neuroscience / Adrian Johnston
and Catherine Malabou.
p. cm. — (Insurrections)
Includes bibliographical references and index.
ISBN 978-0-231-15830-5 (cloth : alk. paper) — ISBN 978-0-231-15831-2 (pbk. : alk. paper) —
ISBN 978-0-231-53518-2 (e-book)
1.   Emotions. 2.   Self. 3.   Psychoanalysis. 4.   Neurosciences. 5.   Psychoanalysis and
philosophy. I. Malabou, Catherine. II. Title.

BF531.J64   2013
J28'.2—dc23
2012036488

Columbia University Press books are printed on permanent
and durable acid-free paper.
This book is printed on paper with recycled content.
Printed in the United States of America

Cover image: © *Illona Wellmann/Trevillion Images*
Cover design: *Lisa Hamm*

References to websites (URLs) were accurate at the time of writing.
Neither the author nor Columbia University Press is responsible for URLs
that may have expired or changed since the manuscript was prepared.

CONTENTS

PREFACE

FROM NONFEELING TO MISFEELING—
AFFECTS BETWEEN TRAUMA
AND THE UNCONSCIOUS

This book is the product of a fortuitous encounter between two people with significantly overlapping interests as well as fundamental convictions and intuitions held in common. Adding to this good fortune is the fact that they bring major differences of perspective to these shared grounds. This combination of agreement and disagreement provides an absolutely ideal foundation for productive exchange and stimulating debate.

Catherine and I met in April 2007 at the annual Theory Reading Group conference hosted by Cornell University. During that weekend of intense discussions, we quickly recognized each other as well-matched interlocutors. Our backgrounds in Hegelianism, concerns with psychoanalysis, and, especially, beliefs in the importance and urgency of engaging with today's life sciences on the basis of Continental European theoretical traditions from Kant to the present all converged to convince us that we needed to build a lasting collaborative relationship. Our feeling of kinship has been further reinforced by an impression of being together in a marginal position vis-à-vis the majority of Continentalists, with their antinaturalist proclivities and preferences, by virtue of our fascination with and enthusiasm for things biological. We remain convinced that no genuine materialist philosophy legitimately can neglect the natural sciences generally and that no authentically materialist theory of subjectivity defensibly can sideline the life sciences specifically.

Within weeks following our time together in Ithaca, Catherine and I hatched a plan via e-mail to coauthor a book. After we paused for deliberation, Catherine proposed the topic of affect as a focus for our joint project, expressing a desire to write about wonder in her half of the text. I happily agreed to this. It gave me the opportunity to revisit and more thoroughly digest problems I had been left to grapple with in the wake of my time spent in psychoanalytic training. The question of whether (and, if so, in what sense[s]) affects can be unconscious strictly speaking persistently perturbed Sigmund Freud throughout his career and has remained an unresolved controversy in the worlds of psychoanalysis ever since. This issue is a big bone of contention, particularly in French psychoanalytic contexts dominated by Jacques Lacan. It entails far-from-negligible consequences for theoretical metapsychology as well as clinical practice. Compelled by a mixture of personal and intellectual reasons, I wanted to try to tackle the enigmatic (non)rapport between affects and the unconscious. By contrast, Catherine clearly intended to push further the challenges to psychoanalysis as a whole posed by her philosophical reflections on the implications of various neuropathologies. As I see it, the main fault line of divergence separating our approaches here is between my more immanent and her more external critiques of the psychoanalytic modeling and handling of the psyche, with our philosophical critiques of analysis nonetheless both being developed in dialogue with neurobiology.

Before continuing to sketch an overview of the differences distinguishing my and Catherine's positions, I will offer a sharper outline of our common commitments, the shared preoccupations that brought us together and continue to cement our fundamental solidarity. For the past several decades, much ink has been spilled by scholars in the theoretical humanities about the intersections of Continental philosophy and the psychoanalytic traditions linked to Freud. However, with a few notable exceptions, Continental philosophers and those scholars in the humanities and social sciences influenced by them have been and remain averse to the prospect of any deep theoretical engagement with the life sciences. Biology as a whole, and the neurosciences in particular, have been largely avoided by such thinkers and writers on the basis of now-outdated (mis)conceptions according to which any such engagement inevitably must result in an ideologically dangerous mechanistic materialism demoting human subjects to the degraded status of mere objectified puppets of an evolutionary-genetic nature. This sort of alibi, speciously justifying an avoidance of philosophically and psychoanalytically responding to the revolutionary advances occurring in the life sciences, is no longer plausible or valid (if it ever was to begin with).

Nowadays, it simply isn't true that one has to sell one's philosophical or psychoanalytic soul in its entirety in order to dance with the neurobiological devil (although Catherine and I have separate views regarding the nitty-gritty details of this). In fact, over the past half century, scientific matters concerning neuroplasticity, mirror neurons, epigenetics, and newly proposed revisions to Darwinian depictions of evolution, among other topics, have destroyed the caricature of biological approaches to subjectivity upon which the ever-more-hollow excuses of a tired old antinaturalism rely, caricatures depicting such approaches as essentially deterministic and reductive. This antinaturalism leans upon the partially obsolete early-twentieth-century critiques of the natural sciences formulated by, to name just a handful of prominent individuals, Edmund Husserl, Georg Lukács, Martin Heidegger, and Jean-Paul Sartre. The time is long overdue for psychoanalysis and the ensemble of established Continental philosophical orientations to begin appreciating and seriously working-through a number of developments in the life sciences. Especially for any conceptual framework that wishes to identify itself as materialist, turning a blind eye to these developments seems unpardonable. A completely antinaturalist, antiscientific materialism is no materialism at all.

What might European philosophy and Freudian-Lacanian psychoanalysis look like if sincere and sustained efforts finally are made to digest the many implications for conceptions of the human mind flowing from cutting-edge neuroscientific research? There is very little presently available in print interfacing psychoanalytic metapsychologies with the neurosciences through the mediation of the rich conceptual resources of primarily French and German philosophy from the seventeenth century through today (especially Hegel-indebted variants of historical and dialectical materialism arising in the nineteenth century). Furthermore, what currently goes by the name of "neuro-psychoanalysis," primarily an Anglo-American clinical endeavor, entirely ignores the ideas of Lacan and the philosophical sophistication of Lacanian analysis, its sophistication being rooted mainly in the legacies of modern philosophy beginning with Descartes.

One of the several fashions in which the two pieces by Catherine and me brought together in this volume complement each other is through their carefully correlated contrasts in terms of philosophically thinking the relations between psychoanalysis and the neurosciences. Simply stated, whereas Catherine's primary agenda is to delineate the constraining limits of psychoanalysis when it is faced with revelations arising from scientific investigations of the brain, my guiding program is targeted at examining how these two fields promise mutually to enrich one another if synthesized with sufficient care. Catherine maintains that analysis can neither theoretically explain nor practically cure the sorts of afflictions at the heart of scientific studies of many neuropathologies; its attempts to do so have to be abandoned and it must rethink radically, in light of the damaged brains examined by neurology, the philosophical concepts and categories of contingency, continuity, event, selfhood, and subjectivity lying at the metapsychological basis of its clinical practices.

I maintain that a genuinely materialist and empirically up-to-date psychoanalysis can and should be arrived at through Lacanianizing non-Lacanian neuro-psychoanalysis. In tandem with this, both the psychoanalytic and neuroscientific sides of this hybrid interdisciplinary formation must be dialectically reworked in parallel with each other. Such a program promises to flesh out a scientifically well-grounded materialist account of how more-than-material subjective structures (such as those at the center of various strains of Continental philosophy and psychoanalysis) arise that come to escape the explanatory jurisdiction of natural-scientific discourses alone.

Furthermore, unlike Catherine, I think that Freudian-Lacanian analysis is in a good position to accommodate and absorb the findings of recent scientific research into the brain, so long as one bears in mind the distinction between the theorizable and the treatable in analysis (in addition to operating with an appropriate philosophical framework for nonreductively interfacing the analytic and the biological). From my perspective, and to be more precise, four categories have to be acknowledged as permutations of this distinction: (1) what analysis can both theorize and treat; (2) what analysis cannot theorize but can treat; (3) what analysis can theorize but not treat; and (4) what analysis can neither theorize nor treat. Whereas the first of these four categories is the most straightforward—what I'm thinking of are the familiar, garden-variety neuroses providing analysts from Freud onward with the daily bread-and-butter work of their clinics—some readers initially might be perplexed by the second of these four categories. However, many clinical analysts openly wonder about the "therapeutic action" of their practices, honestly admitting uncertainty and puzzlement about what it is that they're doing (or not doing) that's responsible for the therapeutic progress of their analysands (i.e., what they're successfully treating without being able confidently to theorize).

The real axes of tension between Catherine and me have to do with the third and fourth categories. I can illustrate what's at stake here with the famous example, dear to the celebrated neuroscientist Antonio Damasio as well as Catherine, of Phineas Gage, the unfortunate nineteenth-century Vermont railway laborer whose left frontal lobe was severely damaged by a workplace accident in which a tamping iron was blown through his skull by an explosion. Gage, who survived this awful incident, could be characterized as ur-patient zero of the neurosciences to the extent that they have relied heavily on human subjects whose brains have been harmed and impaired in specific fashions by disease or injury. These ill-fated subjects enable the methodical pinpointing of "cerebral localizations" in which features of mental life are correlated to specific parts of the central nervous system. The outcome of Gage losing the inhibitory, self-censoring functions evidently arising from the damaged areas of his brain was that, as the story goes, he underwent a dramatic change of personality, going from being a disciplined, respectful, and considerate person before the accident to being the opposite soon after it.

For Catherine, Gage and those like him—this would include other victims of various types of traumas to the head as well as those ravaged by such terrible ailments as Alzheimer's disease—undergo brutally senseless physical ordeals in which they lose their former subjectivities without the possibility of the redemption of meaning. They live on as shadowy husks of their former selves, cruelly transported by the contingent vicissitudes of material reality to unimaginable mental wastelands beyond the reach of psychoanalytic recognition and rescue. In Catherine's eyes, not only is analytic interpretation unable either to comprehend or to cure such patients, but these "new wounded," at the levels of both their pasts and futures, pose external checks on the universal explanatory ambitions of the metapsychologies of the temporally extended psyche put forward by Freud, Lacan, and their followers. She is guided by the firm conviction that these sufferers of a range of neuropathologies definitely belong in the last of the four categories I enumerated above (i.e., what analysis can neither theorize nor treat).

With reference to the examples of Gage and his kind, I am guided by the equally firm conviction that more of these instances than Catherine estimates belong in the third category (i.e., what analysis can theorize but not treat). However, I would concede to her, while wondering whether this concession would oblige psychoanalysis sweepingly to transform itself in a self-critical fashion, that analytic theory doesn't have much to say about extremely advanced Alzheimer's or the severest, most disabling forms of brain damage— unless, if the damage is caused by an injury resulting from an accident, such accidents sometimes qualify as tragic varieties of parapraxis, namely, the "bungled actions" famously analyzed by Freud in his 1901 book *The Psychopathology of Everyday Life* (not to say that understanding these accidents as parapraxes would be of much therapeutic use to their damaged-beyond-repair victims). Returning to nineteenth-century Vermont, Gage likely did not become disinhibited in a generic manner; his posttraumatic personality, however drastically different from his pretraumatic one, probably exhibited distinctive, idiosyncratic details in terms of the specifics of his (foul) language, (impulsive) behavior, and so on. It seems implausible to me that myriad conscious and unconscious elements of his complex ontogenetic life history predating the trauma, elements distributed across many more still-functioning regions of his brain than just the wounded left frontal lobe, abruptly ceased to play any explicable role whatsoever in his existence in the aftermath of the event. Analytic interpretation, although admittedly therapeutically impotent in this case, would be not without its powers to explore and illuminate the associative chains of continuity shaping the sociosymbolic aspects of the Gage who survived this harsh brush with death as a subject transformed in difficult-to-discern relation, but relation nevertheless, to his prior subjectivity.

Of course, if someone in Gage's circumstances were to arrive in an analyst's consulting room asking about the possibility of starting an analysis, the analyst probably would advise him first to visit a hospital to have the iron rod in his skull removed before thinking about starting analytic work. (Perhaps it is inappropriate to put a somewhat humorous point on this dark example.) Although the early pioneers of analysis in the first decades of the twentieth century tended to overestimate the extent of the curative powers and therapeutic jurisdiction of their young discipline, no reasonable analytic clinicians practicing today believe that analysis is a catch-all treatment suitable and effective for those with cripplingly debilitating brain damage or Alzheimer's. Analysts indeed debate with each other about "width of scope": The wider an analyst's scope, the more sorts of analysands with more severe psychopathologies he/she is willing to put on the analytic couch (and, the *psycho-* here signals that pathologies having more to do with psyche than soma are what is at stake in these intra-analytic debates). But, even those with the widest of scopes almost certainly would refer the types of individuals of concern to Catherine, if and when such persons presented for analyses, to other specialist practitioners of nonanalytic treatment modalities. Perhaps save for a tiny minority of extreme and eccentric exceptions proving the rule, the days of a psychoanalysis making hubristic claims to unqualified universal hegemony are definitely over, for better and worse.

Likewise, certain forms of psychosis (e.g., the schizophrenias) are widely considered by analysts as well as nonanalysts to be triggered by somatic-organic, rather than psychical-historical, causal factors. Analysis cannot treat such conditions in a way that provides a total cure. But, in line with how I argued with respect to Gage, those schizophrenics exhibiting linguistically and conceptually articulated mental content (e.g., elaborate delusions or hallucinations)—content that testifies to their enduring as proper psychical subjects, however disturbed and disturbing—at least can be better heard and understood thanks to the metapsychological theories and interpretive practices of analysis. Analytic assistance, combined with other appropriate means of medical and non-medical support, might even help them to varying degrees short of a full-blown elimination of the pathology's underlying somatic-organic causal triggers; perhaps it could partially address aspects of their multidimensional conditions, especially social and psychical ones. This is to underscore, apropos the four categories I listed earlier, the difference between my favoring the third category (i.e., what analysis can theorize but not treat [in a way that provides a total cure]) and Catherine's favoring the fourth category (i.e., what analysis can neither theorize nor treat) as regards an overlapping set of pertinent examples.

Catherine explores the future of psychoanalysis as it is interrupted and cut short by the neurosciences. I explore the future of psychoanalysis as it is enriched and carried forward by these same sciences. Despite this division, we agree that neither psychoanalysis nor the neurosciences (nor philosophy, for that matter) can remain unchanged in passing through these ultimately unavoidable disciplinary intersections. Similarly, in response to wary, skeptical questions demanding justification for why philosophers and psychoanalysts should pay attention to the biology of the brain, our answer is simple: ignoring the impressive advances of neurobiology lands the theorist of subjectivity in either metaphysical dogmatism or factual error—intellectual bankruptcy either way. What's more, clinicians risk blundering about in partial darkness, irresponsibly and perhaps dangerously, if they willfully deprive themselves of potential sources of information further illuminating the minded subjects that are the objects of their practices.

Another manner in which Catherine's and my pieces dovetail with each other has to do with our choices of which emotions to focus on analyzing, with affect serving as the topic in relation to which we both weave together philosophy, psychoanalysis, and the neurosciences. Catherine zooms in on wonder and I on guilt. The former affect, as per Aristotle, lies at the motivating basis of theoretical philosophy (i.e., epistemology, ontology, metaphysics, logic, and so on); the latter affect plays a key role in practical philosophy (i.e., ethics, morality, and politics). Hence, taken together, our texts revisit the Western philosophical tradition's vexed, ambivalent relationship with its affective sources—emotions and feelings have been perennially problematic phenomena for philosophy since Socrates—equipped with the combined resources of psychoanalysis and new scientific studies of the brain. Moreover, the place of affect in accounts of embodiment and subjectivity has been a hotly disputed topic particularly in Continental philosophy from the mid-twentieth century up through the present. Between phenomenology, structuralism, post-structuralism, feminism, and deconstruction, to name some of the main trajectories shaping the history of this philosophical tradition, a plethora of debates remain unresolved about what affects are and the extent of their importance in shaping the objects of philosophical investigation. We each reframe these debates in light of the neurosciences.

In "Go Wonder: Subjectivity and Affects in Neurobiological Times," Catherine pushes off on the basis of a philosophical platform consisting in, from the early modern period, the Continental rationalists René Descartes and Baruch Spinoza and, from the postwar period, the French poststructuralist philosophers Gilles Deleuze and Jacques Derrida. She anchors her reflections in a consideration of the deconstructive thesis according to which the self-presence of the modern philosophical subject's "autoaffection" (i.e., its reflexively being in touch with itself, so to speak) actually amounts to a "heteroaffection" (i.e., being touched by another, by the foreignness of an alterity-to-self). Catherine asks about the relative radicalism of the deconstructions of (affective) subjectivity pursued separately under the banners of contemporary philosophy, psychoanalysis, and the neurosciences when compared with one another. Her text builds toward proposing that today's nonreductive neurobiological investigations into selfhood and emotional life, especially Damasio's work in these areas (including his neuroscientific reevaluations of Descartes and Spinoza), "think the unthought," as Heidegger would put it, of both the philosophical and psychoanalytic deconstructions bearing upon heteroaffected subjective identity. The "synaptic self" (to employ Joseph LeDoux's phrase) of current neurobiology is a subject not only exposed to constant mediation by others (as per heteroaffection), but also vulnerable to traumatic occurrences of disruption that erase it and leave behind an utterly different subject (or even nonsubject) in its vanished place.

Such inflicted breaks of total and complete discontinuity in the organism's life history sometimes result, as numerous tragic case studies illustrate, in what Catherine calls a "hetero-heteroaffection," through which heteroaffection, as the subject's capacity to be affected, itself is affected by the event of trauma qua the *hetero-* of a certain sort of alterity or otherness. The sad result, whose sadness cannot be registered by the victim of an intrusive happening affecting his/her brain thus, is a "dis-affected" subject, a subject deprived of the ability to be affected so as to experience emotions and feelings. According to Catherine, neither Freudian-Lacanian psychoanalysis nor Derridean deconstruction and allied trends in postwar French philosophy rise to the task of trying to envision and explain such posttraumatic neuro-subjectivity, a subjectivity confronting its witnesses with the unsettling, upsetting spectacle of human beings who biologically survive the ordeal of the deaths of their prior forms of personal identity. Catherine's contribution seeks to remedy this lacuna.

Whereas Catherine is interested in an affecting (i.e., neurological trauma) that negates the potential of being further affected emotionally, I am fixated upon the seemingly paradoxical notion of unconscious affects (i.e., feelings that aren't felt as such). As I remarked previously, the relation (or lack thereof) between the unconscious and affective life is an issue that haunts psychoanalysis from its inception with Freud onward. Despite Freud's tendency to dismiss unconscious affective phenomena as self-contradictory impossibilities—it apparently makes no sense to speak of unfelt feelings—certain observations pertaining in particular to individuals' guilt repeatedly nudge him over the course of his intellectual itinerary to speculate about the existence of affects affecting the psyche without being consciously registered as what they really are in (repressed) actuality *an sich* (such as repressed guilt being self-consciously [mis]experienced as free-floating anxiety). Operating with metapsychological theory, clinical practice, and German and French textual details simultaneously in view, I reread the history of this persisting problem in the development of psychoanalysis from Freud through Lacan to very recent analytic and philosophical orientations, a problem with both theoretical and clinical ramifications. I argue against Lacan's insistence that Freud categorically denies the reality of unconscious affects, interpretively uncover a more sophisticated metapsychology of affect in Lacan's teachings than is usually suspected (even by Lacan himself) to be there, critically intervene in post-Freudian and post-Lacanian controversies over these topics, and bring the results of all this to bear on my effort to forge a Lacan-influenced neuro-psychoanalytic account of affective subjectivity.

Based on a tripartite distinction between affects, emotions, and feelings that I extract from readings of Freud and Lacan, I analyze affective phenomena as complex constellations of multiple tiers and dimensions, rather than as elementary, unitary experiences of a self-evident nature incapable of further analytic decomposition. This analysis is profoundly inspired by a Hegelian philosophical outlook. Insofar as feelings are always feelings of feelings (i.e., mediated experiences of the second order or greater), the phenomena of "misfelt feelings," generated through the interference of defense mechanisms functioning unconsciously within and between different strata of psychical structure, become thinkable possibilities, possibilities not yet thought through by philosophy and psychoanalysis. Contemporary affective neuroscience (à la Damasio, LeDoux, and Jaak Panksepp, among others) is requisite for doing justice to the lingering difficulty of the topic of unconscious affect via the idea of misfelt feelings, with the latter involving distorted conscious registrations of unconscious affects that aren't consciously felt for what they truly are, but are felt all the same. In the process, I undertake formulating a novel vision of the relationships between, on the one hand, the sciences of nature, and, on the other hand, both psychoanalysis and Continental philosophy.

Those interested in European philosophy and its history will appreciate this book's wide-ranging conceptual recasting of affective phenomena with reference to theories of subjectivity. Those interested in psychoanalysis will appreciate this book's balance between, on one side, delineating the explanatory and therapeutic limitations of analysis vis-à-vis neuropathologies and, on another side, its opening up of fresh paths for productive collaboration between analysts and neuroscientists. Those interested in the neurosciences will appreciate this book's encouraging invitation to them to bring their knowledge into cooperative connection with the subtleties and complexities of state-of-the-art philosophical and psychoanalytic thought.

Catherine forges the concept of hetero-heteroaffection. I introduce the concept of misfelt feelings. Both of us, through our ways of triangulating philosophy, psychoanalysis, and the neurosciences, seek to push readers to reconsider significantly their senses of each of these three fields as well as to imagine exciting new alliances among them full of promising potentials.

Adrian Johnston

ACKNOWLEDGMENTS

I warmly thank Adrian Johnston for the trouble he has taken to reread, correct, and sometimes translate the texts that follow.

I thank equally the students at the Department of Rhetoric at the University of California, Berkeley, who, in the spring of 2008, were the first auditors of the seminar that is at the origin of my contribution to this work.

CM

⁂

To begin with, I would like to express what a sheer joy it's been to get to know and to collaborate with Catherine Malabou. I hope and believe that this project marks the start of an enduring cooperative relationship between us.

Wendy Lochner and the staff at Columbia University Press have been fantastic to work with on this book. I greatly appreciate Wendy's care and guidance generously provided throughout the publication process. I also am profoundly grateful to the editors of the Insurrections series for their support of this project: Clayton Crockett, Creston Davis, Jeffrey W. Robbins, and Slavoj Žižek.

Richard Boothby and Tracy McNulty were amazing as external readers of the manuscript. Their incredibly thoughtful feedback was absolutely invaluable to me as I edited and revised pivotal portions of the manuscript.

Moreover, Rick's and Tracy's friendship and support is very dear to me. Additionally, I owe Tracy an enormous amount of gratitude for her having organized a reading group at Cornell University centered on this manuscript, in which I participated via a Skype video link. This group selflessly furnished me with ideas and insights that proved to be crucial to the final version of this text. For this, I thank Karen Benezra, Shanna Carlson, Aaron Hodges, Ryan Jackson, Fernanda Negrete, and Brad Zukovic. Bruno Bosteels, also at Cornell, offered me very helpful suggestions apropos the topic(s) of *honte* and *pudeur* in particular.

I had several wonderful opportunities to present and discuss aspects of this work in a number of venues. Audiences and interlocutors at the following events were extremely helpful to me: the 2009 Second Annual Spring Conference of the Psychoanalysis Reading Group at Cornell University; the 2009 conference on "Concept and Form: The *Cahiers pour l'Analyse* and Contemporary French Thought" at the Centre for Research in Modern European Philosophy (now at Kingston University); and a one-day seminar on this book hosted by the Department of Comparative Literature at Emory University in 2011.

So much of what I have to say here about psychoanalysis is an outgrowth flowing from what I learned and underwent while a research fellow and clinical training candidate at the Emory Psychoanalytic Institute from 2002 to 2006. The people who played key roles in my experience there are too numerous to list. I imagine they know who they are and want them to be aware of just how much I appreciate everything they gave me.

Finally, and as always, I wish to proclaim the profundity of my debts and thankfulness to, and love for, my partner in everything, Kathryn Wichelns. Not only is she the very center of my being, but with her caring brilliance, she's taught me more than anyone else about emotional life in all its subtle richness and complexity.

I appreciate the editors of the journals in which earlier draft versions of some of the chapters of my text appeared for allowing these to reappear in revised form here: "Affects Are Signifiers: The Infinite Judgment of a Lacanian Affective Neuroscience," *Nessie*, ed. Fabien Tarby, no. 1, 2009, nessie-philo.com/Files//adrian_johnston___affects_are_signifiers.pdf; "The Misfeeling of What Happens: Slavoj Žižek, Antonio Damasio, and a Materialist Account of Affects," in "Žižek and Political Subjectivity," ed. Derek Hook and Calum Neill, special issue, *Subjectivity* 3, no. 1 (April 2010): 76–100; "Affective Life Between Signifiers and *Jouis-sens*: Lacan's *Senti-ments* and *Affectuations*,"

Filozofski Vestnik: What Is It to Live?, ed. Jelica Šumič-Riha, 30, no. 2 (2010): 113–141; "*Affekt, Gefühl, Empfindung*: Rereading Freud on the Question of Unconscious Affects," *Qui Parle? Critical Humanities and Social Sciences* 18, no. 2 (Spring/Summer 2010): 249–289.

For Dr. Grant

AJ

SELF AND EMOTIONAL LIFE

PART I.

GO WONDER

SUBJECTIVITY AND AFFECTS
IN NEUROBIOLOGICAL TIMES

※ ※ ※

CATHERINE MALABOU

INTRODUCTION

FROM THE PASSIONATE SOUL
TO THE EMOTIONAL BRAIN

C urrent neurobiology is engaged in a deep redefinition of emotional life. The brain, far from being a nonsensuous organ, devoted solely to logical and cognitive processes, now appears, on the contrary, to be the center of a new *libidinal economy*. Such a vision is not only displacing the relationship between body, mind, and the psyche. It also disturbs disciplinary boundaries and induces secret networks between sciences (biology and neurobiology) and the humanities (philosophy and psychoanalysis). A new conception of affects is undoubtedly emerging.

Many neurobiologists today insist upon the role of the "emotional brain." This leads them to elaborate a new theory of affects that is rooted in the traditional one, but whose conclusions transgress the frame of the philosophical analysis of passions, and even the frame of deconstruction.

The general issue I address here is the following: Does this new conception produce a genuinely different approach to emotions, passions, and feelings? Or, by contrast, does it consist in a mere reformulation of the traditional approaches to these topics? Is current neuroscience just a repetition or is it engaged in an unprecedented material and radical deconstruction of affects, feelings, and emotions—and, hence, in a new deconstruction of subjectivity? The problem is knowing whether emotions and affects are still considered rooted in an originary process of autoaffection of the subject—where the subject has to touch itself in order to be moved or touched by objects—or if the study of the emotional brain precisely challenges the vision of a self-affecting subjectivity in favor of an originary *deserted* subject, a subject that is definitely not present to itself.

This issue is all the more difficult if we consider that psychoanalysis, as well as contemporary Continental philosophy, has attempted precisely the production of a strong critique of autoaffection and its supposed priority. What, then, does the conception of a specifically *neural* libidinal economy introduce into the field of this critique? Does it just confirm this critique or does it dramatically metamorphose it?

The following intervention involves a confrontation between three approaches—philosophical, psychoanalytical and neurobiological—to the same issue: the origin of affects, an origin that is not and can no longer be determined by and as the primordial gesture of a subject meeting up with itself. We will see how, from this shared question, the responses vary to the point of producing perhaps insurmountable divergences. It is in pushing off from a reading of the theory of the passions in Descartes and Spinoza that Antonio Damasio, in his books *Descartes' Error* and *Looking for Spinoza*, has presented his studies of the relations between the brain and emotion—with these studies also seeming to have the consequence, in his eyes, of leading to a new definition of affects. It has appeared to me pertinent to set off again from this theory in order to establish a dialogue or, perhaps, its impossibility. I will confront here Derrida's reading of Descartes, Deleuze's and Damasio's readings of Spinoza, and Damasio's work on these two major philosophers. The psychoanalytic theory of affects will be examined from a transversal point of view, appearing *through* the other discourses, as both a necessary benchmark and a controversial reference.

Affects and Autoaffection: Definitions

Let's borrow the definition of the term *affect* from Deleuze who, in one of his lectures from 1978 on Spinoza's *Ethics* (January 24, 1978), declares:

> I begin with some terminological cautions. In Spinoza's principal book, which is called the *Ethics* and which is written in Latin, one finds two words: *affectio* and *affectus*. Some translators, quite strangely, translate both in the same way. This is a disaster. They translate both terms, *affectio* and *affectus*, by "affection." I call this a disaster because when a philosopher employs two words,

it's because in principle he has reason to, especially when French easily gives us two words that correspond rigorously to *affectio* and *affectus*, that is "affection" for *affectio* and "affect" for *affectus*. Some translators translate *affectio* as "affection" and *affectus* as "feeling" [*sentiment*], which is better than translating both by the same word, but I don't see the necessity of having recourse to the word *feeling* since French offers the word *affect*. Thus when I use the word *affect* it refers to Spinoza's *affectus*, and when I say the word *affection*, it refers to *affectio*.[1]

Deleuze refers here explicitly to book 3 of the *Ethics*, which is entirely devoted to the problem of affects. It is true that the English translators of Spinoza make use of "emotions" instead of "affects," as in the title of book 3 ("Concerning the Origin and Nature of the Emotions" [*De Origine et Natura Affectuum*]) or in definition 3 of that book: "By emotion [*affectus*] I understand the affections of the body by which the body's power of activity is increased or diminished, assisted or checked, together with the ideas of these affections."[2]

Generally speaking, an affect is a modification. Being affected means to be modified—that is, altered, changed—by the impact of an encounter, be it with another subject or an object. But, what, exactly, is modified by this encounter, and why does this modification create an emotional, and not immediately cognitive, phenomenon? This is because the encounter does not trigger any faculty or sense or logical structure; it touches—and thus reveals—the very feeling of existence. Deleuze goes on: "I would say that for Spinoza there is a continuous variation—and this is what it means to exist—of the force of existing or of the power of acting. . . . Affectus in Spinoza is variation (he is speaking through my mouth; he didn't say it this way because he died too young . . .), continuous variation of the force of existing, insofar as this variation is determined by the ideas one has."[3] The force of existing is constant, but it differs from itself all the time, varies in its continuous power. Affects circumscribe precisely this paradoxical transformability of duration and persistence. An affect is thus always related to the feeling of existence itself through the changing of objects. We may call affect every kind of modification produced by the feeling of a difference.

Let's now move to the word *autoaffection*. Apparently, this term is very distant from the Spinozan context to the extent that it was coined by Heidegger in *Kant and the Problem of Metaphysics*. Heidegger makes use of it when he comments on section 24 of *Critique of Pure Reason*. Here, Kant states that the subject is both a transcendental logical form—the form of the "I think" (or transcendental apperception), with no sensuous content—and the empirical form of the subject's intuition, the way in which the subject "sees," "feels," or "intuits" herself. The subject is two in one.[4] The only mode of communication between the "two" subjects is a kind of affect. First, the subject can only represents itself as it appears empirically to itself.[5] Second, the "I think" itself, or the apperception, as soon as it takes itself as an object, loses its formal transcendental determination to become an intuited object (i.e., an object of the inner sense that *affects* it). The subject can only represent itself as affected—altered—by itself. The self has access to itself through its *own* otherness or alterity. The self-representation of the subject is thus always an *autoaffection*.

The process of autoaffection is for Kant time itself. The subject receives its own forms, it perceives its own logical structure, through the way in which it apprehends itself empirically as remaining the same through change and succession. Autoaffection is thus the temporal difference between the self and itself. Heidegger declares: "Time, that is pure autoaffection, constitutes the essential structure of subjectivity."[6] This structure—autoaffection as temporality—is, according to Heidegger, the origin of all other kinds of affects: passions, emotions, and feelings. Autoaffection appears to be the basis, the condition of possibility, of the primary and primordial form of every particular affect. Feelings like love, hatred, envy, and the like are only possible because the very core of our self is primarily autoaffected. The relationship between subjectivity and itself is prior to the relationship between subjectivity and its objects.

It is easy to discover that the motif of autoaffection is closely linked with Spinoza's definition of affects as modifications of the power of existing, or *conatus*. Autoaffection designates the very feeling of existence; the "I" who feels itself is the dominant structure of all affective modification. The very structure of subjectivity, within the metaphysical tradition, was one and the same with the structure of autoaffection, that is, as this kind of *self-touching* through which the subject is feeling its singular presence. If it is true that, according to traditional philosophers, there cannot be any affects without a primary autoaffection, then all affects might be defined as particular touches, as variations of an originary self-touching, the introduction of time within identity. If an affect is a modification produced by the feeling of a difference, the primordial form of emotional modification is produced by the feeling of the subject's own difference from itself. Hence the precise definition of the passions of the soul: in section 27, Descartes declares: "We may define them generally as those perceptions, sensations or emotions of the soul which we refer particularly to it."[7]

How are we then to understand our initial issue? Can we think of affects outside autoaffection, *affects without subjects, affects that do not affect "me"*?

The contemporary authors that we will study all envisage a response to this question. They do so in playing Descartes and Spinoza against each other, in showing that the two philosophers both, each in his manner, already brings out this problem. In the first case (Derrida and Damasio), Descartes is the pure thinker of autoaffection, while Spinoza anticipates the vision of a subjectivity that does not preexist its affects but is, on the contrary, constituted by them. Damasio, for his part, affirms that Spinoza is the first and only philosopher of the tradition to have elaborated a materialist definition of affects that relates them to a primary activity of cerebral cartography and not to the substantial presence of a subject to itself. The Descartes-Spinoza conflict prefigures the contemporary conflict between metaphysics and neurobiology about the definition of the mind and the psyche. For Damasio, if Descartes is the great metaphysician of presence, Spinoza appears, on the other hand, as a "protoneurologist." As for Deleuze, it's a different case, with his recognizing in Descartes a power of surpassing the closure of the subject in on itself. Both Descartes and Spinoza bring to light a certain dimension of affects by which they exceed the pure reflexivity of the "I."

In following the thread of these readings, we will try to situate the locus of a possible dialogue between two conflictual positions, that of philosophy and that of neurobiology. How is it possible to effectively deconstruct autoaffection? Is it by positing the existence of what Derrida identifies as originary "heteroaffection," where the subject is primarily and profoundly alien to itself? Or, is it by affirming, as Damasio does, that a subject is constantly exposed to the potential deprivation of all affects because of brain damage? According to neurobiologists, the possibility of being detached from one's own affects is not a pure and purely external contingency that may happen to a healthy autoaffected subject; it is virtually already inscribed in some way within the process of autoaffection itself.

Damasio, by elaborating the theory of "somatic markers," stresses the central importance of emotions in neural regulation. Elementary mechanisms of thought or of reasoning are deeply linked with emotional processes. The principle of decision making, for example, is emotional. In the introduction to *Descartes' Error*, Damasio writes: "I began writing this book to propose that reason may not be as pure as most of us think it is or wish it were, that emotions and feelings may not be intruders in the bastion of reason at all: they may be enmeshed in its networks, for worse *and* for better. The strategies of human reason probably did not develop, in either evolution or any single individual, without the guiding force of the mechanisms of biological regulation, of which emotion and feeling are notable expressions."[8]

Paradoxically enough, it is the impairment of emotional processes—occurring after a brain lesion, for example—that reveals their importance: "the *absence of emotion and feeling* is no less damaging, no less capable of compromising the rationality that makes us distinctively human and allows us to decide in consonance with a sense of personal future, social convention, and moral principle."[9]

I would like to advance here that the notion of an *absence of emotions*, which does not come from a kind of disavowal or any type of psychic strategies, marks the novelty of the current neurobiological point of view on affects. Paradoxically, it is not so much the insistence on the major role of emotion in reasoning or in cognitive processes in general that signals the revolutionary position of some cutting-edge neurobiologists today, but rather the possibility for emotional procedures to disappear after brain damage. Again, this disappearance is a kind of affect (it affects the affective subject) or alteration that challenges the notion of "heteroaffection." The patient is less heteroaffected than *not affected at all*. He has become an other, a new person, a nonsubject.

Is the affected subject, then, someone else, the presence of an other subject within itself? Or, is it just nobody, the absence of a substantial first person?

The Issue of Wonder

In order to narrow the numerous perspectives opened by this polemical dialogue between heterosubjectivity and nonsubjectivity, I will focus my study on a particular affect, which appears to be, for both Descartes and Spinoza, the most fundamental of them all: wonder.

The substantive *wonder* is the English translation of the Latin *admiratio* in Descartes and Spinoza. In its classical sense, *admiratio* must not be understood as the modern word *admiration*, but rather as the capacity to be amazed. The Latin *admiratio* comes from *mirari*, which means to be astonished or surprised. According to the dictionary, "wonder," as a noun, characterizes a feeling of surprise and admiration caused by something beautiful, unexpected, or unfamiliar. It also designates a person or thing that causes such a feeling.[10] As a verb, *to wonder* means to be curious, to feel amazement and admiration, to feel doubt or to inquire about something ("I wonder if . . .").

For both Descartes and Spinoza, wonder is what attunes the subject both to the world and to itself. It is an affective opening that at the same time marks the origin of affects. According to Descartes, wonder (*admiration* in French) is the first of the six primitive passions. In *The Passions of the Soul*, we find exposed and presented first wonder, then joy, sorrow, love, hatred, and desire. Descartes gives this definition of wonder: "When our first encounter with some object surprises us and we find it novel, or very different from what we formerly knew or from what we supposed it ought to be, this causes us to wonder and to be astonished at it. Since all this may happen before we know whether or not the object is beneficial to us, I regard wonder as the first of all passions. It has no opposite, for, if the object before us has no characteristics that surprise us, we are not moved by it at all and we consider it without passion."[11] Wonder is this primary affect, deprived of a contrary and of contradiction, that alters the subject's intimacy but reveals it at the same time. Without the capacity to be surprised by objects, the subject wouldn't be able to have a feeling of itself.

In a slightly different way, Spinoza affirms: "As soon as we think of an object that we have seen in conjunction with others, we immediately record the others as well. . . . But in supposing that we perceive in some object something special that we have never seen before we are saying only this, that the mind, while regarding that object, contains nothing in itself to the contemplation of which it can pass on from contemplation of that object. Therefore, the mind is determined to regard only that object. . . . This affection of the mind, or thought of a special thing, in so far as it alone engages the mind is called Wonder (*admiratio*), which, if evoked by an object that we fear, is called Consternation, because wonder at an evil keeps a mind so paralysed in regarding it alone that it is incapable of thinking of other things whereby he might avoid the evil."[12] Here, the philosopher seems to admit that wonder does have a contrary—consternation—but he shares with Descartes the idea that surprise and novelty open the mind to a certain relationship to objects, namely, the capacity to get struck.

Hence the ambiguity of wonder: What are the soul, or the mind, struck by: the surprising object or its own capacity to be surprised? What do the soul or the mind wonder at: the other or themselves? Is wonder open to alterity or is it the very form of autoaffection (a passion *of* the soul, an emotion that the soul "refers particularly" to itself)?

The essential reason for choosing wonder as a central motif is that its ontological and psychic status situates it right *in between auto- and heteroaffection.* Its ambivalence makes all its philosophical interest.

First, then, wonder may be seen as the structure of autoaffection: the subject touching itself as if it were a surprising other. Wonder is the philosophical affect as such. In book 1 of the *Metaphysics*, Aristotle states that philosophy proceeds from wonder: "For it is owing to their wonder that men both now begin and at first began to philosophize."[13] Is not wonder the privileged way in which spirit affects itself, wakes itself up by soliciting itself, the primary way of feeling oneself feel? Less than the ability to be astonished by something external to the subject, wonder is in reality the faculty of self-surprising, the amazement of the mind at itself, its own opening to objects.

Descartes explains that the passions of the soul form a special kind of perception, "the perceptions we refer only to the soul [and] whose effects we feel as being in the soul itself"; they are "passions with respect to our soul," passions for the soul itself.[14] Aren't the passions of the soul for the soul the foundation or the origin of every other kind of affect? Spinoza, for his part, declares: "When the mind regards its own self and its power of activity, it feels pleasure, and the more so, the more distinctly it imagines itself and its power of activity."[15] This description of self-pleasure seems explicit: don't we have to understand that the soul essentially wonders at and about itself and feels pleasure at its own contemplation?

Second, and contradictorily, wonder may well be considered the affect of the other as such. Because it is deeply linked with the ability to be surprised or raptured, wonder appears to be the emotional consequence of the intrusion of alterity into the soul. In that sense, wonder may be seen as the affect of difference, the soul's realization that the self is not alone. This affect of difference as such affects also the other *in me*. If I am able to wonder about or at something, it is because I am not identical to myself, because I am different from myself.

To what extent can we sever wonder from autoaffection and reserve it purely for difference? What would a "heterowonder" be, and can wonder resist its own deconstruction? At the same time, is it possible to deconstruct anything without wondering at or about the very thing we intend to deconstruct? Is it possible to think of any thing in general without wonder, when we know that wonder is a synonym for philosophical thought?

Either it is possible to show that wonder bears in itself the possibility of resisting its own deconstruction, that is, the possibility of transgressing the realm of sheer autoaffection, or we have to admit, on the contrary, that the only effective deconstruction of the relationship between wonder and autoaffection comes from the possibility that wonder may be destroyed, that the capacity to wonder may be definitely impaired. The only effective deconstruction of subjectivity requires in this case a theoretical elaboration of what the *loss* of affects is: the subject's total disconnection from her affects. The second term of this alternative is envisaged today only by neurobiologists, never by philosophers or psychoanalysts.

Again, whatever Derrida may write against Descartes's theory of passions, aiming at deconstructing mainly the Cartesian conception of the couple formed by wonder and generosity in the *Treatise*, a certain notion of wonder is still and always implied in and by deconstruction. For Derrida, there is no deconstruction of wonder without wonder. Heteroaffection is still an affect. The possibility of losing the very ability for the individual to feel or get affected by something or someone is never envisaged.

One of the major points of discussion between philosophy, psychoanalysis, and neurobiology concerns not only the possibility of heteroaffection, but the possibility of a hetero-heteroaffection (if we may speak thus), that is, an affection of the affects themselves that causes their ruin or their disappearance. A heteroaffected subject is still an affected subject. A hetero-heteroaffected subject is "disaffected." Most of the time, the impairment of emotional processes produces an indifference that coincides purely and simply with a disability to wonder. Damasio states that *the loss of wonder is the emotional and libidinal disease of our time*. After brain damage, the emotional brain is traumatized, and in very serious cases the subject loses any interest in life in general. Surprise, interest in novelty, amazement, astonishment just disappear. Detachment, "cold blood," unconcern determine the patient's behavior. About a patient of his named Eliott, Damasio writes: "He was cool, detached, unperturbed even by potentially embarrassing discussion of personal events. He reminded me somewhat of Addison de Witt, the character played by George Sanders in *All About Eve*."[16] The brain, more than the Freudian psyche, might be seen as the biological intruder that challenges not only autoaffection, but also heteroaffection in its philosophical sense.

What happens to wonder in a neurobiological age? Who is this new subject, stranger to surprise, amazement, and *admiratio*? The analyses to follow here do not constitute a demonstration properly speaking. It's rather about giving to the reader some reference points in suggesting a certain number of important texts, in crossing these texts and making them respond to each other. The aim is to create a network of references and discussions that permits, from the noncognitivist and nonreductionist point of view of Continental philosophy, comprehending the stakes of the redefinition of psychical life and the emotions undertaken by the neurosciences today.

I.

WHAT DOES "OF" MEAN IN DESCARTES'S EXPRESSION, "THE PASSIONS *OF* THE SOUL"?

The distinction drawn by Descartes between "passions in the soul" and "passions of the soul" indicates the ambiguity of *The Passions of The Soul*. If passions proper (affects that cannot be confused with the consequences, "in" and on the soul, of simple bodily movements and reactions) are passions rooted in the intimacy of the soul, does it mean that the structural definition of affect is the autoaffected structure? Or, are these passions that the soul "refers only to itself" the paradoxical name of a specific mode of being of the unity between the body and the soul, in which both are at one with each other's alterity and difference?

General Presentation of *The Passions of the Soul*

Descartes's treatise is divided into three main parts. The first part, which comprises the first fifty paragraphs, presents a general definition of the passions and a description of the union of the body and the soul in passionate behaviors. The second part is devoted to the distinction between the "primitive" and the "derived" passions.[1] Descartes explains that all particular affects derive from the six primitive passions: wonder, love, hatred, desire, joy, and sadness. Part 3, entitled "On Specific Passions," consists in a description of these derived passions. In this third part, we find the famous definition and description of generosity (*générosité*).

The analysis of wonder appears in the two last parts of the treatise.[2] A strong, intimate link binds wonder to generosity and forms what we may call an ethical loop within the *Treatise*. A theory of affects or passions, for Descartes as for all classical philosophers, necessarily leads to the constitution of an ethics.

Passions "in" the Soul Are Consequences of Bodily Movements

The passions *of* the soul constitute a specific kind of affect, which Descartes defines only in paragraph 27 ("Definition of the Passions of the Soul"). The first part of the treatise is divided in three. First, from sections 1 to 27, Descartes characterizes passions in general; then, from sections 27 to 30, he analyses the passions of the soul proper; and then, from sections 30 to 51, he shows that the passions are the very locus of the union of the body and the soul. In the end of this last section, he asks in what way the soul is able to master its passions. Generosity appears at that point.

Descartes distinguishes a general sense of the expression *passions* from a restricted sense. In its general sense, a passion must be understood as a passion *in* the soul: "We should recognize that what is a passion in the soul is usually an action in the body."[3] Passions "in" the soul are the effects of bodily actions. There are two essential kinds of bodily movements: the invisible movements that are internal to the body—circulation of the blood and agitation of the animal spirits—and the movements that provoke visible muscular actions: fear, anger, anxiety, and so on. The major agents of the first kind of movements are the heart and the brain (the locus of the small material particles called "animal spirits"). The two main paragraphs devoted to blood circulation are 7 and 9. Discussing Harvey, Descartes explains:

> All those not completely blinded by the authorities of the ancients, and willing to open their eyes to examine the opinion of Harvey regarding the circulation of the blood, do not doubt that the veins and arteries of the body are like streams through which the blood flows constantly and with great rapidity. It makes its way from the right-hand cavity of the heart to the arterial vein, whose branches are spread out through the lungs and connected with those of the venous artery; and via this artery it passes from the lungs into the left-hand side of the heart. From there it goes to the great artery, whose branches are spread out to the rest of the body and connected with the branches of the vena

cava, which carries the same blood once again into the right-hand cavity of the heart. These two cavities are thus like sluices through which all the blood passes upon each complete circuit it makes through the body.[4]

In section 10, Descartes completes this description in presenting the movement of the animal spirits:

> The finest parts of the blood, which have been rarefied by the heat in the heart, constantly enter the cavity of the brain in a large number. What makes them go there rather than elsewhere is that all the blood leaving the heart through the great artery flows a direct route towards this place, and since not all this blood can enter there because the passages are too narrow, only the most active and finest parts pass into it while the rest spread out into the other regions of the body. Now these very fine parts make up the animal spirits. . . . What I am calling "spirits" here are merely bodies: they have no property other than that of being extremely small bodies which move very quickly, like the jets of flame that come from a torch.[5]

These inner bodily movements, based on the fundamental movement of the blood and activated by the heart-brain loop, are structurally linked to the way in which "external objects act upon the sense organs."[6] The relationship between inner and external affections cause perceptions in the soul. Perceptions are the first kind of passion *in* the soul. They are representations of external objects.

The second kind of bodily movements consists of muscular movements. Animal spirits enter the brain and help it to move the nerves, which in their turn move the muscles, as Descartes explains in the second part of section 7: "Finally, it is known that all these movements of the muscles, and likewise all sensations, depend on the nerves, which are like little threads or tubes coming from the brain and containing, like the brain itself, a certain very fine air or wind which is called the 'animal spirits.'"[7] The muscular movements also produce passions *in* the soul. Descartes gives the example of fear. After positing the existence of the pineal gland, he declares: "Moreover, just as the course which the spirits take to the nerves of the heart suffice to induce a movement in the gland through which fear enters the soul, so too the mere fact that some spirits at the same time proceed to the nerves which serve to move the legs in flight causes another movement in the gland through which the soul feels and perceives this action. In this way then, the body may be moved to take flight by the mere disposition of the organs, without any contribution from the soul."[8] We are then to understand, after this first moment, that passions "in" the soul designate the different modalities of the soul's passivity. The soul is passive when it is affected, on the one hand, by perceptions (the soul *represents* the external objects) and, on the other, by motor actions (the soul *feels* these actions). In both cases, this passivity is caused by the body's activity, to which the soul *reacts*.

Again, this passivity does not characterize passions proper, that is, passions "of" the soul. We still do not know for the moment what they are. In order to articulate them, Descartes first presents the "functions of the soul" (in section 17): "These are of two principal kinds, some being the actions of the soul and others its passions."[9] Analyzing the two categories of activity and passivity is of capital importance, to the extent that, as we will see, passions "of" the soul are somewhere in between activity and passivity. The actions of the soul are "our volitions, for we experience them as proceeding directly from our soul and as seeming to depend on it alone."[10] Some of our perceptions may also be considered to be actions of the soul: "those having the perceptions of our volitions and all of the imaginings or other thoughts which depend on them."[11] Even if these perceptions may be understood as passions, like all perceptions, "we do not normally call [them] 'passions,' but solely . . . 'actions'" to the extent that they are "one and the same thing as the volition" or the imagining. There is then a kind of active passivity (that of cognition and volition in general) distinct from the affective passivity caused by bodily movements.

Descartes posits the necessity of bringing to light a third kind of perception: a perception that differs from those caused by the effect of external objects on the senses as well as those that are in reality actions of the soul. This third kind corresponds to the "passions of the soul" proper. The restricted sense of the word *passions* appears in section 25: "we usually restrict the term to signify only perceptions which refer to the soul itself. And it is only the latter that I have undertaken to explain here under the title 'passions of the soul.'"[12] Then comes the specific definition: "We may define them generally as those perceptions, sensations or emotions of the soul which we refer particularly to it, and which are caused, maintained and strengthened by some movements of the spirits."[13]

Passions of the Soul Are Related to the Soul Alone

These passions may be called "perceptions," but they differ both from volitions and cognitive acts (i.e., from the actions of the soul) and from sensations (i.e., from passions *in* the soul caused by bodily movements). The passions of the soul are effectively related to the body: they are caused by some movements of the spirits, but they are not caused *by* the body; they designate a certain kind of disturbance that appears to characterize *psychical* affects as such. These affects are said to "agitate and disturb [the soul] strongly."[14] They are *emotions of the soul.*[15]

These emotions are provoked by the *union of the body and the soul itself,* as if the soul could then feel itself as united to the body. That is why these passions "move and dispose the soul to want the things for which they prepare the body."[16] This feeling of psychosomatic unity is made possible thanks to the intermediary of the pineal gland, which is the material locus of the union. Descartes states: "There is a little gland in the brain where the soul exercises its functions more particularly than in the other parts of the body." This gland is the "principal seat of the soul."[17] According to the definition of the gland, we clearly see that the seat of passions is not the heart, but the brain. We must then admit that the soul has its own body, the pineal gland, which is located in the brain. And, the passions of the soul are provoked by this particular *soul's body.*

The discussions in Descartes about the metaphysical as well as ethical dimension of the passions focus, as we will see, on the status of this peculiar "body." The brain appears to be the soul's bodily existence. At the same time, such a body may be regarded as paradoxically dis-incarnated and abstract. Is the brain in Descartes the mirror of the soul, another figure of itself, its alter ego in autoaffection? Or is it a genuine other, the presence of alterity in sameness, the bodily breach within the subject's self-determination?

From Wonder to Generosity

These questions form the heart of the inquiry on wonder, the most fundamental of all six primitive passions. Let's recall its definition in section 52: "When the first encounter with some object surprises us, and we judge it to be new, or very different from what we knew in the past or what we supposed it was going to be, this makes us wonder and be astonished at it. And since this can happen before we know in the least whether this object is suitable to us or not, it seems to me that wonder is the first of all the passions. It has no opposite, because if the object presented has nothing in it that surprises us, we are not in the least moved by it and regard it without passion." Wonder is the only passion that involves no evaluation of its object. It merely presents the object as something novel or unusual. A particular object seems so worthy of attention that we marvel at it, without making any judgment about whether it is good or evil. As such, wonder produces no change in the heart or the blood, which would prepare the body for movement. It affects only the brain, rather than the heart and the blood, but it does involve the movements of the animal spirits into the muscles, thereby fixing an "impression" of the object in the brain. And, that explains the function of wonder: to "learn and retain in our memory things of which we were previously ignorant." It is our response to the features of the world that are worthy of our consideration, something useful both for the preservation of the mind-body union and for the soul itself in its pursuit of knowledge.[18]

Wonder is prior to judgment and will. Because it is nonjudgmental, wonder makes no hierarchy regarding what it wonders at. It is pure openness to the extraordinary. But, what is the extraordinary? On the one hand, the extraordinary seems to be alterity as such, everything that is not the soul and interrupts its self-identity. People who are indifferent to wonder and surprise are in that sense locked in themselves, unable for this reason to perceive the uncanniness of the world. This is why they are said to be unable to become philosophers. On the other hand, if wonder is the passion of alterity, why does it restrict bodily movements to their minimum? Why is wonder motionless? Why doesn't it give way to tears, cries of joy, different manifestations of pleasure? Wonder is a silent and striking passion that imposes stillness on the body, as if the novelty and strangeness of objects and of the world in general is reflecting the beauty and extraordinary presence of the soul, its mirroring and reflection in the brain. It defines the philosophical disposition as a passion raised by the sameness between spirit and the world.

This ambiguous function of wonder is pursued and underscored in Descartes's study of generosity. Generosity produces a kind of self-directed wonder, or esteem, grounded in our recognition "that nothing really belongs to us other than the free disposition of our volitions," along with sensing "in ourselves at the same time a firm and constant resolution to use them well." Generous people are those who "are entirely masters of their passions" and limit them to the contemplation of our potentialities.[19] Generosity is esteem for ourselves, an appropriate judgment about our worth that should be developed as a habit. It has the following features: (1) knowing that nothing is really ours except the freedom to control our willing, and that we should only be praised and blamed for using that freedom well or badly; and (2) feeling within ourselves a strong constant resolution to use our free will well, to always have the will to carry out what we think is the best course of action.[20] This is what it would be to pursue virtue in a perfect manner; what we esteem in ourselves is a virtuous will.

Generosity is then a way of overcoming the disruptions of the passions, giving us control over them.

At the same time, people of generosity are "easily convinced" that others also have the same capacity to exercise free will for good or evil ends. Therefore, if we have generosity, we will not prefer ourselves to others.[21] We find the ambiguity already mentioned again. Although generosity is a perception directed at the self, combining a knowledge of what is truly important in and for ourselves with the will to act on the basis of that knowledge, it generates esteem for others: generous people do good without self-interest; are courteous, gracious, and obliging; and live free from contempt, jealousy, envy, hatred, fear, and anger. Generosity is a species of wonder combined with love, which involves having proper pride or rightful self-regard.[22] This self-esteem is thought by Descartes to make it possible to have the right kind of regard for others: if we value ourselves appropriately, then we will respond to others appropriately.[23] We can understand the esteem Descartes refers to as a basic form of respect. In generosity, we recognize the worth of others, so that respect, veneration, and magnanimity follow wonder. Furthermore, generosity strengthens a healthier form of regard for others and prevents hatred, because we regard them as equally capable of a virtuous will.[24] The vices that the virtue of generosity can be contrasted with are pride and vicious humility. Descartes is optimistic that everyone can attain the virtuous will, no matter how weak they are, though ignorance is the greatest obstacle. Generous or noble-minded people find it important to do good for others and disdain their own interests: "They are always perfectly courteous, affable, and of service to everyone" and "entirely masters of their Passions."[25] If we have generosity, we respect people appropriately and have no remorse, because we know that we have done our best. At one point Descartes notes that he prefers the term *generosity* to the term *magnanimity* because "the Schools" do not understand this virtue.[26] Moreover, we have little cowardice or fear: we are self-assured because of our confidence in our own virtue.[27] This explains why generosity is the key to the virtuous life.

The relationship to surprise and otherness initiated by wonder and extended by generosity preserves the union between the body and the soul and is the token for its liveliness. Wonder is surprise at the extraordinary, and it is the ideal way to regard others because it is prior to judgment and thus free of prejudice. Thanks to wonder and generosity, their existence resists assimilation or reduction to sameness or self and we are able to accept dissimilarities in them. At the same time, aren't wonder and generosity simple projections of our own views or self-understanding onto others, a pure transfer of self-esteem?

2.

A "SELF-TOUCHING YOU"

DERRIDA AND DESCARTES

One may think that the very notion of passions *of* the soul implies a conception of the self-touching of subjectivity that confirms the very structure of autoaffection. We saw that passions of the soul appear to be disturbances of the soul that make it feel alive or existent. The passionate soul has a proper kind of emotion, raised by the most intimate and sensual dimension of the mind-body union. Is this sensuality reducible to a purely spiritual affectivity in which body and space are evacuated? This is the general orientation of Derrida's interpretation of Descartes.

Autoaffection and Self-Touching

Derrida's thought may be regarded, as a whole, as a long and continuous deconstructing gesture of autoaffection in the name of heteroaffection. Derrida never opposes autoaffection to heteroaffection. He shows, on the contrary, that these two structures are intimately linked. In that sense, they appear inseparable. Derrida does not challenge autoaffection as such—there is an unmovable autoaffective dimension of subjectivity—but he criticizes the way in which philosophers always present it as pure (i.e., as purified of any heteroaffection). The incontestable existence of autoaffection cannot occult the fact that there is no such thing as a pure autoaffection. Instead of affirming the existence of an originary autoaffection, Derrida asks, "shouldn't one rather distinguish between several types of auto-hetero-affection without any pure, properly pure, immediate, intuitive, living, and psychical auto-affection at all?"[1]

How does Derrida understand autoaffection? In "To Speculate—on 'Freud,'" he explains that it must be understood as "related to the auto-affective structure of time . . . such as it is described by Husserl in *Lectures on Internal Time Consciousness* or in Heidegger's *Kantbuch*. . . . [This structure] concerns the oneself which apostrophizes itself and calls (to) itself as an other in auto affection."[2] Autoaffection coincides with the "inner voice" and the possibility of hearing oneself speak. According to Derrida, autoaffection is a kind of touch: an autoaffected subject is a subject that solicits itself, calls and answers itself, as if there were two persons in one. The traditional concepts of "consciousness" or the "soul," essential to the definition of subjectivity, are structured as a two-sided instance, one that acts or speaks, the other that receives or listens.

Derrida shows that autoaffection is a transcendental structure that is always presented, in traditional philosophy, as the primordial means, for the subject, to experience its being alive or to feel its own existence. To this extent, autoaffection coincides with life itself: "Auto-affection is a universal structure of experience. All living things are capable of auto-affection. And only a being capable of symbolizing, that is to say of auto-affecting, may let itself be affected by the other in general. Auto-affection is the condition of an experience in general. This possibility—another name for 'life'—is a general structure articulated by the history of life, and leading to complex and hierarchical operations."[3] Once again, Derrida does not criticize this notion for itself; he states that it is not originary, that the self doesn't exist before the movement of heteroaffection.

Heteroaffection means *the affect of the other*, in the double sense that (1) the one who is affected in me is always the other in me, the unknown "me" in me, a dimension of my subjectivity that I don't know and don't perceive, and that (2) what affects me is always somebody other that myself, something else than the feeling of my ownness. Even when I have the feeling of self-existence, for example, the I that feels and the existence that is felt are not exactly the same; they differ. There is always a third term, an unknown instance between me and myself. In the end, we have a series of "you"s instead of a double I. Therefore, autoaffection may be regarded as a self-touching, but this self-touching is always, as Jean-Luc Nancy declares, a "self-touching you" (*un "se toucher-toi"*).

Commenting on this formula, Derrida affirms: "At the very moment when 'I' makes its entrance, . . . it signs the possibility or the need for the said 'I' (as soon as it touches itself) to address itself, to speak to itself, to treat of itself (in a soliloquy interrupted in advance) *as an other*. No sooner does 'I [touch] itself' than it is itself—it contracts itself, it contracts with itself, but as with another. . . . *I* self-touches spacing itself out, losing contact with itself, precisely in touching itself."[4] The feeling of the difference between the self and itself is then never present to itself, never conscious but always, and right from the start, "disarticulated."[5] The difference that lies at the heart of the "I" is the difference between me and an "intruder," the other of me in me, "the heart of the other": "touching, in any case, touches the heart and on the heart, but inasmuch as it is *always* the heart of the other."[6] For that reason, "no one should ever be able to say 'my heart,' my own heart. . . . There would be nothing and there would no longer be any question without this originary exappropriation and without a certain 'stolen heart.'"[7]

The word *exappropriation* is important here, since it insists upon the interruption of ownness or property. All affects proceed from a disappropriation, not from an intuitive synthesis, of the ego. Heteroaffection, more exactly autoheteroaffection, is then the real source of all affects.

A Nonspatial Space

Whereas Derrida, until the 1990s, defined logocentrism as the privilege of voice and speech over writing and distance in general, the sense of touch becomes, in later works like *On Touching*, the most metaphysical of all senses, surpassing vision and hearing in its attachment to presence. In *Of Grammatology*, autoaffection is clearly defined as "hearing oneself speak." In *On Touching*, autoaffection is characterized as the subject's structural self-touching. Following deconstruction's development and evolution, we have then moved from logocentrism to "haptocentrism" (from the Greek *haptein*, "to touch").

Descartes is, according to Derrida, the paradigmatic thinker of this primordial self-contact that defines subjectivity as such. Is not the passionate soul one of the most convincing examples of such a structure? To undertake such an interpretation, Derrida stresses what appears to him to be a major contradiction in *The Passions of the Soul*. This contradiction concerns the status of the pineal gland. Thanks to this gland, the soul, "which has no elation to extension,"[8] acquires a kind of spatial existence, a kind of "body," as we previously said.

In paragraph 30 of *The Passions of the Soul*, Descartes claims that the soul is united to the *whole* body: "The soul is united to all parts of the body conjointly."

At the same time, Descartes affirms that the union of the soul and the body is circumscribed by one part of the body only, to a single point, the pineal gland: "There is a little gland in the brain where the soul exercises its functions more particularly than in the other parts of the body."[9]

Descartes explains: "We need to recognize also that although the soul is joined to the whole body, nevertheless there is a certain part of the body where it exercises its functions more particularly than in all the others. . . . The part of the body in which the soul directly exercises its functions is . . . the innermost part of the brain, which is a certain very small gland situated in the middle of the brain's substance and suspended above the passage through which the spirits in the brain's anterior cavities communicate with those in its posterior cavities."[10]

Derrida asks: If there is a spatiality of the soul, how can it be reduced to a point? Does not the idea of a punctual spatialization of the mind, which corresponds to the site of the union, amount to a pure and simple absence of spatiality (of the mind as well as of the union itself)? Thinking of extension as a point is highly contradictory. The soul's spatiality, and consequently its bodily existence, appears then to be an ideal—and not a material—one. This problem is also what allows Damasio, as we will see, to consider that, despite the affirmation of the mind-body union, the Cartesian mind is a "disembodied" one.

According to Derrida, the "innermost part of the brain" where the pineal gland is situated appears to be only a metaphorical space, not an effective one. Such a space plays the part of an ideal hand by means of which the soul touches itself and feels itself as united to the body. The pineal gland is the soul's hand, the nonspatial space of the soul's self-touching. Instead of opening itself to alterity, the passionate soul is first autoaffected and self-centered, to the extent that it has to touch itself first to be able to touch and be touched by the other.

What does "to touch itself" mean? The treatise's title, *The Passions of the Soul*, in fact means *The Difference Between the Soul's Actions and Passions*. The ideal space metaphorically incarnated by the pineal gland is the space of the soul's self-differentiation, this self-differentiation coinciding with two modes of being of the soul: activity and passivity. All the Cartesian developments concerning the actions of the body and the actions of the soul tend toward the final characterization of the space in which the very difference between activity and passivity is felt as such. Touching, writes Derrida, "situates the locus of equilibrium between action and passion. . . . Touch at the same time fulfills it and covers the entire field of experience, every interval and every degree between passivity and activity. . . . Touch, as such, occupies a median and ideal region of effort poised between passivity and activity."[11] It is also, for that reason, "the name of all the senses."[12]

Every affect is like a finger of the hand that evaluates the ideal difference between the soul's activity and passivity. The pineal gland can thus be characterized as a transcendental locus for the soul's self-differenciation, a prefiguration of the Kantian distinction between apperception and the empirical subject.

In this general context, wonder can only mean the way in which the soul is touched or moved by itself, a kind of emotion of the self for itself. Of course, it involves surprise and openness to the unknown or the unfamiliar, but these feelings are caught in a loop that ties the soul to itself. A striking aspect of the book *On Touching* is that the deconstructive undoing of this loop itself takes place within a tribute paid by Jacques Derrida to his friend Jean-Luc Nancy, a tribute in which Derrida repeats his admiration (wonder) and respect for him. May something like a non-autoaffected wonder exist? May the subject's self-touching be interrupted? May the metaphysics of touching be breached at some point?

Syncope

Jean-Luc Nancy has written at length about the possibility of bringing to light a nonmetaphysical sense of touch. His most explicit book on that topic is *Corpus*.[13] What are the main characteristics of this deconstructive touching? Derrida answers: "*Continuity and indivisibility*: two traits that could help us to formalize the whole metaphysics of touch, which is often an expressly spiritualistic metaphysics, sometimes a matter of 'humanisms.' Nancy seems to break away from haptocentric metaphysics, or at least to distance himself from it. His discourse about touch is neither intuitionistic nor continuistic, homogenistic, or indivisibilistic. What it first recalls is sharing, parting, partitioning, and discontinuity, interruption, cæsura—in a word, syncope. In accordance with a 'my body' that finds itself involved from the outset with a *techné* irreducible to 'nature' as to 'spirit' and according to a sense of touch that Nancy describes as 'local, modal, fractal.'"[14]

A nonmetaphysical touch is a touching *that structurally loses contact with itself*. "Discontinuity, interruption, cæsura, syncope" express this loss. The subject's self-touching is always discontinuous—absent to itself, as it were—as if it were the touching of an other: heteroaffection as such. This interruption marks a moment, a node, a fold, in the continuity: it performs a hinging, both breaking the continuity and letting it appear. In medicine, *syncope* is the temporary loss of consciousness experienced by a quick drop in blood pressure or a blockage of the blood to the brain. This last definition cannot be irrelevant, given Nancy's stress on the body and on his own body and heart in the essays "The Intruder" and "Corpus."[15]

The "syncope" is not a continuous touch between the body and the soul; it is not a punctual touch either as it is in Descartes with the pineal gland. This is a touch that doesn't know about itself. An affect touches me but I don't know what "me" means. This interruption between me and myself appears to be a "spacing," which is the genuine spatiality of the breached affected subject. "At the very moment when 'I' makes its entrance," Derrida writes, "it signs the possibility or the need for the said 'I' (as soon as it touches itself) to address itself, to speak to itself, to treat of itself (in a soliloquy interrupted in advance) *as an other*. No sooner does 'I [touch] itself' than it is itself—it contracts itself, it contracts with itself, but as with another."[16] This kind of originarily interrupted touch, this heteroaffection, is also called "to self-touch you" or the "self-touching-you."[17] Because the primordial affect (the affect of the self for itself) is always interrupted by the intrusion of alterity, all particular affects (love, hatred, joy, sadness, wonder, or generosity) are also constantly syncoped, interrupted, and discontinuous.

"Ontological Generosity"

This non-self-centered origin of affects displaces the very definition of affects themselves. Derrida stresses the possibility of elaborating a new, non-Cartesian meaning of both wonder and generosity, a wonder and generosity that wouldn't know or be aware of their own openness. A genuine generosity would be a pure gift, unconscious of itself, unable to feel itself give: "Generous?" Derrida asks. "Yes, generous: this word is all the more compelling since a certain 'generosity of being' becomes the ultimate justification of his 'experience of freedom.' This generosity is no longer simply a virtue of a subject, of what Descartes might have grasped by this word. This generosity allows one to *configure*, and think together, the *gift* (or rather the *offering*), *decision, spacing*, and *freedom*."[18]

Wonder and generosity are still to be understood as fundamental ethical affects. But, because they don't proceed from a self-touching of the subject, their source is not "selfish" in the literal sense. They are not *my* affects; they are *given* to me. Such gifts can come only from being—hence the expression "generosity of being." An affect is a gift that comes from the absolute outside of being. This "outside" or exteriority of being is characterized again as a "space" or a "spacing" that has no interiority but marks the irretrievable distance between being and the subject.

The problem with the Cartesian ethics of wonder and generosity is that when a subject consciously gives something (is effectively and consciously generous), it is not really an offer. It is the subject's decision, and thus always a form of calculation. To give out of generosity because one can give is no longer to give. The opening cannot be my decision but an ontological movement, impersonal and anonymous. It is existence itself that gives me the feeling of existence, not "me."

Therefore, the affective opening of the self cannot signify autonomy or autoaffection any longer. It is to be thought, each time, as an event: something coming from outside, from the other. Heteroaffection might then be defined as an affect which doesn't touch me to the extent that it doesn't touch itself. Such would be the "generosity of nonsubjective freedom."[19]

3 ·

THE NEURAL SELF

DAMASIO MEETS DESCARTES

T he questions raised by Derrida concerning the impossibility of a presentation of the self to itself, as well as those regarding affect as an
accident modifying a given subjective autoaffected structure, seem
strikingly to coincide with the problems that are currently addressed by the
neurobiological redrawing of the self. If neurobiologists acknowledge the existence of autoaffection, they define it as a nonconscious structure.

Following Damasio's reading of Descartes, the present chapter will bring to
light the deconstructive aspects of the neurobiological (or "neuro-psychoanalytic") redefinition of the subject. It will also show the irretrievable differences
and distances between these approaches. The notion of the "neural self" will be
at the center of our analysis.

Brain and Subjectivity

Plasticity Versus Fixity

In *Descartes' Error*, Damasio declares: "I am convinced that neurobiology
can begin to approach the subject."[1] Neurosciences today allow us to consider
subjectivity not as a biologically determined, fixed instance. On the contrary,

neural subjectivity is a plastic structure in which the emotional dimension plays a major role.

In his foreword to Mark Solms and Oliver Turnbull's book *The Brain And the Inner World*, Oliver Sacks declares: "Neurology [has] evolved, from a mechanical science that thought in terms of 'fixed' functions and 'centers,' a sort of successor to phrenology, through much more sophisticated clinical approaches and deeper understandings, to a more dynamic analysis of neurological difficulties in terms of functional systems, often distributed widely through the brain and in continual interaction with each other. Such an approach was pioneered by A. R. Luria in the Soviet Union."[2] Luria shows that the nervous system is organized through different functional systems, which implies that functions such as emotion and memory as well as consciousness itself are not localized *in* any of the component structures, but rather between them.[3] The nervous system is then a distributed structure, acentered and with shared receptivity. Disturbance—that is, the malfunctioning or rupture of neuronal connections—causes the entire system to malfunction. That is why the ensemble formed by functional systems is said to be plastic. There is an internal law of mutual compensations between these particular systems. The entire structure has to maintain itself through a constant cooperation in order to be able to receive internal or external modifications without being destroyed. Disturbance begins when the force or the impact of events are stronger than the brain's capacity to bear them.

The well-known metaphor of the brain as a computer has become absolutely obsolete, as is shown in a great number of neurobiological developments. We may consider, as an example, Ramachandran's statements in *Phantoms in the Brain*: "Popularized by artificial intelligence researchers, the idea that the brain behaves like a computer, with each module performing a highly specialized job and sending its output to the next module, is widely believed. In this view, sensory processing involves a one-way cascade of information sensory receptors on the skin and other sense organs to higher brain centers. But my experiments with [my] patients have taught me that this is not how the brain works. Its connections are extraordinarily labile and dynamic. Perceptions emerge as a result of reverberations of signals between different levels of the sensory hierarchy, indeed across different senses."[4]

This account of neural plasticity helps us to understand that emotional and affective mechanisms are not predetermined. Experience plays a major part in forming neural connections. These connections are highly modifiable—their shapes change—which shows that the brain is not a rigid structure, closed in on itself. On the contrary, it is open to external influences and affects. Plasticity means a new kind of exposure of the nervous system to danger and, consequently, a new definition of what "event," "suffering," and "wound" mean. When the brain is damaged, it is our whole "self," our subjectivity itself, which is damaged or altered.

In *The Brain and the Inner World*, Mark Solms affirms: "There is a predictable relationship between specific brain events and specific aspects of who we are. If any of us were to suffer a lesion in a specific area, we would be changed and we would no longer be our former selves. This is the basis of our view that anyone with a serious interest in the inner life of the mind should also be interested in the brain, and vice versa."[5] "Brain events" are intimately linked with our identity. We may even say that they constitute them. That is why there is a profound correspondence between the brain and subjectivity, between the brain and the "inner life." We have to understand today the way in which the brain "produces" our subjective mental life. This subjective mental life appears to be a new name for the psyche.

Neuro-Psychoanalysis

These new definitions of the relationship between the brain and subjectivity, or between the brain and personal identity, put Freud's conception of "psychic events" into question. Confronting Freud's definition of events, accidents, and traumas with their current neurological definitions and asking ourselves how and to what extent the psyche is open to what occurs (and, more specifically, to changing and destruction) has become necessary.

Before articulating this confrontation, let's remark that this neurological challenge to Freud does not imply a rejection of psychoanalysis. On the contrary, a new trend in neurology, "neuro-psychoanalysis," is gaining influence and power. In the 1990s, Solms founded a small group that explored neuro-psychoanalysis, or "depth neuro-psychology." This group became the International Neuropsychoanalysis Society.

On the society's webpage, one can read a quotation from one of the society's members: "Freud, in his 1895 'Project for a Scientific Psychology,' attempted to join the emerging discipline of psychoanalysis with the neuroscience of his time. But that was a hundred years ago, when the neuron had only just been described, and Freud was forced—through lack of pertinent knowledge—to abandon his project. We have had to wait many decades before the sort of data which Freud needed finally became available. Now, these many years later, contemporary neuroscience allows for the resumption of the search for correlations between these two disciplines." A statement of the society's purpose follows the quotation:

> Neuroscientists have begun to investigate various topics that have traditionally been the preserve of psychoanalysts, which has produced an explosion of new insights into numerous problems of vital interest to psychoanalysis.
>
> Because neuroscientists are tackling these complex psychological problems for the first time, they have much to learn from a century of psychoanalytic inquiry. A need for sustained scientific rapprochement between researchers and clinicians is essential to learning about and enhancing each other's perspectives and knowledge on matters of mutual interest.[6]

The clinical neuro-psychoanalytic approach is dual. First of all, it is necessary "to make the most detailed neuro-psychological examination of patients with brain damage and then to submit them to a model psychoanalysis." Second, the therapist must "bring the mechanisms of the brain and the inner world of the patient together." It is then within the perspective of a reconciliation which intends to bridge the two approaches that the neurological critique of Freud takes place. Solms adds: "People who suffer brain tumors, strokes and so forth are *people* just like ourselves—they have developed personality, complex histories, and rich internal worlds. Since these things are the stuff of psychoanalysis, these people can be studied psychoanalytically just like anyone else. In this way, basic clinico-anatomical correlations can be drawn, directly linking psychoanalytic variables with neurological ones and thereby integrating them with each other on a valid empirical . . . basis."[7]

Brain Events Are Not Enough

These developments help us set the frame for the general discussion that I intend to conduct here. They indicate that the current neurobiological analyses of the relationship between the brain and subjectivity do not involve a reductionist approach and that it is not a question of founding emotions and affects upon sound material principles. Another proof of this fact is given by Damasio when he refuses to reduce "brain events" to purely biological data. To reduce the body to the "brain" appears also as another attempt to "disembody" subjectivity! Isn't it what happened with Descartes himself? Damasio writes: "There may be some Cartesian disembodiment also behind the thinking of neuroscientists who insist that the mind can be fully explained solely in terms of brain events, leaving by the wayside the rest of the organism and the surrounding physical and social environment—and also leaving out the fact that part of the environment is itself a product of the organism's preceding actions."[8]

Descartes's so-called error resides, of course, in the mind-body dualism. But, in a more subtle way, it consists in delegating to the brain (and to the brain only) the task of uniting mind and body (think of the pineal gland). The brain, as it is presented in *The Passions of the Soul*, becomes then a kind of logical link or "software" that bridges the soul and the body without unifying them in a system or in a genuine organism. Taking the whole body as well as its natural and social environments into account entails that we develop a new approach to the brain according to which the brain appears as an open structure, but, once again, as a fragile one. The brain is part of a "biologically complex but fragile, finite, and unique organism."[9] Only if we acknowledge this fragility will we be able to regard and consider the bodily effects of psychological conflicts that are, in other terms, the psychosomatic dimension of brain events.

These relationships between the inside and the outside (between the brain and the body proper, or between organism and environment) help us to articulate the neurobiological determination of the auto- or heteroaffection relationship.

A New Approach to the Self

One of the most striking elements of Damasio's contribution to the current approach to the brain is his affirmation that the brain is primarily a sensuous and affected organ. Affects are older than reason, and all cognitive mechanisms, even the most sophisticated, need to be rooted in emotion to be able to function. Such is the case for reasoning and decision making. Damasio argues against Descartes that consciousness, or the soul, is not a pure activity of reflection that only secondarily gets stained by emotions. He asserts the existence of a constitutive, necessary link between emotion and consciousness: Consciousness itself is an emotional reaction to the intrusion of the outside. Consciousness, at its most elementary, is the awareness of a disturbance of the organism's homeostasis caused by a repeated encounter with an external object. This is why consciousness is inherently emotional. It is an interested reaction to a disturbance.

This point has many consequences for the present discussion. First, it places the issue of affects at the center of the neuroscientific approach to subjectivity. Second, it helps to articulate the problem of neural kinds of auto- and hetero-affection. Third, it challenges the traditional deconstructive approach to these same issues in allowing the emergence of a new definition of the body.

Homeostasis and Autoaffection

According to Damasio, primordial affects or emotions are those that are involved in autoaffection. Here, autoaffection doesn't designate a conscious, subjective "self-touching" procedure; on the contrary, it characterizes the nonconscious homeostatic processes that maintain the living organism. Interestingly, Damasio shows that emotion is deeply involved in homeostatic regulation.

The primordial affects that attach the self to itself are thus nonconscious. In this sense, neural autoaffection may be regarded as a kind of biological hetero-affection to the extent that the "I" which is affected has no idea of "itself." We will have to compare this lack of self-knowledge with the psyche's ignorance of its own extension as per Freud. Let's notice for the moment that such a non-conscious autoaffection leads to a profound redefinition of the "self."

The Structure of the Self

Damasio distinguishes three kinds of self within the self:

(1) the protoself
(2) core consciousness
(3) extended consciousness and the autobiographical self

(1) The protoself is the nonconscious, purely organic-neural self. It is made of the interconnected and coherent collection of neural patterns that, moment by moment, represent the internal state of the organism, that is, the neural "map" the organism forms of itself. This map helps the organism to regulate and maintain its homeostasis, which is continuously disturbed by intruding objects. This preservation of life implies an attachment of the self to itself. Emotion plays an important part in this process.

(2) Then, the conscious *core self* emerges, which is the zero-level form of consciousness (also called "thick consciousness"), the locus of the "feeling of

ourselves." The feeling of existence coincides with the being of an individual. As the first form of subjective ownership and agency, it is a modification of the protoself, which implies the distinction between me and others. The core self may be determined as a pure affective awareness with no cognitive function.

(3) Eventually, the core self is supplemented by the *autobiographical self.* "The autobiographical self," Damasio writes, "is based on autobiographical memory which is constituted by implicit memories of multiple instances of individual experience of the past and of the anticipated future. The invariant aspects of an individual's biography form the basis of autobiographical memory."[10] Contrary to the preceding types, this autobiographical self is conscious.

Insisting upon the nonverbal and even nonpictorial character of the protoself, Damasio asserts: "The basic neural device does not require language. The metaself construction I envision is purely nonverbal, a schematic view of the main protagonists from a perspective external to both. In effect, the third-party view constitutes, moment-by-moment, a nonverbal narrative document of what is happening to those protagonists. The narrative can be accomplished without language, using the elementary representational tools of the sensory and motor systems in space and time. I see no reason why animals without language would not make such narratives."[11] It is very clear for Damasio that there is a self which cannot be identified with consciousness: "The focus on self does not mean that I am talking about self-consciousness."[12]

In using the notion of self, I am in no way suggesting that *all* the contents of our minds are inspected by a central, single knower and owner, and even less that such an entity resides in a single brain place. I am saying, though, that our experiences tend to have a consistent perspective, as if there were indeed an owner and knower for most, though not all, contents. I imagine this perspective to be rooted in a relatively stable, endlessly repeated biological state. The source of the stability is the predominantly invariant structure and operation of the organism, and the slowly evolving elements of autobiographical data.

On Wonder, Fragility, and Impairment

A long chain of affects, linking primordial biological emotions with social emotions and eventually with feelings, accompanies and structures the formation of subjectivity.[13] In this chain, wonder plays a major role because it coincides with the passage from core consciousness to the autobiographical self. Wonder marks the opening of the self to experience. From autoaffection to surprise, curiosity, and the relation to objects in general: this is the normal path followed by the primordial emotions up to conscious feelings. Wonder is, in a way, at the interface between the nonconscious homeostatic attachment of the self to itself and the conscious autobiographical experience.

Why then does Damasio always talk about wonder when it is absent? Why does his description of wonder seem to take place in a negative phenomenology, as if one could speak of it only when it is not there? "Absent," "not there": these expressions refer to the emotional loss that occurs after most serious brain lesions. Damasio's descriptions of some cases of brain damage show that the autoaffective structure may be impaired and that, consequently, the whole emotional process is damaged or altered. It is then possible to lose the ability to wonder, as happens in anosognosia or other pathologies. The patients become "cold."

We will develop more about these cases in a later chapter. What I want to underscore here is that the neurobiological approach to emotions allows us to think *a strangeness or estrangement of the self to its own affects*. I mean this in two senses. First, regarding the nonconscious character of autoaffection, the self knows nothing about it. Second, regarding the possibility, for the self, of being detached from its own emotions after brain damage, the patient becomes indifferent and disaffected.

The "self," as we saw, is a state rather than a substance, a state constituted by different strata both unconscious and conscious. There is no possible awareness of this complexity. It is only *negatively*, when the self is impaired or when the emotional process is seriously altered, that it becomes possible to determine what the self and its affects *are*. Damasio declares: "At each moment the state of self is constructed, from the ground up. It is an evanescent reference state, so continuously and consistently *re*constructed that the owner never knows it is being *re*made unless something goes wrong with the remaking. . . . Our self, or even better, our 'metaself,' only 'learns' about that 'now' an instant later."[14]

※ ※ ※

There is no direct access for the self to itself. In normal situations, this access is only delayed ("an instant later"). In pathological cases, this access is impossible: patients suffering from anosognosia, for example, are unable to refer their trouble to their self. We understand why Damasio considers brain lesions as constituting a kind of "method." They allow the scientist to approach negatively, in the absence of the phenomenon that one seeks to describe, this very phenomenon itself, namely, here, the self, its autoaffective procedure, the way it is rooted in emotion. The neural self can be lost or definitely damaged, and this *possibility* is the only way to give an account of the self. Autoaffection becomes sensible only when we lose it or at least when its fundamental mechanism is impaired. Autoaffection, which is the root of all other affects, is subjectively invisible.

It thus seems that the neurobiological approach provides us with a radical concept of heteroaffection. This concept does not follow from the deconstruction of subjectivity; it describes the very essence of subjectivity. The subject is fundamentally, immediately, biologically a stranger to itself, which never encounters itself, which never touches itself.

This type of heteroaffection, unlike that brought out by Derrida, proceeds from a resolutely materialist inquiry. Heteroaffection originally is nothing other than the unconscious character of autoaffection, which places the subject straightaway in the position of being unable to accede to the origin of the feeling of self. This situation is determined by the structure of the brain, and not by that of consciousness, which is derived from the brain.

4.

AFFECTS ARE ALWAYS AFFECTS
OF ESSENCE

BOOK 3 OF SPINOZA'S *ETHICS*

We will now introduce, after Descartes, Derrida, and Damasio, the fourth participant in our discussion: Spinoza. Why this order? What is striking when we read book 3 of the *Ethics* is that no individual subject properly speaking ever appears to be the locus of affects. It is not a *subject*—the word is not used by Spinoza—who is affected. The processes of affections and emotions take place at an entirely ontological level that does not require the power or the autonomy of human subjectivity.

In his preface, Spinoza precisely develops a critique of Descartes's conception of passions considered as affects of the human subject proper, a subject that exists as an independent substance "outside Nature." Spinoza writes: "Most of those who have written about the emotions (*affectibus*) and human conduct seem to be dealing not with natural phenomena that follow the common law of Nature but with phenomena outside Nature. They appear to go so far as to conceive man in Nature as a kingdom within a kingdom. . . . They assign the cause of human weakness and frailty not to the power of Nature in general, but to some defect in human nature."[1] The critique of Descartes becomes explicit a few lines further: "I know, indeed, that the renowned Descartes, though he too believed that the mind has absolute power over its actions, does explain human emotions through their first causes, and has also zealously striven to show how the mind can have absolute control over the emotions."[2] Spinoza contests the idea of an autonomous mind controlling its own defects, which are also its own affects: "But my argument is this: in Nature nothing happens which can be attributed to its defectiveness, for Nature is always the same, and its force and power of acting is everywhere one and the same. . . . Therefore the emotions [affects] of hatred, anger, envy, etc., considered as themselves, follow from the same necessity and force of Nature as all other particular things."[3]

Affects do not belong to the human mind as such but appear as *natural ontological phenomena*, the causes of which have to be rigorously determined. Because there is no such thing as "defect" in nature, affects cannot proceed from a failure; and, the human mind has no independence. This also implies that the mind and body are not two distinct instances, but two expressions of the same substance, which is Nature, Being, or God.[4] This substance expresses itself through its own attributes (thought and extension) and modes (finite beings).

If affects are affects of Nature, if they do not belong to the human subject as such, and if Nature is equivalent to God and therefore to Being, it implies that *affects are always affects of Being*. This is exactly what Deleuze says when he declares: "Be it as it may, every affection [affect] is affection of essence. Thus the passions belong to essence no less than the actions; the inadequate ideas [belong] to essence no less than the adequate ideas."[5]

Are we facing, with Spinoza, an "ontological generosity" (to use Derrida's phrase) that is not related to human subjectivity? Are we confronted with a genuine theory of heteroaffection? It seems that Deleuze and Damasio agree on that point: the Spinozist theory of affects exceeds the realm of consciousness and subjectivity. Deleuze brings to light a theory of a nonsubjective autoaffection in Spinoza, an element that seems to confirm the similarity of his reading to Damasio's. There is a deconstructive gesture in Spinoza before "deconstruction."

Damasio's and Deleuze's readings differ nevertheless on many points. First, Deleuze's reading is not anti-Cartesian, but insists, on the contrary, upon a certain unexpected proximity between Spinoza and Descartes. Second, and more profoundly, the ontological value of affects in Spinoza is not interpreted in the same way by these two authors. For Deleuze, analyzing affects at the ontological level means that every being, including God, is affected in some way, which blurs the importance of human subjectivity and locates affectivity at the very heart of essence and ideas. For Damasio, "ontological" is another name for "biological." To situate affects at an ontological, nonsubjective level is the prefiguration of the neutral and anonymous biological processes of mapping body and mind together through neuronal activity.

General Structure of Book 3

Book 3 of Spinoza's *Ethics*, "Concerning the Origin and Nature of the Affects," comprises two parts. The first part comprises the fifty-nine propositions; the second is formed by a conclusion entitled "Definitions of the Emotions [Affects]."[6]

Affects and Conatus's Variability

Propositions 1–5

The three first definitions characterize (1) what an "adequate cause" is (a cause whose effect can be clearly and distinctly perceived, in opposition to situations when the effect is not clearly and distinctly perceived as belonging to a cause, which are "inadequate causes"); (2) the distinction between passivity and activity; (3) what an affect is. "By emotion (*affectus*)," Spinoza writes, "I understand the affections of the body by which the body's power of activity is increased or diminished, assisted or checked, together with the ideas of these affections."[7]

The link between inadequacy, affects, and passivity, induced by these three propositions, has to be understood in a way totally different than that of the traditional mode of understanding passions. Again, we should not regard passions as weaknesses in and of human nature. In that sense, if we have to admit a certain passivity due to affects, it cannot be the result of movements of the body, inadequately caused, on the soul. An action of the body cannot be regarded, contrary to what Descartes affirms, as a passion *in* the mind. It is equally useless to try to isolate a specific kind of passion that is a passion *of* the soul, or mind, proper.

Our body is a determined set of relations of movement and rest, and our mind is the idea of our body. Body and mind are two expressions of the same nature, one expressed through the attribute of extension, the other through the attribute of thought. It is hence impossible to consider actions of the body as causing effects in the mind. The same argument prevails when it comes to ideas: We have clear ideas and confused ideas, says Spinoza in proposition 9. But, if we say that our confused ideas come from our bodies, then we go back to Descartes's explanation of passions as defects that have to be referred to the weakness of human nature. Body and mind are always affected together and in the same way.

How can we understand this point? The theory of the conatus answers this issue. Its presentation makes the difference between Spinozist and Cartesian developments of affects and passions even clearer and stronger. Here is the definition of the conatus: "Each thing, in so far as it is in itself, endeavors to persist in its own being." The conatus is an ontological tendency that implies persistence and perseverance in one's being: "The *conatus* with which each thing endeavors to persist in its own being is nothing but the actual essence of the thing itself."[8] This tendency is one and the same with life itself, with the drive to survive and the preservation instinct. Both the body and the mind endeavor to persist in their own being, as Spinoza shows in proposition 9. This tendency is common to them both. The conatus, however, is not to be regarded as a third term, contrary to the Cartesian theory of the soul-body union as a third substance. The conatus is one tendency that can be envisaged differently if one looks at it from the bodily side or from the mind's side. There is therefore no such thing as an inner feeling of the unity between body and mind; the conatus is never subjectivated.

How, then, can we define affects? We saw that they could not be regarded either as bodily actions causing the mind to be passive or as passions of the mind alone. What is it, then, that is affected? If the conatus is an ontological tendency of the mind and the body jointly, affects cannot be actions of the body or passions of the soul. They are necessarily affects of the conatus itself in its entirety. They therefore have to be considered *variations of intensity in and of the conatus.*

The conatus appears as the "power of acting" of a "thing." This power— one would say today "empowerment"—is variable; it can be increased or diminished, assisted or checked. Whatever its disposition, our conatus is always affected in a certain way, always *attuned*. "Whatsoever increases or diminishes, assists or checks, the power of activity of our body, the idea of the said thing increases or diminishes, assists or checks the power of thought of our mind," writes Spinoza.[9] Therefore, passions cannot be considered as defects but as different degrees of variation of our power of acting.[10] In effect, this tendency is modulable depending on what causes desire and on what kind affective echo accompanies this cause. Inadequate ideas are those that diminish the power of acting; adequate ideas, on the contrary, increase and strengthen it.

Propositions 11–52: Joy and Sorrow

How can we understand the variability of the conatus? There are two fundamental modalities of attunement, from which all other affects are derived, joy
(*laetitia*) and sorrow (*tristitia*).[11] Joy characterizes the active affects, those that
allow the passage to a "greater perfection." It means that joyful affects cause a
greater desire and confer on the individual strength, courage, curiosity, *wonder*,
and the will to act and to think. Sorrowful affects, by contrast, imply bore-
dom, hatred, envy, anguish, and melancholy; they alienate the power of acting
and check it in various ways: nostalgia, depression, despondency. Again, the
conatus is not a rigid instance or a blind drive. On the contrary, it "undergoes
considerable changes."

We are now able to understand what Spinoza calls "passivity." Passivity
proceeds from sorrowful affects and the reduction of our empowerment. As
Deleuze writes: "If we manage to produce active affections, our passive affections will be correspondingly reduced. And as far as we still have passive affections, our power of action will be correspondingly 'inhibited.'"[12] Hence, what
constitutes the capacity to be affected and the locus of affects themselves is the
difference between acting and suffering, a difference open to their inversely
varying proportion. Affirmative or negative affects are not affects of a subject,
but modifications of an ontological structure, which implies that it is not an
"I" that is passive or active, but the conatus that, like a musical instrument, is
played with more or less intensity.

In "Definitions of the Emotions," at the end of book 3, Spinoza summarizes:
"Joy is man's transition from a state of less perfection to a state of greater perfection. Sorrow is a man's transition from a state of greater perfection to a state
of less perfection."[13] Spinoza admits the continuous change of the power of
acting, which he also defines as the "force of existing." Now, what causes joyful
and sorrowful affects? How can we explain their difference? We are, of course,
always affected by objects, or, more precisely, by "encounters."
Deleuze declares:

Spinoza employs a Latin word that is quite strange but very important: *occur-
sus*. Literally this is the encounter. To the extent that I have affection-ideas I
live chance encounters: I walk in the street, I see Peter who does not please
me.... When I see Peter who displeases me, an idea, the idea of Peter, is given
to me; when I see Paul who pleases me, the idea of Paul is given to me. Each

one of these ideas in relation to me has a certain degree of reality or perfection. I would say that the idea of Paul, in relation to me, has more intrinsic perfection than the idea of Peter since the idea of Paul contents me and the idea of Peter upsets me. When the idea of Paul succeeds the idea of Peter, it is agreeable to say that my force of existing or my power of acting is increased or improved; when, on the contrary, the situation is reversed, when after having seen someone who made me joyful I then see someone who makes me sad, I say that my power of acting is inhibited or obstructed.

This passage helps us to understand the nature of the conatus as it is common to the mind and the body. To affirm that the mind is the idea of the body means that every movement of the body is translated into the realm of thought as an ideal instance. When I encounter someone I don't like, my body feels a counterreaction, the urge to stop moving, to withdraw or make a detour. This checking of my mobility has its ideal counterpart: the idea of this person has little perfection or reality. There is a strict correspondence between the interruption of movement and a low degree of ideal reality. Sorrow is the very name of this correspondence, as joy signifies the unity between bodily activity and ideal integrity and degree of perfection.[14]

We are determined to look for every kind of encounter that is able to increase the power of acting and to flee from everything that threatens to destroy it. But, we don't know why such and such encounter will have such and such effect. We can only imagine what this effect will be.[15] Therefore, Spinoza declares: "It is clear from the above considerations that we do not endeavor, will, seek after or desire because we judge a thing to be good. On the contrary we judge a thing to be good because we endeavor, will, seek and desire after it."[16] Desire is not our decision. We never know how *extended* it is, how far it can go. Our judgments follow the ontological law of desire, which is never ours but the very mark of an ontological and natural striving toward duration and perfection.

52–59: On Wonder

Wonder comes to appear as the fundamental and most important joyful passion. Surprise and astonishment solicit the power of acting in a very creative way. It is attraction to singularity: "To an object that we have previously seen in conjunction with others or that we imagine to have nothing but what is in common to many other objects, we shall not give as much regards as to that which we imagine to have something singular."[17] The singularity of an object creates a greater desire to look for it; in consequence, it increases the power of striving and thriving. Indifference to novelty and singularity appears, by contrast, as a reactive and depressing trend that restricts the vitality of the conatus.

As in Descartes, but for different reasons, wonder is presented as the key to virtue. The last words of the *Ethics* insist upon the difficulty of leading a virtuous philosophical life: "but all things excellent are as difficult as they are rare [*sed omnia praeclara tam difficilia, quam rara sunt*]," Spinoza concludes.[18] "Excellent" translates the Latin *praeclarus*, which also means famous, beautiful, striking—in other words, and literally, wonderful. "Difficult" things are singular and rare. For Spinoza, "difficult" does not mean complicated. It is not the contrary of simplicity but of easiness and facility. Difficult things are simple: noncomposed, frank, entire, total. Simplicity is not facility, which, on the contrary, means commonness, usualness, and vulgarity. Wonder is the affect that helps us to differentiate simplicity (and, thus, difficulty) from facility. It reveals to us the beauty of difficult things and attunes our mind to their scarcity and rarity. Again, it is not the mind that affects itself and appraises itself through wonder. Wonder is the call of being, the tendency to turn the conatus toward the ontological beauty of the necessity of things.

Definition of the Emotions (Affects)

Still, we cannot be satisfied with our definitions of affects as ontological affects. A particularly important issue remains. We explained the relation between activity and passivity in insisting upon the conatus's variability, and we saw that this variability was not controllable: We never know how far our own conatus is extended. We may therefore consider that we are "heteroaffected" by our conatus. However, these explanations are valid as far as the modes (i.e., finite creatures) are concerned. To affirm, with Deleuze, that an affect is always an affect of essence seems to makes sense only for mortals. If it is true that Nature is everywhere one and the same, that man is not an empire within an empire, and that affects do not proceed from any individual or particular defect, then we have to understand how God himself, or Nature, may also be affected to the extent that there cannot be any variability of infinite desire—and there is, of course, no divine conatus.

Let's go back to the variability of conatus and the power of acting. In *Expressionism and Philosophy*, Deleuze declares: "Spinoza suggests . . . that the relation which characterizes an existing mode as a whole is endowed with a kind of elasticity. What is more, its composition, as also its decomposition, passes through so many stages that one may almost say that a mode changes its body or relation in leaving behind childhood, or on entering old age. Growth, aging, illness: we can hardly recognize the same individual. And is it really indeed the same individual? Such changes, whether imperceptible or abrupt, in the relation that characterizes a body, may also be seen in its capacity of being affected, as though the capacity and the relation enjoy a margin, a limit, within which they take form and are deformed."[19]

How can such an "elasticity" be attributed to God? Is it not the property of the modes only? How can Being be considered as passive, "elastic," that is, *affected*? We started this chapter with the Deleuzian affirmation that an affect, for Spinoza, is always an affect of essence. Do we have to understand that the infinite essence is also changeable? Or, can we reduce its mode of being affected to a pure and simple divine autoaffection? If it is so, finite affects (heteroaffection of the conatus) would be defective copies or reflections of a primary autoaffection—and Spinoza would be more Cartesian that we think!

Maps Between Affects and Concepts

Unless a kind of autoaffection outside any subjectivity can exist, an autoaffection is a movement internal to essence. Such an affection is not a feeling, but rather is the opening of a space in Being, of a map, a surface of inscription. The finite conatus is the finite modality of such an ontological mapping, of this spacing without subject or consciousness. Such will be Deleuze's answer. Damasio also will place the issue of mapping at the center of Spinoza's thought. As we will see, however, the two authors, Deleuze and Damasio, don't understand the terms *maps* and *mapping* in the same way.

5.

THE FACE AND THE CLOSE-UP

DELEUZE'S SPINOZIST APPROACH
TO DESCARTES

Surprisingly enough, Deleuze will bring to light this ontological kind of autoaffection both in Spinoza and Descartes. Instead of opposing the two philosophers, Deleuze—as is obvious in his reading of Descartes presented in *The Movement Image* and in *What Is Philosophy?*[1]—intends to show that the same move leads them both to discover a mapping activity in the economy of affects. Therefore, Deleuze's interpretation of Descartes leads to a conclusion quite different than Derrida's. The Cartesian subject is not autoaffected in the usual way, that is, self-touched. Autoaffection is, of course, present in Descartes's thought as it is in Spinoza's, but surprisingly, it does not designate the loop of subjectivity, namely, its self-reflexivity in the traditional sense.

From Spinoza to Descartes

Let's go back to Spinoza for a moment. Again, according to Deleuze, affects are primarily ontological affections. He declares that, for Spinoza, "not only are all the passions affections of essence, but even among the passions, sadnesses, the worst passions, every affect affects essence! I would like to try to resolve this problem. This is not a question of discussing one of Spinoza's texts; we must take it literally. It teaches us that, be that as it may, every affection is affection of essence. Thus the passions belong to essence no less than the actions; the inadequate ideas belong to essence no less than the adequate ideas."[2]

There are, as we know, three kinds of ideas for Spinoza, which coincide with three kinds of knowledge.[3] Knowledge of the first kind is divided into two parts. The first consists in knowledge from random experience (*experientia vaga*). This is knowledge "from singular things which have been represented to us through the senses in a way which is mutilated, confused, and without order for the intellect." The second consists in knowledge from signs (*ex signis*), "for example, from the fact that, having heard or read certain words, we recollect things, and form certain ideas of them, like those through which we imagine the things."[4] What links both of these forms of knowledge is that they lack a rational order.

With the second kind of knowledge, reason (*ratio*), we have ascended from an inadequate to an adequate perception of things. This type of knowledge is gained "from the fact that we have common notions and adequate ideas of the properties of things."[5] What Spinoza has in mind here is the formation of adequate ideas of the common properties of things and the movement by way of deductive inference to the formation of adequate ideas of other common properties. Unlike in the case of knowledge of the first kind, this order of ideas is rational but remains unaware of the immanent necessity of this rationality.

The third kind of knowledge (*scientia intuitiva*) "proceeds from an adequate idea of the formal essence of certain attributes of God to the adequate knowledge of the [formal] essence of things."[6] This type of knowledge gives insight into the essence of some singular thing together with an understanding of how that essence follows of necessity from the essence of God. Furthermore, the characterization of this kind of knowledge as intuitive indicates that the connection between the individual essence and the essence of God is grasped in a single act of apprehension and is not arrived at by any kind of deductive process.

According to Deleuze, all three kinds of ideas or knowledge entail a determined relationship between passivity and activity, affects and concepts. All three are, in their own way, affections of the substance, that is, of the essence of reality. We have to understand that some affects are caused by external objects, and others by internal solicitations. "When ... I am raised," Deleuze writes, "to ideas of the third kind, these ideas and the active affects that follow from them belong to essence and are affections of essence, this time insofar as essence is in itself [*en soi*], is in itself [*en elle-même*], in itself and for itself, is in itself and for itself a degree of power [*puissance*]." It is when we reach the ideas of the third kind that we come across the motif of autoaffection: "Ideas of the third kind are affections of essence, but it has to be said that, following a word that will only appear quite a bit later in philosophy, with the Germans for example, these are autoaffections. Ultimately, throughout . . . the ideas of the third kind, it's essence that is affected by itself. Spinoza employs the term *active affect* and there is no great difference between autoaffection and active affect. . . . The power of being affected of an essence can be as well realized by external affections as by internal affections."[7]

The Deleuzian notion of autoaffection does not refer to what Derrida calls the subject's self-touching. First of all, even in the third kind of knowledge, affects never interiorize an external solicitation. Autoaffection is not the reflection of an internal or immanent movement. When essence affects itself, be it through passions or through its own capacity of referring to itself, this self-encounter always occurs as a spacing. In other words, the reflexivity of essence over and on itself is never immediate, but creates a material and spatial surface. Each kind of idea creates, by introjection and projection at the same time, a space of encounter between thought and its object. This encounter between thought and being may be immanent, as in the case of the third kind of knowledge, but it gives way to a surface creation nonetheless. Deleuze calls this surface—exterior or interior—a "plane of immanence." It also appears in Deleuze's texts as a "map": "The map is open and connectable in all its dimensions; it is detachable, reversible, susceptible of constant modifications."[8] In that sense, autoaffection does not arouse any feeling, but is comparable to an artistic creation, as if the ideal solicitation were painting or imaging itself.

Descartes

The emergence of such a "plane" or "map" is also, according to Deleuze, present in Descartes's *Passions of the Soul*. Contrary to Derrida, who affirms that there is no internal spacing of the soul or the psyche in Descartes, Deleuze shows that the Cartesian theory of affects implies such a spacing, a spacing that prevents autoaffection from being a simple self-touching of the subject, a closure of subjectivity upon itself.

In his reading of *The Passions of the Soul*, Deleuze concentrates on the end of part 2. These paragraphs are devoted to the external signs of the passions. As Descartes explains, "The external signs of these passions: . . . I have yet to deal with the many external signs which usually accompany the passions—signs which are much better observed when several are mingled together, as they normally are, than when they are separated. The most important such signs are the expressions of the eye and the face, changes in colour, trembling, listlessness, fainting, laughter, tears, groans and sighs."[9] As we can see, these external signs appear mostly on the *face*. That is why, according to Deleuze, the face becomes the Cartesian plane of immanence par excellence, as if the soul's internal spacing is projected itself on it.

That is why Deleuze shows, in *Cinema I*, that Descartes, in a way, would have invented the "close-up."[10] The face and its passionate expression are the very site of autoaffection understood as the creation of a determined surface of interaction or an encounter between the affecting and the affected instances. Autoaffection must then be interpreted as a kind of spatial phenomenon. Even if this spatiality of autoaffection does not occur in the same way as in Spinoza, its mechanism is, from a structural point of view, the same.

Deleuze gives an interpretation of the two fundamental kinds of movements caused by the action of animal spirits. The first causes action in the muscles and limbs. Deleuze calls it the "movement-action." The second causes specifically the passions of the soul and has effects on the face. This kind of movement, invisible in its source, becomes visible at the surface of the body. This becoming-visible of the passionate movements is called by Descartes himself the inscription of signs on the face. The face thus becomes a surface of inscription or a writing tablet.

These movements of inscription are called by Deleuze "expressive movements" or "movements of expression." Deleuze explains that the first and main meaning of a face in general is social. When the face becomes expressive because of passions, it transcends its social role and stops playing its identificatory part. Affects interrupt or suspend the normal behavior and meaning of the face. When the face expresses an affect, it becomes a surface or a plane that coincides with the affect itself. It loses its autonomous existence to become a "pure" affect. Deleuze writes: "The face must get rid of its individual and social aspects in order to emerge as what it is in reality: the 'affect-face.' . . . If the face is in reality the 'affect-face,' it is clear that it has nothing to do with the individuation or social function of a person."[11]

The affect face is a reflexive surface of inscription. The face, as it coincides with the affect, becomes a pure quality or pure intensity. It then reveals its ontological dimension. It is as if being itself came to the surface through the face. That is why the face is said to express the essence of the face; the "visage" becomes "visageity" (*visagéité*). About the movements of expression, Deleuze affirms: "The moving body has lost its movement of extension, and movement has become movement of expression. It is this combination of a reflecting, immobile unity and of intensive expressive movements which constitutes the affect. But is this not the same as a face itself? The face is this organ-carrying plate of nerves which has sacrificed most of its global mobility and which gathers or expresses in a free way all kinds of tiny local movements which the rest of the body usually keeps hidden. Each time we discover these two poles in something—reflecting surface and intensive micro-movements—we can say that this thing has been treated as a face [*visage*]: it has been 'envisaged' or rather 'faceified' [*visagéifiée*], and in turn it stares at us [*dévisage*], it looks at us."[12] This is the emergence of the "icon."

In this becoming "pure affect" of the face, wonder plays a major role. Deleuze places stress upon this role in *The Passions of the Soul*: "Descartes will develop a theory of passions starting with—how can I say that—a degree zero. This degree zero coincides with the fundamental passion. The most originary passion is like this degree zero. Degree zero of what? The degree zero of the expressive movements. . . . Descartes calls this originary passion 'Wonder.'"[13]

Wonder is the least expressive of all passions, but it is at the same time the very site of conversion of physical needs into ontological signs. That is why, as is clear in English, wonder is intermediary between passion and thought. *Admiration* (wonder) "marks a minimum of movement for a maximum of unity, reflecting and reflected on the face. . . . There are two sorts of questions which we can put to a face, depending on the circumstances: what are you thinking about? Or, what is bothering you, what is the matter, what do you sense or feel? Sometimes the face thinks about something, is fixed on to an object, and this is the sense of admiration or astonishment that the English word *wonder* has preserved. In so far as it thinks about something, the face has value above all through its surrounding outline, its reflecting unity which raises all the parts to itself."[14] The wondering face does not express something intellectual; it reflects the affect of thinking as such.

In both cases, the wondering face becomes a "close-up": "There is no close-up of the face. The close-up is the face."[15] The close-up suspends individuation or social roles. Descartes's theory of passions thinks of the splitting-off of the individual subject from itself and its transformation into an impersonal surface. Affects are impersonal. From Griffith to Eisenstein, cinema will explore this becoming-neutral, becoming-intensive, and becoming-spatial of the face: "a nudity . . . much greater than that of the body, an inhumanity much greater than that of animals. The kiss already testifies to the integral unity of the face, and inspires in it the micro-movements that the rest of the body hides. But, more importantly, the close-up turns the face into a phantom."[16]

Descartes would have thus described, in *The Passions of the Soul*, the framing and cutting in the composition of the close-up, the assemblage of the face with itself in passion, and particularly in wonder, which suspends the face from its own flesh and materiality. In this sense, passions are the movie of the soul.

A Nonmetaphysical Philosophy

Again, there seem to be two possible readings of Descartes. The first one is the deconstructive one, which shows that the Cartesian thought of affects belongs to the traditional metaphysical thought of subjectivity, conceived as a process of autoaffection and self-touching. The second consists in leading or pushing Descartes out of this trend, to show that Descartes belongs to another tradition, which Deleuze calls "Philosophy," and which is quite different from "metaphysics." In *What Is Philosophy?*, Deleuze articulates this nonmetaphysical concept of philosophy. According to this concept, philosophy is thought of as a way of inscribing events on a certain kind of surface. This surface is precisely what Deleuze calls the plane of immanence. Every philosopher has his own conception of this plane. We saw that, in Descartes, the face is the plane of immanence of the cogito.

The events that are inscribed on the plane of immanence are what Deleuze calls "Concepts." These are not just ideas; they are forms, figures, shapes, and even characters—"conceptual personae," as is very clear with Nietzsche's *Thus Spoke Zarathustra*. The Cartesian subject is in itself such a concept. Contra what we usually think, there is no constituted subject in the first place and neither is there the affected subject that would have come afterward. On the contrary, the affects produce subjectivity as such as a "personage," a figure.

"Concepts are events, but the plane is the horizon of events," writes Deleuze in *What Is Philosophy?*[17] The encounter of concepts and events determines the emergence of conceptual personae, which are incarnations of the philosopher: "I am no longer myself but thought's aptitude for finding itself and spreading across a plane that passes through me at several places. The philosopher is the idiosyncrasy of his conceptual personae."[18] The subjectivity escapes its traditional definition.

We now face two concepts of affects and autoaffection: a traditional one, according to which the subject is affected by an object and by itself first of all;

and a different one, according to which affects come before subjectivity as such, as events, points of impact of these events on a surface, like colors on a canvas. If we follow this second line of interpretation, affects and autoaffections are heteroaffections to the extent that they separate the human subject, the "I," from itself. The I becomes an "icon," that is, nobody in particular, a nonsubstantial instance, just like in a close-up, where the actor disappears as an individual to become "the" face.

6.

DAMASIO AS A READER OF SPINOZA

F ollowing up the topics of the plane of immanence, the surface, and the map, we can now turn to Damasio's reading of Spinoza, developed in *Looking for Spinoza: Joy, Sorrow, and the Feeling Brain*.[1] The general purpose of the book is to show that Spinoza, as the "first neurobiologist," insists upon the importance of emotions and feelings in the very process of reasoning. Spinoza's nondualistic conception of the relationship between mind and body implies a definition of the conatus in which the ontological and the biological are intertwined. According to Damasio, Spinoza anticipates the brain's importance as the meeting point between being and life. This meeting point is materialized through the operation of neural "mapping." Here also, there is a projection or a production of *surfaces* and *planes*. I will focus here upon the specific way in which Damasio elaborates the problems of the preservation of life, the relationship between the surface and the event, and the conception of a neural subjectivity.

Toward a Biological Conatus: Emotions and Feelings

In his book, Damasio shows that the ensemble formed by emotions and feelings constitutes the mechanism regulating life and promoting survival. Feelings, which correspond for Damasio to classical philosophical passions (joy, sorrow, pleasure, pain, love, hatred), are more elaborate forms of affects than the basic emotions that are involved in homeostasis. Feelings are also important for survival. "The simple process of feeling begins to give the organism *incentive* to heed the results of emoting."[2]

Emotions determine homeostasis to be the process of the self's attachment to itself. They constitute the elementary form of autoaffection. Damasio defines emotions as simple "internal simulations" with no specific content. Feelings, for their part, transform emotions into what Damasio calls a "concern." Emotions produce self-attachment; feelings produce the concern for self-attachment. In this sense, feelings form the mechanism of attachment for the attachment, the redoubling of autoaffection.

Feeling in general, and wonder in particular, lays the foundation for care, the care of ourselves, the care for ourselves. The systematic unity of emotions and feelings takes place in the brain and remains unconscious for the most part. Damasio undertakes his reading of Spinoza to explore this systematic unity and its importance in the conatus, the regulation of life, and the life of ideas at the same time.

Damasio declares; "Now that I have sketched my main purpose, it is time to explain why a book dedicated to new ideas on the nature and significance of human feelings should invoke Spinoza in the title. Since I am not a philosopher and this book is not about Spinoza's philosophy, it is sensible to ask; why Spinoza? The short explanation is that Spinoza is thoroughly relevant to any discussion of human emotion and feeling. Spinoza saw drives, motivations, emotions and feelings—an ensemble Spinoza called *affects*—as a central aspect of humanity. Joy and sorrow were two prominent concepts in his attempt to comprehend human beings and suggest ways in which their lives could be lived better."[3]

This insistence upon the role of affect in the development of our ideas implies, of course, the biological regulation of life. This is what Spinoza critiques in Cartesian dualism. For Spinoza, mind and body, or thought and extension, are, as we know, parallel attributes of the same substance—hence the idea that the mind is the idea of the body. Damasio concludes that "Spinoza might have intuited the principles behind the natural mechanisms responsible for the parallel manifestations of mind and body. . . . I am convinced that mental processes are grounded in the brain's mappings of the body, collections of neural patterns that portray responses to events that cause emotions and feelings."[4]

The unity of the body and mind determines a conception of bodily manifestations of mental processes. These manifestations coincide with what are called today neural maps, that is, sorts of material surfaces upon which all kinds of events, both mental and affective, inscribe themselves. These inscriptions, in their turn, give way to feelings, which are superior forms of social emotions: embarrassment, shame, guilt, contempt, indignation, sympathy, compassion, awe, wonder, elevation, gratitude, pride.[5]

Deprived of such emotions or feelings, humanity wouldn't have been able to survive. This point leads Damasio to consider the importance of the notion of the conatus in Spinoza: "For Spinoza, organisms naturally endeavor, of necessity, to persevere in their own being; that necessary endeavor constitutes their actual essence. Organisms come to being with the capacity to regulate life and thereby permit survival. Just as naturally, organisms strive to achieve a 'greater perfection' of function, which Spinoza equates with joy. All of these endeavors and tendencies are engaged unconsciously."[6]

Because of this extremely modern conception of the conatus, Spinoza may be regarded as a "protobiologist." There are, according to this conception, "four" Spinozas: the religious scholar, the political thinker, the philosopher, and the fourth one, "the protobiologist." Damasio writes: "There is a fourth Spinoza; the protobiologist. This the biological thinker concealed behind countless propositions, axioms, lemmas, and scholia."[7]

In order to study or discover this fourth Spinoza, it is necessary, again, to stress the importance of the conatus. "It is apparent that the continuous attempt at achieving a state of positively regulated life is a deep and defining part of our existence—the first reality of our existence as Spinoza intuited when he described the relentless endeavor (*conatus*) of each being to preserve itself. Striving, endeavor, and tendency are three words that come close to rendering the Latin term *conatus*, as used by Spinoza in Propositions 6, 7 and 8 of the *Ethics*, Part III. In Spinoza's own words; 'Each thing, as far as it can by its own power, strives to persevere in its being' and 'The striving by which each thing strives to persevere in its being is nothing but the actual essence of the thing.'"[8]

Damasio shows that the different actions of self-preservation hold the different parts of a body together and maintain the unity of the whole. Fighting against external threats of destruction allows the unity of the individual being to take shape and helps the constitution of the body scheme or schema. Despite the transformations due to age or experience, the conatus remains the same all through life because it respects the same structural design. The conatus is a process of repetition or recurrence of the self. This repetition as such is the very origin of personal identity. Emotions and feelings play a major role in this repetition process. The more the organism increases its power of acting—by feeling joy—the more the different parts of the organism fit together and stick to their unity.

"Armed with this revised conception of human nature," Damasio continues, "Spinoza proceeded to connect the notions of good and evil, of freedom and salvation, to the affects and to the regulation of life."[9] The ontological and ethical meaning of affects is rooted in this biological tendency to survive. Being itself is survival, or endeavor. God, or Nature, is *within* ourselves. Ontology thus means the immanent presence of nature in us. Can we deduce that this immanence gives way, in Damasio as in Deleuze, to the construction of *planes* of immanence?

Mappings

The title *Looking for Spinoza* may be read in two ways. It first means "in search of Spinoza." But, it may also signify looking "in his place," in Spinoza's place, trying to see something that he was not able to see or to look at himself—being his eyes for him. What Spinoza was not able to see clearly by himself, because of the limited state of scientific observation, discovery, and experiment in his time, was the architecture of the nervous system. Damasio helps Spinoza to see more distinctly what Spinoza only had a sense of without exactly measuring the importance of such a discovery: "We can fill in the brain details and venture to say for him what [Spinoza] obviously could not."[10]

For the neurobiologist, the most striking and insightful statement of the *Ethics* is formulated in proposition 13 of book 2: "The object of the idea constituting the human Mind is the Body." This statement is elaborated in other propositions too: "The human mind is the very idea or knowledge of the human body"; "the Mind does not have the capacity to perceive . . . except in so far as it perceives the ideas of the modifications (affections) of the body"; "The human mind is capable of perceiving a great number of things, and is so in proportion as its body is capable of receiving a great number of impressions."[11]

Damasio affirms: "Spinoza is not merely saying that mind springs fully formed from substance on equal footing with the body. He is assuming a mechanism whereby the equal footing can be realized. The mechanism has a strategy; events in the body are represented as ideas in the mind. There are representational 'correspondences,' and they go in one direction—from body to mind. The means to achieve the representational correspondences are contained in the substance. The statements in which Spinoza finds ideas 'proportional' to 'modifications of the body,' in terms of both quantity and intensity, are especially intriguing. The notion of 'proportion' conjures up 'correspondence' and even 'mapping.'"[12]

What Spinoza was not able to see by himself is thus the neural activity of "mapping." Mapping characterizes the way in which events in the body are represented as ideas in the mind. As "representational 'correspondences,'" the coincidence between ideas and bodily events draws neural maps that, looking apparently very much like the Deleuzian "planes of immanence," inscribe bodily messages on an internal projective surface.

Spinoza "could not say that the means to establish ideas of the body include chemical and neural pathways and the brain itself. Of necessity, Spinoza knew very little about the brain and about the means for body and brain to signal mutually. . . . He carefully avoids mentioning the brain when he discusses mind and body, although we can be certain from statements elsewhere that he saw brain and mind as closely associated. For example, in the discussion that closes Part I of *The Ethics*, Spinoza says that 'everyone judges of things according to the state of his brain.'"[13]

Damasio proposes to substitute the term *image* for idea. Images emerge from neural patterns, or neural maps, formed in populations of neurons that constitute neural networks or circuits. Emotions and feelings play a major role in the way in which our brain forms these images. They render the mind-body correspondence easy or uneasy. Here again, Spinoza sensed this point in developing his conception of joy and sorrow. "The maps associated with joy signify states of equilibrium for the organism. Those states may be actually happening or as if they were happening. Joyous states signify optimal physiological coordination and smooth running of the operations of life. They not only are conducive to survival but to survival with well-being. . . . We can agree with Spinoza when he said that joy (*laetitia* in his Latin text) was associated with a transition of the organism to a state of greater perfection. . . . The maps related to sorrow, in both the broad and narrow senses of the word, are associated with states of functional disequilibrium. The ease of action is reduced. . . . If unchecked, the situation is conducive to disease and death."[14] The variability of the conatus is induced by the modulation of the instinct of survival. The ontological tendency to endeavor in one's own being is interpreted in terms of life drives. In that sense, wonder is the very expression of these vital impulses.

The Third Person's Perspective

If mind and body are two aspects of the same thing, if they mirror or reflect each other, then it is not even useful to use the terms *mind* and *body* any longer; it is not even useful to refer to their unity as a conscious subject. The term *organism* designates them both. It is the organism as a whole that is capable of wondering, that persists in life. We thus have to admit the existence of an impersonal *admiratio*.

Considering the neural patterns that constitute the biological basis of subjectivity, we can state that there is a process of heteroaffection in autoaffection because the feeling of oneself speaks and refers to itself in the third person. If autoaffection can be described here as the mutual mirroring of mind and body, then it is clear that something remains nonsubjective in this process. Something remains nonconscious and nonreferable to an "I" or a first person. The maps, or the neural drawing of an internal space of correspondence, is the space of heteroaffection.

This nonsubjective state can nonetheless be emotional because, as we just saw with Spinoza, it is linked with the conatus and its joyful and sorrowful variations. What we have to study now is what happens when the process of mapping is interrupted, when this auto-heteroaffection is impaired as a consequence of brain damage. In effect, to declare that passions are originarily nonsubjective means that they can be materially, empirically cut off from the subject.

7.

ON NEURAL PLASTICITY, TRAUMA, AND THE LOSS OF AFFECTS

The Two Meanings of Plasticity

The brain's exposure to accidents directly involves its plasticity. Under the term *neural plasticity* hides, in fact, two plasticities. One is positive: It characterizes the formation process of neural connections and the fact that these connections may be transformed during our lifetimes under the influence of experience and of the kind of life we are leading. Every brain has its own form and there is no such thing as two identical brains. So, in the case of the healthy plastic brain, every kind of event is integrated into the general form or pattern of the connections, and the series of events of our lives constitute the autobiographical self. There exists a second kind of plasticity, however, which refers to brain damage and its destructive power. This negative plastic power consists in the transformation of the patient's previous personality and in the emergence of a new individual proceeding from the explosion of the former identity. We see clearly here that plasticity appears as an accurate balance between the ability to change and the resistance to change.

Damasio states that "the circuits are not only receptive to the results of first experience, but repeatedly pliable and modifiable by continued experience."[1] This "good" plasticity, so to speak, can be interrupted by what neurobiologists call "disconnection." A lesion that occurs in a brain region "does more than gashing a hole in this region. It removes this region from the whole brain organization. . . . Cerebral lesions are always disconnections."[2]

Why should we call the destructive work of disconnection plastic? Isn't plasticity an inappropriate name here? To answer this issue, I refer to the famous case of Phineas Gage, which is related by Damasio in *Descartes' Error* and by Mark Solms in *The Brain and the Inner World*:

> In the 1840s, an unfortunate man by the name of Phineas Gage was laying railways tracks in the midwestern United States. He was pressing down a charge of dynamite into a rock formation, using a tamping rod, when the charge suddenly exploded. This caused the tamping rod to shoot through his head, from underneath his checkbone into the frontal lobe of his brain and out through the top of his skull. Partly because the rod passed through so rapidly, probably cauterizing the tissue on its way, the damage to Gage's brain was not very widespread; only a relatively small area of frontal tissue was affected. . . . Gage did not even lose consciousness, and he made a rapid physical recovery. His physician, however, reported some interesting changes when he published the case in a local medical journal a few years after the incident. Dr Harlow noted that, despite the good physical recovery and the relatively small extent of the brain injury, his patient was radically changed as a person; his personality was changed. . . . Let's read a passage from Doctor Harlow's report: "he is fitful, irreverent, indulging at times in the grossest profanity (which was not previously his custom), manifesting but little deference for his fellows. . . . In this regard his mind was radically changed, so decidedly that his friends and acquaintances said that he was 'no longer Gage.'"[3]

Let's focus on the statement that "his mind was radically changed." The specific operation of such a "radical" change cannot be of the same type as the one fulfilled by the plastic power of experience upon neural connections. Why not? First of all, a brain lesion interrupts all kinds of experience. The events that cause the pathological "radical change" are purely contingent, external, and totally unanticipated. They cannot be assimilated or interiorized by the psyche or by the brain. Second, the sort of transformation that occurs in such cases is not a partial modification but a complete metamorphosis of the personality. In Gage's case, there is no existential phantom limb phenomenon. The previous personality is totally lost and there is no remainder. Of course, some aspects of this personality are preserved: language, cognition, and reasoning. These faculties are strangely intact. But the emotional brain has been badly injured and this causes a dramatic change. Even if some capacities remain untouched, the patient is unrecognizable. Such a transformation may nevertheless be said to be plastic in the sense that it *forms* and *sculpts* a new identity.

The two plasticities are two different kinds of relationships between events and affects. When brain damage occurs, it interrupts the economy of our affects. Solms declares: "In our clinical work as neuropsychologists we have met hundreds of Phineas Gages, all with damage to the same part of the brain. This is a fact of obvious importance for anyone with an interest in personality. It suggests that there is a predictable relationship between specific brain events and specific aspects of who we are. If any one of us were to suffer the same lesion in that specific area, we would be changed in much the same way that Gage was, and we, too, would no longer be our former selves. This is the basis of our view that anyone with a serious interest in the inner life of the mind should also be interested in the brain and vice versa."[4]

The destructive plasticity forms what it destroys. It is not a simple annihilation or suppression to the precise extent that it has a result. This result is the formation of "someone else," a new self, a self that is not able to recognize itself. The accident appears to be the plastic explosion that erases any trace and every memory, and that destroys any archive. And yet, such a damaged mind is still alive. It is a kind of survival that absolutely renounces the possibility of redemption or salvation.

The event of the brain damage occurs without presenting itself and forever stays out of access, out of interiorization, remaining exterior to any "becoming-subject." Destructive plasticity is a biological deconstruction of subjectivity. All the questions Derrida raises under the name of heteroaffection—the impossibility of a presentation of the self to itself, of the I to itself, the impossibility of regarding the event as an accident belonging to the subject—all these questions seem to coincide precisely with the problems that are addressed in the neurobiological redrawing of the self.

The Loss of Affects

Brain damage is also a theoretical accident that happens to the very idea of the accident in its traditional definition. All the cases of brain damage that Damasio exposes are cases of absent subjectivity. Such a subjectivity is absent to itself and to its essence as well as to its accidents—a subjectivity *without* affects, the extreme form of heteroaffection.

The "survivors of neurological disease," as Damasio calls them in *The Feeling of What Happens*,[5] lead a life that is sometimes almost totally destroyed in its temporality and its structure. All these survivors share something in common: they all endure a profound change of personality caused by this destruction: "Prior to the onset of their brain damage, the individuals . . . affected had shown no such impairments. Family and friends could sense a 'before' and an 'after,' dating to the time of neurologic injury."[6] The loss of the previous self almost always leads the patients to indifference, coldness, and a lack of concern, "a marked alteration of the ability to experience feelings."[7]

All the cases that Damasio examines show this characteristic, which he calls "disaffectation" and, sometimes, "cold blood." One of the first examples of this phenomenon is exposed in *Descartes' Error*, in chapter 3, "A Modern Phineas Gage." This modern Phineas Gage is named Elliot. He was suffering from a brain tumor that had to be removed. "The surgery was a success in every respect, and insofar as such tumors tend not to grow again, the outlook was excellent. What was to prove less felicitous was the turn in Elliot's personality. The changes, which began during his physical recovery, astonished family and friends. To be sure, Elliot's smarts and his ability to move about and use language were unscathed. In many ways however, Elliot was no longer Elliot."[8] Damasio continues:

> Bit by bit the picture of this disaffectation came together, partly from my observations, partly from the patient's own account, partly from the testimony of his relatives. Elliot . . . seemed to approach life on the same neutral note. I never saw a tinge of emotion in my many hours of conversation with him: no sadness, no impatience, no frustration with my incessant and repetitious questioning. I learned that his behaviour was the same in his own daily environment. He tended not to display anger, and on the rare occasions when he did, the outburst was swift; in no time he would be his usual self again, calm and without grudges.
>
> This was astounding. Try to imagine it. Try to imagine not feeling pleasure when you contemplate a painting you love or hear a favorite piece of music. Try to imagine yourself forever robbed of that possibility and yet aware of the intellectual contents of the visual or musical stimulus, and also aware that once it did give you pleasure. We might summarize Elliot's predicament as *to know but not to feel*.[9]

The mechanism of mapping seems to be separated from all emotional processes. The attachment of the self to itself, or concern, does not take place any longer. There is no possible healing of such a disaffection: "Elliott seemed beyond redemption, like the repeat offender who professes sincere repentance but commits another offense shortly after."[10]

Another case is that of "L": "The stroke suffered by this patient, which I will call L., produced damage to the internal and upper regions of the frontal lobe in both hemispheres. An area known as the cingulate cortex was damaged, along with nearby regions. She had suddenly become motionless and speechless. . . . The term *neutral* helps convey the equanimity of her expression, but once you concentrated on her eyes, the word *vacuous* gets closer to the mark. She was there but not there. . . . Again, emotion was missing."[11]

A third example is even more serious and concerns cases of anosognosia (from the Greek *nosos*, "disease," and *gnosis*, "knowledge"). Anosognosia denotes the inability to recognize a state of disease in one's own organism: "No less dramatic than their oblivion that anosognosic patients have regarding their sick limbs is the lack of concern they show for their overall situation, the lack of emotion they exhibit, the lack of feeling they report when questioned about it. The news that there was a major stroke . . . is usually received with equanimity, sometimes with gallows humor, but never with anguish or sadness, tears or anger, despair or panic."[12]

Anosognosia is a lack of perception of damage. It is also known as Anton's Syndrome. Anton was an Austrian physician living at the end of the nineteenth century. In a talk he gave to the Society of Physicians of Austria, he described these patients as "soul-blind for their own blindness." Anton's Syndrome is the inability to make a certain functional loss available for conscious experience. The patients who suffer from this syndrome lose any ability to wonder about anything. The feeling of wonder itself has disappeared from both their body and their mind. This disappearance is a total one, not a partial loss. In what case is the deconstruction of autoaffection the more radical: when wonder proceeds from heteroaffection, or when affects are definitely impaired? Do we have to think of a heteroaffected subject or of a nonaffected subject to complete or accomplish the deconstitution of traditional subjectivity?

Freud and the Event

Freud wouldn't agree to consider that an emotion or an affect may totally disappear. In the psyche, he says, "nothing that has once come into existence will have passed away."[13] This capacity to preserve the past is precisely called plasticity. Freud compares the psyche to the city of Rome, in which every strata of the past is still present: every memory is still alive in the psyche. He insists upon the impossibility of total oblivion in psychic life. Every memory is thus like a monument.

In the development of the mind, says Freud in "Thoughts for the Times on War and Death,"

> every earlier stage persists alongside the later stage which has arisen from it; here succession also involves co-existence, although it is to the same materials that the whole series of transformations has applied. The earlier mental stage may not have manifested itself for years, but none the less it is so far present that it may at any time again become the mode of expression of the forces in the mind, and indeed the only one, as though all later developments had been annulled or undone. This extraordinary plasticity of mental developments is not unrestricted as regards directions; it may be described as a special capacity for involution—for regression—since it may well happen that a later and higher state of development, once abandoned, cannot be reached again. But the primitive stages can always be re-established; the primitive mind is, in the fullest meaning of the word, imperishable.
>
> What are called mental diseases inevitably produce an impression in the layman that intellectual and mental life have been destroyed. In reality, the destruction only applies to later acquisitions and developments. The essence of mental disease lies in a return to earlier states of affective life and functioning. An excellent example of the plasticity of mental life is afforded by the state of sleep, which is our goal every night. Since we have learnt to interpret even absurd and confused dreams, we know that whenever we go to sleep we throw out our hard-won morality like a garment, and put it on again next morning.[14]

We clearly see that Freud only stresses the positive meaning of plasticity. Plastic means imperishable, resilient, possessing the ability to cure or to heal. The metaphor of the city of Rome shows that psychic space, thought in reference to architectural extension, is always capable of exhibiting its memory and overcoming wounds and loss. The psyche can be both extended and positively plastic or indestructible.

Neurobiology puts this so-called psychic immortality into question. The formation of a "new" identity after a brain lesion shows that the primitive psyche is not imperishable, as Freud states; it can be damaged without any return to a previous state. The patients are not allowed to regress or to seek shelter in their own history or their own past.

The value of Freud's "excellent example of the plasticity of mental life" (i.e., dreams) seems to be put into question by some kinds of brain damage that destroy the very process of dreaming. Mark Solms shows that damage caused to sites specializing in mental imagery provokes a disturbance in the ability to dream: "If the patient loses the ability to generate a mental image, the inability to dream seems a logical consequence."[15] Three areas are involved in the process of imagery. When these areas are affected, visual experiences cease. For example, these patients lose the ability to perceive color or movement, or they lose the ability to recognize specific objects or faces. What are the effects of these lesions on dreaming? "Damage to the primary visual cortex, Zone 1, has (perhaps surprisingly) no effect on dreaming at all. Although these patients cannot see in waking life, they see perfectly well in their dreams. . . . Damage to the middle zone of the system, Zone 2, causes exactly the same deficits in dreams as it does in waking perception: these patients continue to dream in various sense modalities, especially somatosensory and auditory, but their visual dream imagery is deficient in specific respects. For example they no longer dream in color, or they dream in static images (loss of visual movement), or they cannot recognize any of the faces in their dreams. Damage to the higher zone, . . . Zone 3, on the other hand, produces complete loss of dreaming."[16]

What does the Freudian definition of the plasticity of mental life mean to people who have lost their ability to dream, to people who cannot see what they are dreaming of? In what sense is their sleep a return to a previous state? What is there to find? These patients indeed do have a psychic life. We must ask ourselves what this kind of psychic life means when there is no return, no regression, no attachment to the past, and no detachment from the past either.

A neurological accident is hopeless, unpredictable, and never consumable, an accident that cannot be integrated by the psyche, that cannot make sense for it, that cannot form a moment of a personal history. This is a purely destructive event, which provokes the total disappearance of a psychic formation, or of a brain region, or of affects, particularly wonder.

CONCLUSION

The main issue of this study was the following: Is it possible to develop a philosophical or theoretical approach to affects that does not determine them to be simple consequences of an originary autoaffection? Is the way in which the subject affects itself the definitive foundation of all affects?

We saw that autoaffection, which coincides, according to Derrida, with the inner voice and the possibility of hearing and feeling oneself, is defined as a kind of self-touching. For this autoaffective structure of the subject, Derrida substitutes several types of heteroaffection, or auto-heteroaffection, stating that there is no pure, properly pure, immediate, intuitive, living, and psychical autoaffection at all.

Can we follow such a path and think of affects as belonging to an originary structure of heteroaffection? We characterized heteroaffection as the affection of the other, in the double sense of the genitive: the affection coming from the other, from the utterly other, without any expectation or anticipation, and my being affected by the other in me, as if affects affected someone else in me other than me.

Wonder, the "philosophical" affect as such, tends both to erase and to underscore the border between auto- and heteroaffection. To the extent that it is a kind of surprise or astonishment, it appears to be the affection of the other, the unexpected. At the same time, wonder seems to be the privileged way in which spirit feels and enjoys itself. Spinoza himself declares: "When the mind regards its own self and its power of activity, it feels pleasure, and the more so, the more distinctly it imagines itself and its power of activity."[1] Wonder is thus an ambivalent affect.

For Derrida, Deleuze, and Damasio as readers of Descartes and Spinoza, the approach to affects in general and wonder in particular, in its ambivalence, determine three things: first, a concept of alterity; second, a privileged metaphor; and, third, a specific notion of spatiality.

In Derrida, the concept of alterity coincides with a definition of subjectivity as a relationship between an "I" and a "You," a "self-touching you." The way in which the intruder or the other affects me is a gift that comes from nowhere; it is given. This is what Derrida calls, contra Descartes, ontological, as opposed to subjective, generosity. Wonder always comes from the other wondering in me. Derrida's privileged metaphor is the *graft*. The psyche's extension provides us with a new concept of spatiality.

In Deleuze, affects are always affects of an *essence*, not of a subject. His privileged metaphor is the *face*. Spatiality is understood as the *plane of immanence*. Wonder coincides with the interruption of the social part of the individual. The face becomes a sign.

According to Damasio, there is a fundamental biological alterity of the self to itself to the extent that autoaffection (homeostasis) remains nonconscious. Damasio's privileged metaphor is that of *cold blood*. The spatiality is that of *maps* or *neural patterns*. Wonder means interest in the world and desire for acting. But it cannot be thought outside of its opposite, namely, the absence of wonder: coldness, detachment, indifference.

Who brings to light heteroaffection in the most radical way? In order to answer this question, let's confront three texts. Each of them presents an essential aspect of heteroaffection. The first one (by Derrida) could be entitled "The Two Lovers," the second (by Deleuze) the "Becoming-Non-Human," and the third (by Damasio) "I Am in Pain But I Don't Feel It."

In *On Touching*, Derrida imagines a very specific case of separation:

Imagine: lovers separated for life. Wherever they may find themselves and each other. On the phone, through their voices and their inflection, timbre, and accent, through elevations and interruptions in the breathing, across moments of silence, they foster all the differences necessary to arouse a sight, touch, and even smell—so many caresses, to reach the ecstatic climax from which they are forever weaned—but are never deprived. They know that they will find ecstasy again, ever—other than across the cordless cord of their entwined voices. A tragedy. But intertwined, they also know themselves, at times only through the memory they keep of it, through the spectral phantasm of ecstatic pleasure— without the possibility of which, they know this too, pleasure would never be promised. They have faith in the telephonic memory of a touch. Phantasm gratifies them. Almost—each in monadic insularity. Even the shore of a "phantasm," precisely, seems to have more affinity with the *phainesthai*, that is, with the semblance or shine of the visible.[2]

In his lectures on Spinoza, Deleuze affirms:

The affect goes beyond affections. . . . The affect is not the passage from one lived state to another but man's nonhuman becoming. Ahab does not imitate Moby Dick. . . . It is not resemblance, although there is resemblance. . . . It is a zone of indetermination, of indiscernability, as if things, beasts and persons . . . endlessly reached that point that immediately precedes their natural differenciation. This is what is called an *affect*. In *Pierre, or The Ambiguities*, Pierre reaches the zone in which he can no longer distinguish himself from his half-sister, Isabelle, and he becomes woman. . . . This is because from the moment that the material passes into sensation as in a Rodin sculpture, art itself lives on this zone of indetermination.[3]

Damasio establishes a distinction between pain and emotion caused by pain:

In short, pain and emotion are not the same thing. You may wonder how the above distinction can be made, and I can give you a large body of evidence in its support. I will begin with a fact that comes from direct experience, early in my training, of a patient in whom the dissociation between *pain as such* and *emotion caused by pain* was vividly patent. The patient was suffering from a severe case of refractory trigeminal neuralgia, also known as tic douloureux. This is a condition involving the nerve that supplies signals for face sensation in which even innocent stimuli, such as a light touch of the skin of the face or a sudden breeze, trigger an excruciating pain. No medication would help this young man who could do little but crouch, immobilized, whenever the excruciating pain stabbed his flesh. As a last resort, the neurosurgeon Alamida Lima, offered to operate on him, because producing small lesions in a specific sector of the frontal lobe had been shown to alleviate pain and was being used in last-resort situations such as this.

I will not forget seeing the patient on the day before the operation, afraid to make any movement that might trigger a new round of pain, and then seeing two days after the operation, when we visited him on rounds; he had become an entirely different person, relaxed, happily absorbed in a game of cards with a companion in his hospital room. When Lima asked him about the pain, he looked up and said quite cheerfully that "the pains were the same," but that he felt fine now. I remember my surprise when Lima probed the man's state of mind a bit further. The operation had done little or nothing to the sensory patterns corresponding to local tissue dysfunction The mental images of that tissue dysfunction were not altered and that is why the patient could report that the pains were the same. And yet the operation had been a success. . . . Suffering was gone. . . . This sort of dissociation between "pain sensation" and "pain affect" has been confirmed in studies of groups of patients who underwent surgical procedures for the management of pain.[4]

These three texts have something in common. Each of them challenges the possibility for the self to touch itself, or to coincide with itself. They all state the impossibility of what Merleau-Ponty calls the "touching-touched" relationship between me and myself: "When my right hand touches my left," Merleau-Ponty writes, "I touch myself touching: my body accomplishes a 'sort of reflection' and becomes a 'subject-object.'"[5] In each case, we find, in a way, two subjects: (1) the two lovers, which can also be read as two expressions of the self-subject, as a staging of the impossibility of autoaffection, and which are the difference of the subject and his own affects that escape him; (2) the subject feeling pain but not being affected by it. We always find two subjects in one. But, there is an infinite distance between them.

The "telephonic memory of a touch" presupposes the existence of a touch without presence. If two lovers can stay together without ever being able to see each other, beyond joy and sorrow, it is because there is no presence of the self to itself, no mirror, no self-reflection. There is no difference between the feeling of myself and the feeling of the other. In both cases, what I experience is separation, parting, discontinuity, and interruption.[6] The opening of the self to itself or to the other does not come back to itself, does not form a loop. Wonder remains without closure.

Deleuze takes three examples of affects, which correspond to the three kinds of ideas in Spinoza: first, the affect caused by the effect of the sun on the body; second, the affect caused by the effect of the sun on a painter's canvas; third, the affect caused by the essence of the sun on the mind. In each case, there is no reflection; the sun (the affecting or touching power) is not reflected by the surface that it touches. The touching and the touched are driven out of themselves. They form a block that exceeds the material locus of their contact: the body, the canvas, and the mind. That is why Deleuze says that percepts go beyond perceptions, affects beyond affections, reaching this zone of indetermination that is the nonhuman.

Affects, including autoaffection, separate the human subject, the "I" from itself. I am not affected. In *What Is Philosophy?*, Deleuze writes, referring to Merleau-Ponty's schema of both touching and touched hands: "The difficult part is not to join hands but to join planes."[7] The different kind of affects and affections in Spinoza, the sun on my body, the sun on a canvas, the solar self, or autoaffection of essence are mediated by a "plane of immanence," a projective surface that prevents immediate contact. There is always the space of a difference between the touching and the touched, which is clear even in the case of essential autoaffection.

According to Damasio, the most intimate and elementary part of our neural self is, as we saw, the "protoself." The protoself is made of the interconnected and coherent collection of neural patterns that, moment by moment, represent the internal state of the organism, that is, the neural "map" that the organism forms of itself. This map helps the organism to regulate and maintain its homeostasis, which is continuously disturbed by intruding objects. Homeostasis is not a merely mechanistic or logical process. It produces the first form of attachment of the self to itself.

To the extent that this attachment is nonconscious, the subject is anonymous. If we could have a look at our internal neural processes, Damasio says, it would always be from the third-person perspective. In the case of the suffering patient, what happens is not exactly the loss of emotion, but the loss of conscious emotion. The surgery provokes the dissociation of two strata of the subject that are usually unified: the protoself and the conscious self. The third person, involved in homeostatic processes, and the first person, involved in conscious procedures, are disconnected and can look at each other at a distance.

Sometimes, the opposite situation occurs. After certain sorts of brain damage, some patients loose their feelings and emotions, but not their first-person perspective, not their consciousness. Those people, as Damasio says, act in cold blood. Because of their disease, they are led to indifference, coldness, and a lack of concern, to "a marked alteration of the ability to experience feelings."[8]

※ ※ ※

It is time now to return to the initial issue: Who thinks autoaffection in the most radical way? All the questions raised by Derrida—the impossibility of a presentation of the self to itself, the impossibility of regarding the affects as rooted in conscious autoaffection—appear precisely to coincide with the problems that are addressed by the neurobiological redrawing of the self. We also know that Deleuze devotes a whole chapter to the brain at the end of *What Is Philosophy?*

In fact, this apparent proximity between our three authors hides a genuine discrepancy. It seems that the thought of affects in Deleuze and the thought of heteroaffection in Derrida always require the thought of a heterobody, that is, of a nonorganic body or of body without organs.

To bring to light the originary process of heteroaffection, Derrida and Deleuze need to delocalize the natural body. The absence of organs, for Deleuze, means the lack of organization, as if our flesh, our blood, our brain were suspected of being the material expressions of metaphysics, as substance, system, presence, and teleology are such expressions. The "Body Without Organs" remains a body but it only presents itself as a surface to slip over or bounce off. It is a plane. Derrida also needs to think of a kind of nonnatural surface, a nonbiological bodily extension, which allows for the encounter with the other. What he calls the "subjectile" is such a surface, which "stretches out under the figures that are thrown upon it" and lies "between the subject and the object" without any biological determination.[9]

This exclusion of the body also appears in *On Touching*: "No one should ever be able to say 'my heart,' my own heart, except when he or she might say it to someone else and call him or her this way. . . . There would be nothing and there would no longer be any question without this originary exappropriation and without a certain 'stolen heart.'"[10] Why is that? Why shouldn't we say "my heart"? Why this moral injunction "shouldn't"? Is it necessary to transcend biology to articulate a concept of affects that is not related to subjectivity or to its self-touching? Or, on the contrary, doesn't it seem that this is one of the most striking lessons of neurology today: that the organic neural organization is radically deconstructive, that a deconstruction of subjectivity is at work in our neurons?

We may wonder whether the critique of phenomenology, of the phenomenological body, of "flesh" and "fleshism," does not lead Derrida and Deleuze to dematerialize, in their turn, the process of affects. When I clasp my hands, is it two planes that I join? Is it certain that two lovers can resist the absence of bodily pleasure and be satisfied with fantasm? Why is it necessary to look for the outside outside of the body? Why put the body at a distance, at a distance from its own organs?

% % %

This leads us to examine Freud's puzzling statement about the psyche's spatiality. On August 22, 1938, he wrote on a single sheet: "The psyche is extended, knows nothing about it [*Psyche ist ausgedehnt, weiss nichts davon*]."[11] If this were the case, space, like time, would be outside the realm of consciousness and knowledge. Amazingly, when discussing psychic time and space, Freud refers to Kant's definition of the forms of intuition. If our unconscious does not know anything about its own temporality and spatiality, it is because their structure is analogous to that of a transcendental apparatus. We must admit time and space to be pure forms of the psyche, in the same way that Kant speaks of the pure temporal and spatial forms of our intuition. Freud writes: "At this point I shall venture to touch for a moment upon a subject which would merit the most exhaustive treatment. As a result of certain psychoanalytic discoveries, we are today in a position to embark on a discussion of the Kantian theorem that time and space are 'necessary forms of thought.'"[12]

By the time that Freud came to write *Beyond the Pleasure Principle*, he had formulated many spatial metaphors to represent his hypotheses about the psychical apparatus and its components, to represent spatially the structural hypotheses of id, ego, and superego and the topographical concepts of consciousness, preconscious, and unconscious. We can think, for example, of the passage from *The Ego and the Id* where Freud affirms that "the ego is first and foremost a body-ego. It is not merely a surface entity, but is in itself a projection of a surface."[13]

This spatial character of the psyche stays forever unconscious. Commenting on Freud's statement, Derrida declares: "Psyche the untouchable, Psyche the intact: wholly corporeal, she *has* a body, she *is* a body, but an intangible one. Yet she is not only untouchable for others. She doesn't touch *herself*, since she is wholly extended *partes extra partes*."[14] Inaccessible to subjectivity and reflexivity, the spatiality of the psyche incarnates the impossibility of self-touching and appears as the very structure of heteroaffection.

Such a space, such a body, is nonempirical and nonbiological. As we know, when Freud uses the word *topic*, or when he represents the psychic apparatus as a series of strata or layers, it is always metaphorical. The psyche's spatiality is imaginary; it does not exist as such. Freud would have, of course, refused to consider an organ like the brain to be the extension and material ground for psychic phenomena. That is also why Freud does not admit the idea of a total destruction of any part of the psychic apparatus. The unconscious is indestructible because it has an abstract, unreal spatiality, something that can be blurred but not physically impaired.

To declare that the unconscious, and the psyche in general, are indestructible amounts to saying that affects and emotions themselves are always present, even when they are negative, even when they belong to what Spinoza calls sorrowful instincts. How would it be possible to envisage an emotionless psyche?

If we are allowed to consider that Freud and Lacan elaborate a vision of a psyche that, contrary to the classical philosophical subject, is never autoaffected, but seems always affected from outside, without any possibility of appropriating this alterity, it seems that the principle of this heteroaffection cannot be destroyed.

The issue of wonder may be assimilated, in Lacan, to the problematic of the gaze, on the one hand, and to the problematic of the *agalma*, on the other. *Agalma* is an ancient Greek term for a pleasing gift presented to the gods as a votive offering. The *agalma* was intended to woo the gods, to dazzle them with its wondrous features and so gain favor for its bearer. The *agalma*, therefore, was endowed with magical powers beyond its apparent superficial value. Over time, the term *agalma* has come to mean an iconic image, something beautiful, an object to be treasured. Lacan introduced the term in his seventh seminar (1960–1961), lecturing on Plato's *Symposium*. The *agalma* is defined by love; it is the inestimable object of desire that ignites our desire. Relating this to the analytic setting, Lacan proposes that the *agalma* is the treasure that we seek in analysis, the unconscious truth we wish to know.[15]

Looking for this treasure would be impossible if we didn't feel *gazed* at during this search. The psychoanalyst gazes at the subject at the same time that the subject wonders at him as at a desirable treasure. To gaze means: "to stare in wonder and in admiration." The French translation of this word, in the Lacanian context, is "fascination." The transference relationship requires both the *agalma* and the gaze as a double direction of wonder: gazing at and being gazed at. Looking at the *agalma*, the inestimable object of desire, becomes for the analysand the catalyst agent of the transference relationship. This look (which does not come from any eyes, as Lacan firmly states) is in itself a response to the feeling of being looked at, of feeling oneself "*sous le regard*" or "*sous la fascination*" (under the gaze). Because the gaze and the *agalma* are not the works of any given subjectivity, and because their very structure has much to do with fantasy, the affects they generate (love, fascination, idealization, and the like) do not proceed from an autoaffective process of the psyche. They are heteroaffections to the extent that they come from the other. Still, this being affected by the other cannot itself be affected, that is, altered to the point that it can disappear or be totally destroyed.

The same thing happens in Derrida's philosophy. Wonder and affects in general may be deconstructed, but their deconstruction does not amount to their possible destruction or disappearance. A subject cannot be cut off from its own affectivity or libidinal disposition. We saw that Deleuze also doesn't seem to envisage the end of wonder, the possibility for a face to not express anything, to lose its capacity to become a surface of inscription or a plane of immanence.

% *%* *%*

For neurobiologists, psychic spatiality is not ideal, abstract, or transcendental. It coincides with the brain and is exposed to its possible material destruction. In most cases, a brain injury is a type of wound that cannot be anticipated and that, in opposition to the Freudian definition of the psychic event, cannot be explained by the personal history or destiny of the subject. A brain injury most of the time has no other cause than an accidental or an external cause. In this sense, it is "the utterly other."

If Solms has a right to claim that there is a coincidence between brain events and the inner life of subjective experience, brain injuries cannot then be considered as mere physiological or organic lesions. Rather, they also appear as *psychic* lesions. The brain today appears as the space of and for the neuronal unconscious.

The emergence of a new type of unconscious and psychic life that is entirely destructible has important consequences for the general theory of death and destruction drives. A major form of brain and psychic disturbance today is, as we saw, emotional indifference and "flatness." Studying some particular cases of brain lesions such as agnosia or anosognosia, Damasio notices that the people who suffer those kinds of diseases are "absent without leave." Oliver Sacks, in *The Man Who Mistook His Wife for a Hat*, describes "The Lost Mariner's Case." The patient "was strongly built and fit, he had a sort of animal strength and energy, but also a strange inertia, passivity, and (as everyone remarked) 'unconcern'; he gave all of us an overwhelming sense of 'something missing,' although this, if he realised it, was itself accepted with an odd unconcern."[16]

Damasio links those cases of the loss of emotion with criminal psychological types such as serial killers and with all kinds of social withdrawal. It appears that a philosophical approach to these neurological analyses of injury, indifference, and criminality is necessary in order to understand what we should call a new state of mind of the psyche, determined by a neural death drive, indifferent to love or wonder, indifferent even to its own power of destruction or its own aggressiveness.

The time has come to elaborate a new materialism, which would determine a new position of Continental philosophy vis-à-vis neurobiology, and build or rebuild, at long last, a bridge connecting the humanities and biological sciences. Instead of proposing a substantial vision of subjectivity, current neurobiology is exploring the absence of the self to itself. There could be no power of acting, no feeling of existence, no temporality without this originary delusion of the first person. Such a position might help in radicalizing the notions of heteroaffection, the nonhuman, or the death drive, which remain, in their actual state, remnants of the metaphysical tradition because of the contempt that both philosophy and psychoanalysis have expressed with regard to the biological in general and the brain and the neurosciences in particular.

As the cognitivist Thomas Metzinger writes: "Nobody ever was or had a self. . . . No such things as selves exist in the world: Nobody ever *was* or *had* a self. All that ever existed were conscious self-models that could not be recognized *as* models. The phenomenological self is not a being, but a process—and the subjective experience of *being someone* emerges if a conscious information-processing system operates under a transparent self-model. You are such a system right now, as you read these sentences. Because you cannot recognize your self-model *as* a model, it is transparent: you look right through it. You don't see it. But you see *with* it. . . . As you read these lines you constantly *confuse* yourself with the content of the self-model currently activated by your brain."[17] The transparency of the self-model and the anonymity of the emotional brain are the disenchanted wonders of the new psychosomatic and libidinal space.

PART II.

MISFELT FEELINGS

UNCONSCIOUS AFFECT BETWEEN
PSYCHOANALYSIS, NEUROSCIENCE,
AND PHILOSOPHY

❦ ❦ ❦

ADRIAN JOHNSTON

8.

GUILT AND THE FEEL OF FEELING

TOWARD A NEW CONCEPTION OF AFFECTS

P sychoanalysis is organized around its distinctive conception of the unconscious. Moreover, analysis is, of course, not only a set of philosophical and metapsychological theories regarding this peculiar object of its inquiries; it's also an arsenal of therapeutic techniques for treating specific forms of mental suffering and anguish. Particularly as regards the phenomena confronting working analysts in their clinical consulting rooms day in and day out, the powerful and moving manifestations of affective life, manifestations spanning the full spectrum from the pleasurable to the painful, seem to be of a degree of significance and weight to analysis comparable to that enjoyed by the unconscious itself.

And yet, starting with the founder of psychoanalysis, the question of how to situate the unconscious and affective life vis-à-vis each other consistently has been a controversial matter provoking an array of disparate, and often clashing, responses within and beyond analytic circles. The crux catalyzing the controversy is the basic, fundamental question of if it makes sense to posit feelings that aren't consciously felt (at least as the feelings they presumably really are). As I soon will show in detail, Freud himself repeatedly and markedly vacillates apropos the question of whether or not (and, if so, how) affects can be (and sometimes are) unconscious in a meaningful analytic manner. Additionally, and to paint in broad brushstrokes at this early introductory stage of my exposition, those who follow in Freud's footsteps typically take diverging paths in relation to this issue. At one extreme, certain Anglo-American post-Freudian currents sometimes give the impression that, for them, affects are the alpha-and-omega targets of analytic interpretation—and this in the general absence of a philosophically rigorous metapsychological account of how affects are able to be unconscious, an account resolving the unresolved problems that plagued Freud in thinking about this topic. At another extreme, Lacan is virtually unwavering in his claim that a Freud to whom analysts should remain steadfastly faithful categorically rules out the possibility of unconscious affects as a contradiction in terms—and this on the basis of an exegetically and philosophically sophisticated, albeit quite debatable, reading of Freud's writings and overall metapsychological framework. In my estimation, neither extreme represents a satisfying solution to the riddle of the rapport between the unconscious and affective life.

For analysis, the ramifications of this riddle are both metapsychological and clinical. On the metapsychological side, conceptions of what the unconscious is and how it functions are up for grabs. Do repression and related intrapsychical defense mechanisms operate solely on ideational representations (i.e., linguistic and conceptual mental contents), leaving affects to be pushed and pulled to and fro on the planes of conscious experience as mere superficial appearances? Do the formations of the unconscious comprise exclusively bundles and webs of structured symbolic materials? Or, alternately, do subterranean surges of emotions and feelings pulse through the associative networks of defended-against dimensions of psychical life? How, if at all, do defense mechanisms interfere with or inflect affective phenomena? On the clinical side, the core concern is what analysts' ears, attempting to attune themselves to the murmurings and outbursts of the unconscious, should be listening for from patients on their couches. This concern shapes in turn the techniques practicing analysts deploy in their ways of hearing, interpreting, and intervening in relation to their analysands. When, if ever, are expressions of affect to be taken at face value? How honest or dishonest are emotions and feelings to be regarded? Which affects, if any, ought to draw special attention from the analyst? How should analysts respond to various upsurges of passions and sentiments during the analytic hour? Are certain affective responses on the part of analysands indicative of interpretive or therapeutic success (or failure)? The questions I've raised in this paragraph highlight just a few of many metapsychological and clinical issues in play around the intersection (or lack thereof) between things unconscious and affective.

Having initiated my intervention by outlining the psychoanalytic origins and stakes animating it, I want to continue easing into the topic of unconscious affects from a more philosophical angle. If, as Aristotle famously declares in the *Metaphysics*, wonder is the source driving philosophizing,[1] then a complementary specification immediately should be added to this: Wonder, a compelling, captivating feeling that is experienced as a light, gentle yearning or exhilaration, is the affective motor behind the speculative endeavors of theoretical philosophy. That is to say, if wonder is a fundamental philosophical affect, it's fundamental primarily to those parts of philosophy moved principally by a "desire to understand" (i.e., epistemology, ontology, metaphysics, logic, and the like). But, what about the significant other half of philosophy? In other words, what about practical philosophy (i.e., ethics, politics, and the like), which is concerned not so much with "What can I know?" (expressing the wondering of theoretical philosophy), but rather with "What should I (or we) do?" Guilt is one of the main candidates for being to practical philosophy what wonder is to theoretical philosophy, namely, a foundational affect that is a catalyst for the deliberations, decisions, and deeds of concern to philosophy's prescriptions in addition to its wonder-driven descriptions.

Before proceeding further along these lines, I need briefly to indicate that my focus on guilt is not dictated by the reasons and worries of practical philosophy. That is to say, my exploration of affective life at the crossroads of philosophy, psychoanalysis, and neurobiology isn't steered by ethical or moral interests and agendas. I am much more concerned here with description over prescription (to resort hesitantly in passing to a problematic and unstable dichotomy). I dwell on guilt in particular because it's the one affect above all others to which Freud almost always refers when he speculates about the possibility of affects being unconscious. This pride of place in Freud's texts is what leads to the prominence of guilt as a paradigmatic example in my discussions.

Regarding the preceding philosophical thread, if guilt indeed is a fundamental philosophical affect in relation to ethics—at least in Kant's shadow, it certainly seems to be—then Freud's psychoanalytic discoveries and their aftershocks (both within post-Freudian psychoanalytic movements and in wider circles without) introduce some serious complications. These complications have to do with both the consciousness of guilt (as conscience) and affective mental dynamics more generally. To begin with, analyses of the workings of conscience are part of what prompted Freud to undertake a massive revision of his basic theoretical framework in the middle of his mature career (in *Beyond the Pleasure Principle*, published in 1920), a revision in which the pleasure principle is dethroned from its previously central position as the inviolable law of psychical life. Self-inflicted suffering in the form of conscience-induced guilt is somewhat more difficult to explain under the pre-1920 metapsychological regime (i.e., the "first topography" or "topographical model" of conscious, preconscious, and unconscious), which is centered on the hegemonic pleasure principle. Along with this sweeping shift "beyond the pleasure principle," Freud after 1920, in *The Ego and the Id* (1923), introduces the agency of the superego as part of the new triumvirate (including the id and ego) of the "second topography" (or "structural model"). The outlines of this agency already are foreshadowed in the seminal paper "On Narcissism: An Introduction" (1914), in which an intrapsychical function of surveying and supervising the ego's position vis-à-vis the ego-ideal (i.e., what the ego aims to be), identified by Freud as "conscience," is highlighted.[2] However, despite Freud's employment in 1914 of the everyday word *conscience* for this mental ministry of judgment and punishment, it soon becomes apparent to him that his later renaming of this as *superego* amounts to more than the superficial semantic substitution of technical for quotidian language.

One of the crucial philosophical upshots of the Freudian conception of the superego is that not all of conscience is conscious. With the transition from the first to the second topographies in Freud's thinking in the early 1920s, the triad of the conscious-preconscious-unconscious isn't simply dislodged and replaced by that of the id-ego-superego; moreover, for numerous reasons, one cannot legitimately establish one-to-one correlations here such as "consciousness = ego" or "unconscious = id" (which are based on the erroneous notion that the transition between topographies involves nothing more than simple substitutions). Instead, the three terms of the first topography change from being nouns (designating metaphorically spatial sectors within a map of the psyche's regions) to operating as adjectives. As adjectives, they modify the three agencies of the second topography. Specifically apropos both the ego and superego, this means that there are unconscious as well as conscious dimensions to these two agencies.[3] Considering this, Freud declares, in connection with the psychoanalytic positing of an unconscious side of conscience, that "the normal man is not only far more immoral than he believes but also far more moral than he knows."[4] If much of the content composing the superego (i.e., injunctions, prohibitions, and the like) is inaccessible to self-conscious introspection, circumstances easily can arise in which someone unknowingly has violated a command or rule to which he/she holds him-/herself accountable without being cognizant of this hidden standard. Put somewhat more straightforwardly, a person can disobey his/her conscience without being conscious of doing so. As Freud sees it, although the conscious ego isn't aware of the infraction, the intrapsychically omniscient superego certainly is. And, there are consequences.

But, what, exactly, are these consequences? The most common and, for psychoanalytic metapsychology, least problematic consequent phenomenon is a consciously experienced feeling of seemingly groundless, irrational guilt, a sense of culpability minus the awareness of a transgression as a preceding cause. (This situation sometimes results in what Freud characterizes as individuals becoming "criminals from a sense of guilt," that is, precipitously acting out in transgressive manners so as paradoxically to create a definite cause for a preceding, already-felt sense of indefinite guilt that is free floating:[5] in 1916, Freud discusses these sorts of individuals as instances of typical "character types" dealt with in analyses.) In the case of seemingly inexplicable guilt feelings, consciousness of guilt as an affect is cut off from its appropriate ideational correlates, from its corresponding representations (*Vorstellungen* that, in this instance, remain unconscious). This sort of guilt-in-search-of-a-crime is indeed a phenomenon encountered in analytic work. More generally, analysts from Freud onward consider the occurrence of affects split off from their real representational partners to be ubiquitous phenomena regularly surfacing within the four walls of the consulting room. However, as I will demonstrate later, other potential consequences of driving a wedge between conscience and what is conscious via the hypothesis that there are unconscious dimensions of the superego generate theoretical problems for both Freud and subsequent psychoanalytic theorizing, problems that, arguably, have yet to be satisfactorily resolved at the level of coherent metapsychological conceptualizations.

In connection with the affect of guilt, one can get a preliminary sense of the difficulties Freud comes to face through considering the following questions: Does guilt actually feel different when one is cognizant of its true cause as compared with how it feels when one isn't cognizant of this? Is the latter experience always going to register itself consciously as a feeling that could or would be called "guilt," at least by he/she who registers it? If not, what other feelings, if any other than a clear sense of culpability, will arise instead? Additionally, is it possible for someone to feel guilty without being (fully) conscious of feeling this way? If so, what justifies, both clinically and conceptually, supposing that one can feel without feeling that one feels, namely, that there can be, so to speak, unfelt (or, more accurately, misfelt) feelings?

Interestingly, as I indicated earlier, guilt is the primary affect Freud mentions when entertaining speculations about the existence of unconscious affects in certain of his patients. A standard scholarly story about this topic is that, until the second topography, Freud dismisses the notion of unconscious affects as incoherent and self-contradictory. If feelings, as feelings, always are felt, then how could it make sense to speak of affects as anything other than experiences transpiring within consciousness? Then, so the story goes, with the developments of the second topography as regards the topic of the superego, Freud is compelled to reconsider, if not wholly abandon, his prior metapsychological conviction that affects must be conscious phenomena. As will be seen herein shortly, matters are much more complicated.

As early as 1907, Freud muses about the need to posit the existence of "an unconscious sense of guilt."[6] Hence, one should note that this notion occurs to Freud well before the foundational manifesto of the second topography published in 1923 (*The Ego and the Id*). More importantly still, this occurs to him before the metapsychological paper on "The Unconscious" (1915). Therein, in the third section, "Unconscious Emotions" ("*Unbewußte Gefühle*"), Freud appears categorically to rule out the theoretical legitimacy of hypothesizing affects that aren't conscious.[7] And yet, there are arguments to be made to the effect that this section of "The Unconscious" has been repeatedly misinterpreted by numerous commentators (Lacan included): if, in 1907, Freud already entertains ideas about unconscious emotions, then maybe his remarks in 1915 about this topic need to be carefully reread in light of this generally overlooked textual fact. What's more, this rereading, to be carried out subsequently, reveals Freud to be, once again in yet another fashion, quite ahead of his time. In particular, his metapsychological distinctions, contained in the third section of "The Unconscious," between "affective structures" (*Affektbildungen*), "affects" (*Affekte*), "emotions" (*Gefühle*), and "feelings" (*Empfindungen*)[8]—he also points to how these phenomena might be "misconstrued" by those experiencing them[9]—foreshadow the insights and results of the latest cutting-edge research in affective neuroscience (especially the work of Antonio Damasio, but also that of such researchers as Joseph LeDoux, Jaak Panksepp, and Mark Solms, among others).

So, at this juncture, perhaps it sounds as though what is to be done in the present context is merely to integrate this subcomponent of the Freudian apparatus more thoroughly into the overarching framework of contemporary neuropsychoanalysis. However, what goes by the name "neuro-psychoanalysis" these days is an English-speaking orientation whose psychoanalytic components are drawn almost exclusively from Anglo-American strains of post-Freudianism (i.e., ego psychology, object-relations theory, and so on). Save for such remarkable exceptions as Slavoj Žižek, François Ansermet, Gérard Pommier, and Catherine Malabou, few thinkers versed in Lacanian (and, more broadly, French) styles of psychoanalytic theorizing have made attempts at reconciling Lacan's concepts with the discoveries of the neurosciences. There is as much additional work to be done here as there is resistance to the pursuit of such labors. The historical, cultural, political, institutional, theoretical, and other reasons for this resistance are myriad; an attempt at exhaustively delineating the multifaceted background behind the deeply ingrained hostility to the life sciences so pervasive within the relatively recent intellectual traditions rooted in Continental Europe is something for another occasion.[10] For now, suffice it to say that, as will be argued here (and as I argue elsewhere),[11] the deliberate, principled neglect of biology and related fields is no longer justified or defensible, psychoanalytically or philosophically, on either Lacanian or non-Lacanian grounds. Moreover, both Lacanian psychoanalysis and neuro-psychoanalysis stand mutually to benefit from being interwoven in ways motivated by a meticulous reconsideration of Freudian theories of affect in conjunction with data from the scientific investigation of the emotional brain. In particular, various yet-to-be-resolved difficulties plaguing Freudian-Lacanian metapsychology, including the problem of unconscious affects bequeathed by Freud to his successors, can be reconsidered now in a new, more empirically sound manner. *A priori* fist banging and foot stamping about these issues has ceased to be effective, credible, or necessary.

Of course, not only is Lacan's apparent allergy to the life sciences well known; he is notorious, particularly among those of a poststructuralist bent, for allegedly ignoring affects altogether.[12] A chorus comprising Lacanianism's discontents tirelessly rehearses the charge that Lacan, going against what is said to be essential to the psychoanalytic endeavor both within and beyond the clinical setting, neglects everything that won't be squeezed into the confines of the conceptual boxes constructed along the lines of classical structuralism. The tyranny of the signifier ostensibly imposed by Lacan is, from this perspective, to be countered through recovering and reemphasizing Freud's energetics, including his reflections on affective dynamics (but not through engaging in the least with what the sciences have to say regarding these matters).

Admittedly, Lacan is not without his own direct responses to this line of criticism. His reaction to this charge of affect neglect consists in a mixture of questionable consistency involving both protests of innocence (à la "I devoted the entirety of my tenth seminar of 1962–1963 to the topic of anxiety") and aggressive counterattacks targeting the foundational assumptions of his critics (à la "Freud himself stipulates that the unconscious, as the proper object of psy-choanalysis, is woven solely of *Vorstellungen*, and not affects"). The latter pre-dominates: Lacan and his followers repeatedly appeal to Freud's remarks from 1915 in "The Unconscious" regarding affects to defend their being relatively downplayed in Lacanian psychoanalysis. (The Lacanian analyst Colette Soler reiterates this line in her book on *Les affects lacaniens*, published in 2011.)[13] If this appeal to Freudian authority is undermined by a reexamination of Freud's texts (i.e., another "return to Freud," conducted at least in the spirit of Lacan, if not to his letter) as already outlined in preview, then what are the ramifications for the Lacanian handling (or, maybe, mishandling) of affective life? Is Lacan's sole remaining fallback option his discussion of anxiety in the tenth academic year of *le Séminaire*?

The tenth seminar indeed deserves sustained attention in the context of this discussion of affects. Additionally, a flurry of recent activity by various nota-ble Lacanians latches onto remarks made by the later Lacan regarding shame (*honte*) in the seventeenth seminar of 1969–1970. As with anxiety, here too there seems to be exculpatory evidence in favor of Lacan against accusations of ignoring affects. Additionally, Lacan's articulations concerning *jouissance* and related notions perhaps harbor resources for addressing productively the worries and reservations of his poststructuralist critics. I will be making fur-ther moves pushing off from this later. For instance, an illuminating contrast between *honte* and *pudeur* (both sometimes are translated somewhat mislead-ingly into English as "shame") will be highlighted and deployed so as to bring into sharper relief core features of the hybrid psychoanalytic-neuroscientific-philosophic account of affects to be formulated by me in the present project. This clarifying distinction between *honte* and *pudeur*, although implicit within Lacan's oeuvre, has been left thus far unthematized and unelaborated by both Lacan and his readers. Its implications dovetail in surprising ways with the neglected nuances of Freud's oft-misunderstood metapsychology of affects both conscious and unconscious.

At the broadest of levels, there's a real irony in Lacan's treatment of the psychoanalytic (in)significance of affects in light of his depiction of what is truly revolutionary in Freud's discovery of the unconscious, which is distinct from this concept's earlier historical forerunners and precursors. Lacan sees an unconscious capable of highly elaborate and complex cognitive maneuver-ings, and not a simple nonconscious domain of raw, unthinking animalistic instincts acting as brute, stupid mechanisms.[14] For instance, in his 1960 *écrit* "The Subversion of the Subject and the Dialectic of Desire in the Freudian

Unconscious," Lacan appropriately corrects Freud's self-misunderstanding of the status and implications of his subversive breakthrough. As is common knowledge, Freud compares his decentering of human beings' mental lives away from consciousness, a decentering according to which "man is no longer master in his own house," to the steps taken by such explorers as Copernicus and Darwin before him.[15] According to Freud, just as heliocentrism evicts humanity's earth from the center of a universe-become-centerless, and just as evolution turns the transcendent crown of creation into an immanent by-product of contingent monkey business tracing back to the muck of a primordial ooze, so too does the psychoanalytic doctrine of the psychical primacy of the unconscious inflict yet another wound on human beings' narcissism, their sense of somehow being at the central helm of things, if only within the limited realms of their own minds. But, Lacan observes, Freud's emphasis on this wounding effect of such Copernican-style revolutions, however accurate it may be in particular respects, risks leaving silently passed over, and certainly involves no mention of, a powerful narcissistic secondary gain (to put it in Freud's own terms) accompanying such upheavals in knowledge. Although the discoveries of Copernicus and Darwin lead individuals to reconceive of themselves as insignificant, smaller-than-specks blobs of cosmic dust floating in a disorientingly vast void of incomprehensible dimensions, these same individuals at least can take some pride and joy in knowing that they are blobs who know just how miniscule and meaningless they are.[16] In a very different context of concerns, Pascal already expresses this well: "Man's greatness comes from knowing he is wretched: a tree does not know it is wretched" (*La grandeur de l'homme est grande en ce qu'il se connaît misérable. Un arbre ne se connaît pas miserable*).[17] He continues: "Thus it is wretched to know that one is wretched, but there is greatness in knowing one is wretched" (*C'est donc être misérable que de [se] connaître misérable; mais c'est être grand que de connaître qu'on est misérable*).[18] What Lacan succeeds at revealing is that Freud's comparison of his psychoanalysis with Copernicus's heliocentrism and Darwin's evolution is misleading insofar as it obscures from view a more profound injury to humanity's sense of itself, an injury covered over by the superficial picture of the narcissistic wound of intellectually acknowledging certain scientifically revealed decenterings. This injury afflicts knowledge itself, the source of the Pascalian feeling of "greatness in wretchedness" spontaneously secreted as a salve for human beings' narcissism by the very same wounding breakthroughs with which Freud inaccurately compares his own advances.

From Lacan's perspective, Freudian psychoanalysis, unlike heliocentrism and evolution, subverts the figure of the traditional subject of knowledge, of knowing being anchored in the psychological phenomena of a transparent-to-itself self-consciousness. One of the implications of Freud's barring of any straightforward equivalence or synonymy between the mental and the conscious is that one can think without thinking that one thinks, that one can know without knowing that one knows. (This equivalence is a long-standing assumption in the philosophical tradition that Freud had to fight fiercely against and that nowadays has been utterly invalidated by a deluge of facts uncovered by other, nonpsychoanalytic approaches to the mind.) Hence, knowledge itself, rather than remaining as a comforting narcissistic secondary gain alongside Freud's mislabeled Copernican revolution, is threatened to various extents, cast into a morass of doubts in the shadow of the psychoanalytic unconscious. But, what is the previously mentioned irony in the Lacanian depiction of affective life in relation to his critique of the Copernican metaphor for the Freudian revolution? Whereas Lacan insists that one can think without thinking that one thinks and that one can know without knowing that one knows, he nowhere, not even for the briefest of fleeting moments in connection with Freud's vacillations apropos whether affects can be unconscious, entertains the idea that maybe one somehow can feel without feeling that one feels. The key question is: why not?

To summarize simply a much longer and more complicated theoretical narrative—I will tell this tale at greater length in what ensues—Lacan accepts as self-evident the early Freud's assumption that feelings, as feelings, must be felt consciously (with a parallel neglect of the early Freud's overt, albeit hesitant and rare, speculations regarding unconscious affects). Linked to this acceptance is a corresponding endorsement of a fundamental Freudian dichotomy between, for lack of better terms, energy and structure. In the case of the Lacanian metapsychological articulation of emotional life, this is translated into an opposition between, on the one hand, affects (as necessarily conscious) and, on the other hand, signifiers (as representational structures participating in and constituting the unconscious). In tandem with going back to the lingering Freudian enigma of unconscious affects in light of recent research in affective neuroscience, perhaps it is time both to reconsider Lacan's Freud-inspired dualism strictly partitioning signifiers and affects and, consequently, to reformulate the psychoanalytic metapsychology of ideational representations (*Vorstellungen*). These are two of the endeavors that I will attempt to carry out in what follows.

Overall, the main thesis to be pursued by this project is that affects are reflexive, second-order phenomena (in a way similar to what Lacan, in the opening session of the seventh seminar of 1959–1960, asserts regarding desire: "it is always desire in the second degree, desire of desire").[19] That is to say, instead of being elementary givens that are irreducibly immediate experiences of phenomenal consciousness, the phenomena of affective life involve filterings, foldings, mediations, and redoublings that make these phenomena much more complex and much less self-evident than is usually suspected. One fashion of putting this loosely is that feelings are always the feelings of feelings. And, unconscious forces and factors subsist and operate in the gap between feelings and the feelings of feelings. Advancing and developing this thesis will require combining the resources of Freudian-Lacanian psychoanalysis and affective neuroscience in fashions forcing important modifications of both these fields. It also will require repudiating not only Descartes's (as well as countless other philosophers') equation of the mental with the conscious[20]—this repudiation obviously is foundational for psychoanalysis as a whole—but furthermore the Descartes who, when comparing sensory perceptions (as potentially misleading) to affective passions in *The Passions of the Soul*, declares, "we cannot be misled in the same way regarding the passions, in that they are so close and so internal to our soul that it cannot possibly feel them unless they are truly as it feels them to be."[21]

Contra this Cartesian immediacy and its correlates in quotidian intuitions, my analytically indebted depiction of affects as compound, hybrid, and mediated facets of the lives of psychical subjects, facets capable of becoming far from self-evident, is partially Hegelian in inspiration. Hegel arguably is the greatest and harshest critic in the entire history of philosophy of immediacy in all its guises. He convincingly proves again and again that unrecognized and misrecognized structures and dynamics of intricate, nuanced mediations immanently move within what appears to be the simple straightforwardness of supposedly isolated, self-sufficient givens of a purportedly stable, rock-bottom nature said to be incapable of further analytic decomposition. In manners symptomatic of their occupational tendencies and the preoccupations of their discipline, subsequent philosophers exploring Hegel's criticisms of various versions of immediacy have tended to devote much less attention to affective phenomena than to those more "cognitive" topics dealt with by Hegel that have pointedly direct epistemological, ontological, and sociopolitical upshots. To take a prominent contemporary example, the Anglo-American neo-Hegelian philosopher John McDowell, proudly walking in the footsteps of his Analytic philosophical predecessor Wilfrid Sellars,[22] develops a powerful Hegel-inspired reconsideration of perception according to which the mediation of active conceptual spontaneity always already functions within the (ostensible) immediacy of passive perceptual receptivity; McDowell's concerns, by his own admission, are primarily of an epistemological sort.[23] My account of affective life herein fairly could be characterized as, in part, an extension of McDowell's Hegelian epistemology of perceptual experience (qua cognitive) into the motivational and emotional realms of affective experience.

A perhaps controversial aspect of my notion of misfelt feelings is its clearly implied claim that there is a truth to certain feelings at odds with what the first-person conscious awareness of the feeling subject takes these feelings really to be and be about. In other words, this concept of mine commits me to the thesis that feelings actually can be other than what they're (mis)taken to be by the person having them, that people can be in error about their emotional lives. However disconcerting and counterintuitive this initially might be to some readers, it's a fundamental lesson of psychoanalysis.

The Marxist tradition (as represented by, for instance, Georg Lukács)[24] similarly wagers that sharp discrepancies can and do separate the actual subjective consciousness of a socioeconomic group from what this (lack of) awareness should, could, and would be transformed into if this group were to achieve "class consciousness" based upon a correct comprehension of the objective truth of its social-historical-economic situation. (I am proposing that the latter consciousness, class consciousness strictly speaking, is analogous to, in psychoanalysis, the real feel of feeling masked by the conscious misfeeling of this same defended-against feeling.) Psychoanalysis and Marxism not only both cast weighty doubts on the authority and veracity of the experiences of individual and collective subjective consciousness, thereby rendering the appeals of such consciousness highly suspect; these two orientations share in common a confidence in there being truths to be grasped nonetheless amid these experiences they darken with their suspicions. The traditions launched by Marx and Freud thus come to find themselves moving against the prevailing winds of a postmodern *Zeitgeist* liquidating everything in the confusing verbiage of cheap relativisms and truthless game-playing.

Additionally, the very origins of analysis in Freud's pioneering early work with female hysterics hinge on the idea that there are indeed reasonable and rationally explicable factors underpinning even seemingly unreasonable and intellectually baffling affective phenomena. Freud took these women seriously and listened for the solutions to their problems in what they themselves had to say, unlike his colleagues and contemporaries, who generally and unsympathetically dismissed them as utterly irrational or labeled them as manipulative malingerers. Freud came to contend that the apparently inappropriate, excessive, and out-of-place affective outbursts of hysterics (e.g., intense anxiety or overwhelming disgust) were, in fact, quite appropriate responses to traumatic past experiences. However, realizing this required the deciphering work of analytic interpretation, in which these repressed traumas were raised to the light of consciousness out of the unconscious and brought into explicit, integrated connection with the conscious patient's emotions and feelings. The crucial Freudian hypothesis here is that what the hysterical subject misfeels in such telling forms as phobias and psychosomatic conversion symptoms is, so to speak, madness with a method—namely, a rationally explicable distortion (distorted by intrapsychical defense mechanisms) of an originally reasonable affective response to an extremely painful past experience. Uncovering and revisiting past traumas reveals true feelings behind misfeelings. Freud lays down central components of the foundations of psychoanalysis by, in relation to his early hysterics, risking the hypothesis that there are latent and understandable truths behind these subjects' manifestly incomprehensible and frustrating affects.

In the spirit of Lacan's reinterpretation of what is revolutionary in Freud's discovery of the unconscious, which was glossed earlier, it could be maintained that one of the things psychical subjects know without knowing that they know (apart from signifier-encoded ideational knowledge) is how they "really feel" apart from their consciously registered self-representations of their underlying emotions and affects. Rather than epitomizing a sense of self-certainty (à la "If I know one thing for sure, it's how I feel"), the phenomena of affective life should be recognized as being just as affected by the subversion of the subject of knowledge (i.e., Lacan's "*sujet de la connaissance*")[25] as the mnemic, linguistic, and conceptual components of the psyche's architecture. Not only does the later Freud suggest this possibility in connection with the topic of guilt; the neuroscience of the emotional brain clearly points to the reality of an affective unconscious that can be ignored by Lacanian and post-Lacanian strains of psychoanalysis only at the cost of their empirical soundness. Burying one's head in the sands of theoretical doctrine isn't a real option anymore.

9 .

FEELING WITHOUT FEELING

FREUD AND THE UNRESOLVED PROBLEM
OF UNCONSCIOUS GUILT

A cursory survey of Freud's works seems to reveal two incompatible positions situated in two distinct periods of his theorizing apropos the issue of the overlap (or lack thereof) between the domains of the unconscious and affective life. On the one hand, prior to the second topography, he tends to dismiss the notion of unconscious affects as oxymoronic (the decisive articulation of this stance being located in the third section on "Unconscious Emotions" of the metapsychological paper on "The Unconscious," published in 1915). On the other hand, starting with *The Ego and the Id* (1923), Freud insists upon the existence of at least one unconscious affect, namely, "an unconscious sense of guilt" (*unbewußten Schuldgefühl, unbewußtes Schuldgefühl*).[1] This shift of position on unconscious affects is integrally related to the introduction of the second topography—more specifically, it's connected with this new topography's concept of the unconscious dimension of the psychical agency of the superego. As I already noted (in the previous chapter), there are several serious problems with the simple story of a pre-1923 Freud of the first topography versus a post-1923 Freud of the second topography on the matter of an unconscious side of affective life.

In his paper on "Obsessive Actions and Religious Practices" (1907), Freud refers to a guilt that remains unknown. He states: "We may say that the sufferer from compulsions and prohibitions behaves as if he were dominated by a sense of guilt [*Schuldbewußtseins*], of which, however, he knows nothing, so that we must call it an unconscious sense of guilt [*unbewußten Schuldbewußtseins*], in spite of the apparent contradiction in terms."[2] Several features of this statement deserve attention. To begin with, what testifies to this "sense of guilt" (*Schuldbewußtseins*), despite this German term's link to the word "consciousness" (*Bewußtsein*), is not a self-reflective awareness of an internal feeling-state, but rather sets of interconnected thoughts and actions (i.e., the insistent ideas and ritualized behaviors that are the symptomatic hallmarks of obsessional neurosis). These thoughts and actions exhibit an "as if" association with what one might expect from someone who feels guilty. That is to say, the obsessional neurotic's "compulsions and prohibitions" testify to his/her registering, on one level or another, a conviction that he/she is culpable of something—and this even though an accompanying, affectively charged cognizance of an explicitly thematized knowledge of being guilty can be, and often is, evidently absent. Furthermore, Freud's discomfort with this passing supposition of an affect (guilt) being unconscious is clearly signaled in the quotation: he directly points to "the apparent contradiction in terms" (in line with his view at this time that affects, as feelings, must be felt and, hence, be consciously registered) without explicitly resolving the tension between his prevailing metapsychology of affect from this period of his thinking and this hypothesis from 1907 of there being, at least in certain neurotics, an unconscious sense of guilt. What's more, in German, the "contradiction in terms" Freud feels compelled to resort to is quite glaring, since a more literal English translation of *unbewußten Schuld-bewußtseins* is "unconscious consciousness of guilt."[3] Among other things, Freud's open acknowledgment of this tension indicates that he isn't willing to finesse the problem by recasting this special sort of neurotic guilt allegedly legible in obsessionals as a virtual potential for possibly coming to feel consciously guilty in specific situations. Such a recasting would allow him to stipulate that, because it is unconscious, guilt isn't so much an affect as a protoaffective ideational formation or structure inclining in the direction of a readiness to experience guilt (or related affects like anxiety and shame) under certain conditions at whose psychical or subjective realization analysis aims. (As will be seen in the next chapter, Freud elsewhere, and others after him, flirts with this solution.)

Is there anything else bearing witness to the obsessional neurotic's unconscious sense of guilt other than his/her intrusive, repetitive trains of thought and stylized, idiosyncratic patterns of activity? Immediately following the conjecture regarding an unknown guilt, Freud proceeds to speak of anxiety. He talks about "a lurking sense of expectant anxiety, an expectation of misfortune"[4] (i.e., the obsessional neurotic's vague but convincingly powerful dread that a particular disaster will befall him/her, especially if he/she fails to perform, under a painful, burdensome compulsion, the requisite ritualized defensive behaviors striving to conjure away the imagined danger). Now, this anxious negative affect indeed does constitute a consciously registered feeling-state of which its sufferer is undeniably aware.

Already in 1907, there are grounds for suspecting that Freud's metapsychology of affect, appropriately interpreted, might allow for the occurrence of what I am identifying in this present project as "misfelt feelings." How so? Guilt and anxiety can be considered to be part of a single constellation of family resemblances within the sphere of affective life. Many of the psychical and somatic experiences associated with guilt (e.g., some of the uncomfortable bodily sensations and agitating mental nervousness usually accompanying a cognizance of culpability) are quite similar to those associated with anxiety (something Freud subsequently observes, as will be remarked upon later). Maybe one of the factors that makes for the differences between the self-consciousness of consciously feeling guilty and the self-consciousness of consciously feeling anxious is not so much the psychical and somatic experiences associated with these affects, but instead the ideational parsing of these feelings, a parsing that subtly inflects how feelings feel (assuming the thesis that, contrary to certain deeply entrenched common assumptions, feelings are never immediate, straightforward phenomena, but involve, in the subjectivities of speaking beings, metalevels shaping the feel of feelings). As Freud notes of unconsciously guilty neurotics in "Obsessive Actions and Religious Practices," these neurotics, caught in the pressing grip of their anxious expectations and the defensive activities these expectations provoke, are not conscious of the connections between the ideational representations (*Vorstellungen*) acting as the mental content (i.e., the associations between ideas, memories, symbols, words, and so on) catalyzing their obsessive thoughts and compulsive actions.[5] Hence, due to the lack of a self-aware understanding of these connections, such individuals, although they still consciously feel their guilt, feel it as anxiety rather than as guilt per se. In other words, the guilt per se is not consciously registered, but a being affected by guilt forcefully makes itself (mis)felt in the form of what is self-consciously experienced as anxiety. (Perhaps an aspect of what makes guilt feel like guilt proper is a conscious awareness of a sense of culpability, an awareness bound up with and requiring ideational representations, accompanying the psychical and somatic experiences constitutive of feeling anxious.) Thus, regardless of whether the authorial intentionality of Freud intends anything along these precise lines, maybe one could claim that unconscious affects in the strict Freudian sense are feelings, involving interconnected somatic and psychical states palpably felt by consciousness, as well as reflexively felt by linguistically and conceptually mediated self-consciousness as other than what they are or refer to. (Two examples familiar to clinical analysis of this are selfconsciously experiencing the sensible pangs of inaudible conscience [i.e., the unconscious voice of the superego] as anxiety instead of guilt,[6] and undergoing pleasurable excitement defended against by mechanisms entwined with a given form of restricted consciousness as unpleasurable agitation.) Such a claim obviously gets around the dead end, perceived by Freud, of having to speak in a self-contradictory way of unconscious affects as utterly feel-less feelings. However, further clarifications of these proposals will require not only a much more extensive examination of Freud's observations and comments regarding an unconscious sense of guilt and related issues (including central components of his metapsychological account of affects in general); the resources yielded by neuroscientific investigations into the emotional brain are absolutely indispensable to this task of elucidating what persists as a still-obscure problematic in Freudian and post-Freudian psychoanalysis.

It should be recalled that one of the reasons for highlighting Freud's speculation regarding an unconscious sense of guilt in his relatively early essay "Obsessive Actions and Religious Practices" is to debunk the narrative according to which he ventures this speculation only in the wake of the shift from the first to the second topography. Admittedly, it isn't until 1923, in *The Ego and the Id*, that Freud engages in a sustained discussion of guilt as an unconscious affect (a discussion that I will scrutinize shortly). But, apart from the mention of it in 1907 commented on in the preceding paragraphs, he again, also prior to *The Ego and the Id*, alludes to guilt in the same vein in "Some Character-Types Met with in Psycho-Analytic Work" (1916). Specifically, the third and final section of this paper, devoted to "Criminals from a Sense of Guilt," contains a reference to what is described as an "obscure sense of guilt" (*dunkle Schuldgefühl*).[7] This guilt-in-search-of-a-crime is depicted by Freud in this text as a self-consciously felt feeling of culpability minus a comprehension of why this feeling is felt. But, on the basis of the preceding reflections, it might legitimately be asked whether, at least phenomenologically, there are differences between, on the one hand, the experience of this guilt as "obscure" and, on the other hand, the experience of this "same" guilt if and when its obscured (i.e., repressed) origins are uncovered and appropriated by the guilty subject. Additionally, when, in *The Ego and the Id*, Freud again mentions criminals whose guilt is the cause rather than the effect of their criminality, he describes this affective cause as an "unconscious sense of guilt" (*unbewußte Schuldgefühl*).[8]

The Ego and the Id is a momentously important work in the context of Freud's whole *oeuvre*. As is common knowledge, it constitutes the first comprehensive, systematic elaboration of the metapsychological foundations of the new second topography, a topography centered on the triad of id (*Es* [It]), ego (*Ich* [I]), and superego (*Über-Ich* [Over-I]), instead of, as in the first topography, the triad of conscious, preconscious, and unconscious. For Freud, this compact book consolidates a number of ideas and discoveries that he had only recently had as well as paves the way for further insights and developments in the years to come.

Freud's elaborations in 1923 of the role and workings of the superego in the psyche are of special interest in relation to the present discussion. As I previously observed (in the last chapter), the Freudian superego isn't simply mere psychoanalytic jargon synonymous with the quotidian word "conscience," because, unlike traditional notions of conscience, significant parts of the superego operate below the threshold of explicit, self-conscious awareness; for Freudian psychoanalysis, not all conscience is conscious.[9] Moreover, as with the superego, so also with the ego: there are unconscious portions of it too.[10] And, insofar as the superego is "a grade in the ego, a differentiation within the ego,"[11] these claims about the ego and the superego go hand in hand: if who one is (i.e., one's ego) partly is shaped by who one wants to become (i.e., one's "ego ideal" or "superego")[12] and if some of these ideals and facets of conscience are unconscious, then certain aspects of who one is (i.e., one's ego-level identity) are going to be unconscious as well.

Taking all of this into account as regards the superego's relationship with the ego, four basic structural dynamics of interaction are possible in principle: (1) conscious superego relating to conscious ego; (2) conscious superego relating to unconscious ego; (3) unconscious superego relating to conscious ego; and (4) unconscious superego relating to unconscious ego. The first possibility is easiest to understand, since it corresponds to the everyday sense of conscience in which one consciously hears one's self-evaluations (i.e., in which conscience is conscious, with the voice of conscience being audible in and to self-consciousness, part of its soliloquy). The third could be said to encompass instances of unanchored, seemingly irrational guilt so familiar in the psychoanalytic clinic of the neuroses (i.e., circumstances in which the ego consciously feels some sort of nebulous guilt without know why, in ignorance of its infractions vis-à-vis unknown laws and rules enforced by the unconscious side of the superego). However, the second and fourth possibilities are opaque and perplexing, with Freud apparently not mentioning the second (i.e., conscious superego relating to unconscious ego) but considering the fourth. (As will be seen soon, this fourth possibility [i.e., unconscious superego relating to unconscious ego] is exemplified by what Freud terms "moral masochism" in the essay "The Economic Problem of Masochism.") If guilt is an affective consequence of the superego acting on the ego, then, if (as per the fourth possibility) the unconscious portion of the superego can relate directly to the unconscious portion of the ego, perhaps the result of this fourth possible superego-to-ego structural dynamic is something that indeed could be called "unconscious guilt."

In *The Ego and the Id*, Freud introduces the topic of an unconscious sense of guilt at the end of the second chapter ("The Ego and the Id"). He leads up to this topic thus:

> Accustomed as we are to taking our social or ethical scale of values along with us wherever we go, we feel no surprise at hearing that the scene of the activities of the lower passions is in the unconscious; we expect, moreover, that the higher any mental function ranks in our scale of values the more easily it will find access to consciousness assured to it. Here, however, psycho-analytic experience disappoints us. On the one hand, we have evidence that even subtle and difficult intellectual operations which ordinarily require strenuous reflection can equally be carried out preconsciously and without coming into consciousness. Instances of this are quite incontestable; they may occur, for example, during the state of sleep, as is shown when someone finds, immediately after waking, that he knows the solution to a difficult mathematical or other problem with which he had been wrestling in vain the day before.[13]

These remarks aim at demolishing the presumptions and biases leading people to assume that complex, elaborate mental machinations (including those involved with personal identity and conscience) must be conscious. In the paragraphs that follow, Freud proceeds to mention unconscious guilt:

> There is another phenomenon, however, which is far stranger. In our analyses we discover that there are people in whom the faculties of self-criticism and conscience—mental activities, that is, that rank as extremely high ones—are unconscious and unconsciously produce effects of the greatest importance; the example of resistance remaining unconscious during analysis is therefore by no means unique. But this new discovery, which compels us, in spite of our

better critical judgment, to speak of an "unconscious sense of guilt" [*unbe-wußten Schuldgefühl*], bewilders us far more than the other and sets us fresh problems, especially when we gradually come to see that in a great number of neuroses an unconscious sense of guilt of this kind plays a decisive economic part and puts the most powerful obstacles in the way of recovery. If we come back once more to our scale of values, we shall have to say that not only what is lowest but also what is highest in the ego can be unconscious.[14]

Freud obviously is conflicted here, as elsewhere, about his hypothesis to the effect that guilt sometimes can be an unconscious affect: he is "compelled" to posit this despite his "better critical judgment" as a metapsychologist for whom affects, unlike *Vorstellungen*, cannot be unconscious (a few pages subsequently in the next chapter of *The Ego and the Id*, a hesitant "perhaps" qualifies reference to "an unconscious sense of guilt").[15] He nonetheless immediately puts this uneasy hypothesis to work, assigning it an explanatory function in relation to both the neuroses in general ("in a great number of neuroses an unconscious sense of guilt of this kind plays a decisive economic part") and the more specific intratherapeutic occurrence of what comes to be dubbed "negative therapeutic reaction" ("the most powerful obstacles in the way of recovery").

Early on in the fifth chapter of *The Ego and the Id*, Freud paints a succinct-yet-thorough portrait of what he calls the "negative therapeutic reaction." (This is mentioned subsequently in such texts as *The Question of Lay Analysis* [1926] in connection with which reference is made yet again to the "unconscious sense of guilt" [*unbewußte Schuldgefühl*],[16] and the lecture on "Anxiety and Instinctual Life" from the *New Introductory Lectures on Psycho-Analysis* [1933].)[17] He movingly depicts the sad situation of those neurotic sufferers who cling to their illnesses, whose symptoms get worse rather than better in the face of gains made in the progress of their analyses.[18] Freud's explanation is that these analysands are driven to wallow in their pain and anguish by guilt; on a certain level, they are convinced that they should be miserable, that they don't deserve to be, as it were, relatively happy and healthy. Yet, Freud is careful to stipulate that the guilt underlying cases of negative therapeutic reaction is of a special sort: "But as far as the patient is concerned this sense of guilt is dumb; it does not tell him he is guilty; he does not feel guilty, he feels ill" (*Aber dies Schuldgefühl ist für den Kranken stumm, es sagt ihm nicht, daß er schuldig ist, er fühlt sich nicht schuldig, sondern krank*).[19] One again could argue that this remark lends support to the thesis that unconscious affects, in Freudian metapsychology, are misfelt feelings. In this case, the physical and psychological indicators of a guilty feeling-state consciously are registered and self-interpreted in the guises of the recurring unpleasurable experiences (such as somatic ailments) marking neurotic psychopathologies, for which neurotics frequently don't feel fully and explicitly guilty in a way that makes them also feel culpable or responsible; instead, a much-bemoaned destiny, fate, or bad luck usually bears the brunt of the misplaced blame.

Before proceeding from the particular problem of guilt as an unconscious affect in Freud's work to the larger frame of his overarching metapsychology of affects, those elaborations after 1923 directly tied to the unconscious sense of guilt ought to be touched upon here. These elaborations are contained primarily in two texts: the paper "The Economic Problem of Masochism" (1924) and the volume *Civilization and Its Discontents* (1929). Masochism, construed in a very general fashion, designates a cluster of phenomena that play a major part in pushing Freud to take his step "beyond the pleasure principle" in 1920. In his paper "On Narcissism" (1924), Freud pays attention to how what he then labels "conscience" coerces the ego, through (the threat of) guilt, to maintain an orientation and proximity to the norms and values enshrined within the psychical apparatus in the form of the "ego ideal"; if the ego strays too far away from the horizon defined by the teleological vanishing points embodied in the ego ideal, then conscience inflicts a penalty consisting of unpleasurable negative affect (i.e., guilt, remorse, shame, humiliation, and the like).[20] Earlier versions of the thesis that appears before 1920 according to which the pleasure principle is the dominant law of psychical life are somewhat undercut by the undeniable everyday occurrence of conscience-induced guilt as pain spontaneously inflicted by the psyche upon itself. Ten years later, Freud brings into view an "economic problem" exhibited by what he christens "moral masochism" (an affliction that can manifest itself in such a masochist as excessively brutal self-criticism, inflexibly intolerant perfectionism, and unconsciously arranged setbacks and misfortunes invariably snatching defeat from the jaws of victory). For example, sometimes, when the ego manages to get very close to instantiating the ego ideal, conscience (now, in 1924, identified as the superego) becomes even harsher and more punitive, instead of, as one would expect, rewarding the conscious ego with such pleasures of narcissistic self-satisfaction as senses of confidence, contentment, dignity, and pride (an expectation Freud previously articulates in "On Narcissism"). This unexpected twist occurs in cases of moral masochism, cases in which the internal superego is far more vicious and unforgiving than any external authority figure.[21] (The multitude of psychoanalytic reasons for this superegoistic cruelty—which have to do with the pleasure principle, the death drive [*Todestrieb*], and external reality, among other factors—are too numerous and nuanced to spell out amid the current lines of exegesis and argumentation.)

When first referring to moral masochism as one of three standard varieties of masochism in "The Economic Problem of Masochism" (the other two being "erotogenic" and "feminine" masochism), Freud equates it with "a sense of guilt which is mostly unconscious" (*meist unbewußtes Schuldgefühl*).[22] But, strangely, he qualifies such guilt as "only recently . . . recognized by psychoanalysis."[23] (This is strange insofar as he takes note of the notion of unconscious guilt as early as 1907.) Freud goes on to remind readers of the connection he maintains between the unconscious sense of guilt and the negative therapeutic reaction manifested by particular sorts of neurotic patients in analysis.[24] Then, with respect to this class of analysands, Freud observes:

> Patients do not easily believe us when we tell them about the unconscious sense of guilt [*unbewußte Schuldgefühl*]. They know only too well by what torments—the pangs of conscience—a conscious sense of guilt, a consciousness of guilt [*ein bewußtes Schuldgefühl, Schuldbewußtsein*], expresses itself, and they therefore cannot admit that they could harbour exactly analogous impulses in themselves without being in the least aware of them. We may, I think, to some extent meet their objection if we give up the term "unconscious sense of guilt" [*unbewußtes Schuldgefühl*], which is in any case psychologically incorrect, and speak instead of a "need for punishment" [*Strafbedürfnis*], which covers the observed state of affairs just as aptly. We cannot, however, restrain ourselves from judging and localizing this unconscious sense of guilt in the same way as we do the conscious kind.[25]

Apropos the vexing issue of unconscious affect, it's difficult to know exactly what to make of this passage. On the one hand, Freud appears to appeal to his patients' conscious experiences—what they feel doesn't feel to them (more specifically, to the conscious part of their egos) like guilt—as justification for jettisoning the tension-ridden notion-phrase "unconscious guilt" as "psychologically incorrect" in favor of the supposedly less problematic concept of a "need for punishment." (The concept is less problematic for Freud's metapsychology to the extent that it doesn't require positing a feeling that isn't felt as such—however, one might wonder whether "need" [*Bedürfnis*] is any less problematic for the exact same reasons.) But, on the other hand, he indicates that there's something unavoidable in the purportedly erroneous idea of guilt as an unconscious affect.

Freud proceeds to complicate his analysis of masochism, further refining his description of moral masochism in particular. He distinguishes between moral masochism per se and another variety that he admits to confusing and conflating with moral masochism proper in his preceding reflections on observations derived from the clinical consulting room: In the former (i.e., moral masochism per se), there is a pronounced need for punishment that can be satisfied by either the internal superego or the external world (with this need being mis-recognized by the masochist's self-awareness but testified to by the repeated defeats and miseries that this type of individual unknowingly but predictably visits upon him-/herself). In the latter (i.e., that which seems like, but is to be distinguished from, moral masochism in the strict sense), a sadistic superego, operating below the threshold of consciousness, is invariably the unconscious source of consciously registered suffering (perhaps as a mysterious, perplexing feeling of excessive guilt). Real moral masochists don't necessarily experience a haunting sense of consciously inexplicable guilt-without-a-cause, whereas those previously lumped under this same diagnostic heading are perturbed by guilt-like negative affects arising from the action of unconscious aspects of the superego upon the conscious ego. As Freud puts it, moral masochism per se is centered on the (masochistic) ego's need for punishment (from whoever or whatever, by the superego within or reality without), while that which resembles moral masochism is a suffering generated specifically by the unconscious superego punishing the conscious ego, namely, a suffering driven by the superego's sadism more than the ego's masochism.[26]

The eighth and final chapter of *Civilization and Its Discontents* contains extensive elaborations of Freud's musings about guilt, which I have already glossed. At the start of this chapter, Freud, in response to what he imagines to be his readers' impression that his drawn-out discussions of guilt are a digression in relation to the rest of this book, claims that "the sense of guilt" (*Schuldgefühl*)[27] is "the most important problem in the development of civilization."[28] (Later on in this same chapter, he makes it central to clinical analysis too, surmising that "perhaps every neurosis conceals a quota of unconscious sense of guilt [*unbewußtem Schuldgefühl*], which in its turn fortifies the symptoms by making use of them as a punishment.")[29] Through the development of the superego (a feature of the psychical *Innenwelt* in whose production the historical *Umwelt* of culture and society plays a significant part) and the sense of guilt that the superego makes possible—Freud argues that one can't feel guilty per se unless and until one ontogenetically acquires this psychical structure or agency[30]—the id-level aggressive and sexual impulses of human beings are tamed and domesticated. In fact, the superego represents what one might risk characterizing in roughly Hegelian terms as a symptom of the cunning of civilization's reason, an especially efficacious sublimation in which aggression—which Freud identifies as the gravest threat to the integrity of human collectivities[31]—is "turned inward," away from extraneous others, and discharged through the superego's sadism vis-à-vis the ego.[32] Such a superego-mediated inward discharge is not only innocuous with respect to the concerns of civilization for its own cohesion; such aggression-sublimating self-policing via "conscience" is essential insofar as there will never be anywhere close to enough external policing mechanisms to monitor and control individuals' behaviors (an impossibility involving a potentially infinite regression signaled by the question "who will police the police?"). Matters central to ethics and politics, the two main branches of practical philosophy, are at stake in Freud's handling of guilt; hence, his being at pains to protest that sustained scrutiny of this affect is of the utmost urgent importance in reconsidering arrangements of human collective existence.

After defending the relevance to *Civilization and Its Discontents* of his discussions of guilt therein, Freud turns to talking about "the quite peculiar relationship—as yet completely unexplained—which the sense of guilt [*Schuldgefühls*] has to our consciousness [*Bewußtsein*]."[33] (He already had been struggling to explain this for quite some time.) He says:

> In the common case of remorse, which we regard as normal, this feeling makes itself clearly enough perceptible to consciousness. Indeed, we are accustomed to speak of a "consciousness of guilt" [*Schuldbewußtsein*] instead of a "sense of guilt" [*Schuldgefühl*]. Our study of the neuroses, to which, after all, we owe the most valuable pointers to an understanding of normal conditions, brings us up against some contradictions. In one of those affections, obsessional neurosis, the sense of guilt makes itself noisily heard in consciousness; it dominates the clinical picture and the patient's life as well, and it hardly allows anything else to appear alongside of it. But in most other cases and forms of neurosis it remains completely unconscious, without on that account producing any less important effects. Our patients do not believe us when we attribute an "unconscious sense of guilt" [*unbewußtes Schuldgefühl*] to them. In order to make ourselves at all intelligible to them, we tell them of an unconscious need for punishment, in which the sense of guilt finds expression. But its connection with a particular form of neurosis must not be over-estimated. Even in obsessional neurosis there are types of patients who are not aware of their sense of

guilt, or who only feel it as a tormenting uneasiness, a kind of anxiety, if they are prevented from carrying out certain actions. It ought to be possible eventually to understand these things; but as yet we cannot.[34]

Arguably, "remorse" refers to the intuitive, quotidian notion of guilt as a feeling of the negative affects associated with culpability while, simultaneously, being conscious of a cause or reason for feeling like this; in Freudian parlance, this would amount to conscious components of the ego knowingly being affected by conscious components of the superego. In many instances of obsessional neurosis, as Freud describes it, there are prominent conscious guilty feelings minus an awareness of an appropriate cause or reason for these feelings; in these cases, the conscious parts of the ego are affected by largely unconscious aspects and operations of the superego. (Freud uses obsessional neurosis, insofar as certain obsessional neurotics feel guilty without knowing why, to rule out the hypothesis "that a sense of guilt arising from remorse for an evil *deed* must [*müßte*] always be conscious, whereas a sense of guilt arising from an evil *impulse* may [*könnte*] remain unconscious";[35] such obsessional neurotics, instead of harboring an unconscious sense of guilt for their aggressive or libidinal inclinations, are acutely conscious of guilty feelings, feelings generated behind the scenes available to the inward gaze of the ego by the superego's consciously inaudible condemnations of id-level "repressed impulses.")[36] What's more, whereas in "The Economic Problem of Masochism" Freud indicates that his analysands' inability to comprehend and accept the notion that they harbor an unconscious sense of guilt partially justifies theoretically abandoning this metapsychologically problematic notion and replacing it with the less troubling concept of a need for punishment, he here, in the passage quoted, alters his stance: talking to patients about a need for punishment is more a matter of practical clinical expediency (instead of theoretical and metapsychological accuracy), taking into consideration the unlikelihood that those on the couch could or would work with interpretations appealing to a feeling they don't consciously feel per se. (This same alteration of stance is evident a few years later in the *New Introductory Lectures on Psycho-Analysis*, where Freud once more contends that the consciously unrecognized need for punishment really is an unconscious sense of guilt and not, as indicated in 1924, vice versa.)[37] Additionally, he specifies that not all obsessional neurotics consciously self-interpret their underlying guilt as guilt; some autoreflexively experience it instead as "a tormenting uneasiness, a kind of anxiety." (This again lends support to the thesis that unconscious guilt is still felt, instead of being a paradoxical unfelt feeling; but this guilt is [mis]felt as anxiety rather than culpability strictly speaking.) Finally, Freud confesses to a sense of being in the dark immediately after once more broaching the topic of unconscious affect. (It will be argued in what follows that today's neuroscience of the emotional brain can be of immense help here.)

Freud says further interesting things that elaborate this point in *Civilization and Its Discontents*. Continuing right where the previous quotation leaves off, he remarks:

> Here perhaps we may be glad to have it pointed out that the sense of guilt is at bottom nothing else but a topographical variety of anxiety; in its later phases it coincides completely with *fear of the super-ego* [*Angst vor dem Über-Ich*]. And the relations of anxiety to consciousness exhibit the same extraordinary variations. Anxiety is always present somewhere or other behind every symptom; but at one time it takes noisy possession of the whole of consciousness, while at another it conceals itself so completely that we are obliged to speak of unconscious anxiety [*unbewußter Angst*] or, if we want to have a clearer psychological conscience, since anxiety is in the first instance simply a feeling, of possibilities of anxiety [*Angstmöglichkeiten*]. Consequently it is very conceivable that the sense of guilt [*Schuldbewußtsein*] produced by civilization is not perceived as such [*nicht als solches erkannt wird*] either, and remains to a large extent unconscious [*großen Teil unbewußt bleibt*], or appears as a sort of *malaise* [*Unbehagen*], a dissatisfaction, for which people seek other motivations.[38]

It's incorrect to claim that guilt is the only affect in relation to which Freud speculates about the possibility of unconscious affect, since Freud does connect guilt to anxiety and blurs the lines of demarcation between these closely related states. (In general, demarcating precise, black-and-white categorical borders between affects is rightly quite hard given the hazy, fluid nature of the phenomena in question.) Anxiety, another affect of enormous significance in psychoanalysis, turns out to be relevant to this issue too. Guilt itself is said to be "a topographical variety of anxiety" (i.e., in relation to the second topography of id, ego, and superego, an anxiety specific to the ego vis-à-vis the superego). Freud is "glad" to be able to link guilt to anxiety because it allows him to mobilize his extensively elaborated metapsychological accounts of anxiety as means for resolving the difficulties presented by invocations of an unconscious sense of guilt. Anxiety, Freud here maintains, is a common feature of all of the psychoneuroses (a few pages later in *Civilization and Its Discontents*, guilt is likewise claimed to be a factor in every neurosis).[39] He proceeds to distinguish between felt and unfelt anxiety, only again to repudiate, in the name of "a clearer psychological conscience" for which anxiety, as a feeling, must be (consciously) felt,[40] the latter category (i.e., unfelt anxiety). It's as though he's compelled to play a conflicted game of *fort-da* with the theoretical object called "unconscious affect."

With yet another quick oscillation back in the other direction of speculation, Freud then goes on to distinguish between degrees of unconsciousness as regards guilt, a range including the possibility of it being a misfelt feeling not felt "as such," but instead registered through distorting misperceptions as anxious unease ("*malaise*," "dissatisfaction," and so on.). Freud certainly doesn't seem to feel comfortable with the topic of unconscious affect, apparently being able neither to accept this quasi concept nor simply to abandon it (as the cliché one-liner has it, he can't live with it, can't live without it). Another striking illustration of his conflicting (and conflicted) vacillations apropos this topic can be found in *The Ego and the Id*, wherein, at one point, he defines "the sense of guilt" (*Schuldgefühl*) as "the perception in the ego answering to" the criticisms voiced by the superego.[41] (Since it is, by definition, perceived by the ego, guilt cannot be unconscious; yet, as has been shown, Freud repeatedly appeals to an unconscious sense of guilt elsewhere in *The Ego and the Id*, even declaring therein that, "a great part of the sense of guilt must normally remain unconscious" [*ein großes Stück des Schuldgefühls normalerweise unbewußt sein müsse*].)[42] In the *New Introductory Lectures on Psycho-Analysis* (1933), his ambivalence emerges clearly when he laments, referring to the need for punishment, "If only the words went together better, we should be justified for all practical purposes in calling it an 'unconscious sense of guilt'" (*Würden die Worte nur besser zusammenpassen, so wäre es für alle praktischen Belange nur gerechtfertigt, es 'unbewußtes Schuldgefühl' zu heißen*).[43] Freud never manages to reach a point where he feels that these words can be understood in a sense by virtue of which they sit side by side in a metapsychologically coherent manner. This unresolved difficulty in Freud's corpus, as with so many matters in psychoanalysis, can and should be put to work, in good dialectical fashion, as a productive impasse, as a lingering mystery calling for additional exploration. Such an exploration, which I will undertake now, promises to divulge a number of interesting insights and implications not only for psychoanalysis, but also for theoretical and practical philosophy.

10.

AFFECTS, EMOTIONS, AND FEELINGS

FREUD'S METAPSYCHOLOGIES
OF AFFECTIVE LIFE

The Freudian metapsychology of affects (or, more accurately, metapsy-chologies of affects) is complex in the strict Freudian sense,[1] namely, a dense, tangled knot of a plethora of axioms, concepts, theses, and so on that branch out in all directions and that are ramified from numerous angles in relation to the entire framework of psychoanalysis. In other words, Freud's treatment of affects is far from being a "simple" account capable of be-ing addressed as a self-sufficient whole independent of the rest of his evolving metapsychological apparatus. Insofar as Freud's theories regarding affects are complex or nonsimple in this way, my handling of them cannot claim to be ex-haustive. Similarly, due to limits of time and space, many of the points of over-lap between Freud's metapsychologies of affects and other facets of his wider metapsychological scaffolding must be left to the side here.

At least in the worlds of Lacanian and post-Lacanian psychoanalysis, the first and foremost feature of the Freudian doctrine of affects is the distinction between, as Jean Laplanche and Jean-Bertrand Pontalis put it in their influential psychoanalytic dictionary, "affect" (*Affekt*) and "idea" (*Vorstellung*).[2] This dis-tinction closely parallels the broader fundamental dichotomy between energy and structure, a dichotomy running through the entire span of Freud's writings from start to finish, so starkly visible in the *Project for a Scientific Psychology* (which was composed in 1895, and which is a foundational text for everything that ensues in Freudian metapsychology) in the form of the difference between the structural system of neurons and the energetic quantities of excitation (Q) flowing through this same system.[3] And, a roughly contemporaneous text, the essay "The Neuro-Psychoses of Defense" (1894), explicitly articulates a conception of affect along these precise metapsychological lines. Therein, Freud states: "If someone with a disposition [to neurosis] lacks the aptitude for conversion, but if, nevertheless, in order to fend off an incompatible idea [*Vorstellung*], he sets about separating it from its affect [*Affekt*], then *that affect is obliged to remain in the psychical sphere*. The idea, now weakened, is still left in consciousness, separated from all association. *But its affect, which has become free, attaches itself to other ideas which are not in themselves incompatible; and, thanks to this 'false connection,' those ideas turn into obsessional ideas.*"[4]

By "conversion," Freud means a "*sum of excitation* being *transformed into something somatic*"[5] (à la the conversion symptoms of somatizing hysterical subjects)—that is to say, a channeling of the quota of affective charge emanating from a defended-against *Vorstellung* (as a memory, idea, and so on) into the defiles of the body as a fleshly medium of expressive discharge.[6] It is important to note that the affect thus converted is still felt, albeit (mis)felt, in hysteria's conversion symptoms as unpleasant physical feelings, rather than as a particular affective feeling-state that is a specifically psychical phenomenon (the inseparability of feeling-states from corresponding, associated somatic sensations might explain what makes conversion in this sense a feasible possibility, facilitating the converting transfer). Whereas hysterics can and do employ the option of conversion, obsessionals handle (or, really, awkwardly mishandle) threatening affects by detaching them from their accompanying ideational representations, by removing feeling from these charged *Vorstellungen*. But, as Lacan, following this Freudian trajectory, later puts it, "The affect . . . goes off somewhere else, as best it can."[7] In obsessional neurosis, the withdrawn affect becomes the proverbial lump in the carpet woven of the psyche's interconnected ideational threads (as concepts, symbols, words, and so on—namely, as thoughts). And, this lump is displaced along lines of association between *Vorstellungen*, remaining in the sphere of conscious cognizance by being (re)attached to thoughts distant from but still associated with (however loose this associative link might be) the, so to speak, deaffected thought(s) at issue. The original coupling of idea and affect subjected to the defense mechanisms of obsessional neurosis would be a "true connection," whereas the obsessive trains of thought powered by quotas of defensively displaced negative affect are enabled partly by the free-associative logic of primary-process-style mentation, a logic resulting in what Freud identifies as "false connections" (the already-discussed vicissitudes of guilt in obsessional neurosis in particular provide many examples of "free" affect becoming entangled in such false connections).

A metapsychological ambiguity lurks in the background of this differential diagnosis from 1894 that bears upon the fate of affect in hysteria and obsessional neurosis. On the one hand, the contrast between hysterical conversions and obsessional ideas implies that affect becomes nonconscious in the former case while remaining conscious in the latter. On the other hand, insofar as hysterics with conversion symptoms are acutely conscious of their senses of pain and suffering (as somatically converted negative affect), they too, like obsessionals anxiously haunted by compulsively recurring insistent thoughts, remain conscious of being affected by something (i.e., by affect as that which affects). These hysterics still feel their feelings, although, again, not as the affective states that they are per se, but instead as physical sensations typically associated with these affective states minus what would be, in a typical "nonpathological" instance of (self-)consciously feeling these affects or feelings, the accompanying conceptual-linguistic mediating interpreters parsing them so as to make a given feeling feel like what it is as such. Invoking the notion of the misfeeling of feeling enables this metapsychological ambiguity to be resolved.

Also in the second section of "The Neuro-Psychoses of Defense," Freud extends the implications of his reflections on the affect-idea rapport to speculations regarding the nature of the unconscious in general. He rightly emphasizes that the highly charged neurotic symptoms he's been describing in this essay testify to extremely subtle and intricate mental maneuvers transpiring in the service of managing unpleasant affects without the supervisory oversight of reflexive, self-aware consciousness: "The separation of the sexual idea from its affect and the attachment of the latter to another, suitable but not incompatible idea—these are processes which occur without consciousness. Their existence can only be presumed, but cannot be proved by any clinico-psychological analysis. . . . Perhaps it would be more correct to say that these processes are not of a psychical nature at all, that they are physical processes whose psychical consequences present themselves as if what is expressed by the terms 'separation of the idea from its affect' and 'false connection' of the latter had really taken place."[8] Apart from underscoring the crucial difference between the psychoanalytic conception of the unconscious and the superficially similar pre- or nonpsychoanalytic versions of this notion—the former is much more than a rudimentary deep, dark reservoir of simple energetic urges of a primitive, animalistic sort—this passage ventures the tentative hypothesis that physiological mechanisms may be responsible for (or, at least, involved in) the elaborate regulatory regime governing the psyche's far-from-straightforward, hardly self-evident affective life. This is one of those occasions when Freud finds himself, as he openly acknowledges elsewhere,[9] awaiting potential future confirmations and explanations of clinical analytic observations through the life sciences. As I will argue at length later (in the next two chapters), this Freudian future is now.

Whereas, in 1894, Freud seems to waver slightly apropos the question of whether or not affects can become unconscious in the process of being submitted to the manipulations of psychoneurotic defenses, in 1915 he appears to be unambiguously categorical: affects cannot be unconscious. Such is the standard reading of the third section of the metapsychological paper devoted to the topic of "The Unconscious." However, although there is indeed some support in Freud's text for this widely accepted reading, such an interpretation grossly oversimplifies matters, indefensibly neglecting various highly pertinent conceptual and terminological details contained within this piece of writing. So as not to miss these details and their upshots, close attention must be paid to what Freud actually says, namely, to the precise letter of his text.

At the end of the first paragraph of this section on "Unconscious Emotions," Freud wonders, "We have said that there are conscious and unconscious ideas [bewußte und unbewußte Vorstellungen]; but are there also unconscious instinctual impulses, emotions and feelings [unbewußte Triebregungen, Gefühle, Empfindungen], or is it in this instance meaningless to form combinations of the kind?"[10] In terms of the fundamental energy-structure dichotomy situated at the base of his entire metapsychology as a whole, Freud is asking himself whether energetic or qualitative aspects of psychical life (i.e., "unconscious instinctual impulses, emotions and feelings [unbewußte Triebregungen, Gefühle, Empfindungen]") can be rendered unconscious, as happens with structured and structuring ideational representations (i.e., "conscious and unconscious ideas [bewußte und unbewußte Vorstellungen]"). The latter, according to the contemporaneous metapsychological paper on "Repression," become unconscious by virtue of being submitted to the defensive action of repression (Verdrängung).[11] In other words, repression acts upon mental contents such as mnemic traces and conceptual-linguistic formations, rendering these contents inaccessible to voluntary or spontaneous processes of consciousness. But, Freud inquires, can more "energetic" phenomena also lie below the threshold of explicit self-awareness in a repressed state?

After denying that "drives" (Triebe, consistently and erroneously translated as "instincts" in the Standard Edition) themselves can be unconscious—solely the ideational representations constitutive of the aims and objects of drives, and not their sources and pressures,[12] can be condemned to this psychical state[13]—it sounds as though Freud pronounces the exact same verdict as regards affective things. He declares: "We should expect the answer to the question about unconscious feelings, emotions and affects [*Empfindungen, Gefühlen, Affekten*] to be just as easily given. It is surely of the essence of an emotion that we should be aware of it, i.e. that it should become known to consciousness. Thus the possibility of the attribute of unconsciousness would be completely excluded as far as emotions, feelings and affects [*Gefühle, Empfindungen, Affekte*] are concerned."[14] Already at this point, only those struck with a remarkable exegetical tone deafness could fail to detect the audible manner in which Freud is beginning to paint this position—that affective life is intrinsically conscious insofar as feelings, as feelings, must be felt (i.e., consciously experienced)—as specious. This line of reasoning initially might seem intuitively obvious, especially given that the conventions of natural languages, vulgar common sense, and long-held, deeply entrenched philosophical views all speak with one voice in favor of it. However, Freud continues: "But in psycho-analytic practice we are accustomed to speak of unconscious love, hate, anger, etc., and find it impossible to avoid even the strange conjunction, 'unconscious consciousness of guilt' [*unbewußtes Schuld-bewußtsein*], or a paradoxical 'unconscious anxiety.'"[15] Oddly enough, in Freud's other texts, only guilt and anxiety are referred to as candidates for the theoretically uncertain status of being unconscious affects. And yet, in this paper on the metapsychology of the unconscious, other affects ("love, hate, anger, etc.") receive mention in this vein. If one grants that guilt and anxiety can be unconscious, then it stands to reason that any and every affective hue could be so too.

Soon after in the text, Freud says something that, from the perspective of this particular project, is very interesting: "it may happen that an affective or emotional impulse is perceived but misconstrued" (*Es kann zunächst vorkommen, daß eine Affekt- oder Gefühlsregung wahrgenommen, aber verkannt wird*).[16] In essence, this is an articulation of nothing other than the concept of misfelt feelings (i.e., affective or emotional phenomena that are "perceived but misconstrued") I'm proposing here. (Despite the general thrust of his take on affects in psychoanalytic metapsychology, Lacan, in the seventeenth seminar of 1969–1970, suggests something similar,[17] as does the ex-Lacanian analyst André Green in his book *Le discours vivant*, published in 1973.)[18] The sentence that follows reads: "Owing to the repression of its proper representative [*eigentlichen Repräsentanz*] it has been forced to become connected with another idea [*anderen Vorstellung*], and is now regarded by consciousness as the manifestation [*Äußerung*] of that idea."[19] At this juncture, a tacit contrast arguably becomes visible between two "manifestations" (or one could translate this as "expressions") of the "same" affect: this affect's expression in "true connection" with its "proper representative [*eigentlichen Repräsentanz*]" versus this affect's expression, after the vicissitude of being detached and displaced from its real corresponding ideational representation, in "false connection" with "another idea [*anderen Vorstellung*]" that is a substitutive representational stand-in. (As will be seen in the next chapter, Lacan draws ample attention to these two German terms, *Repräsentanz* and *Vorstellung*, in Freud's texts.) What this project, at this point, adds to the Freudian metapsychology of affects is the supplementary claim (or, at a minimum, the addition of a greater emphasis to the effect) that a "single" affect will feel qualitatively different depending on the ideational representations with which it's connected. Such ideational mediation, always operative in the forms of representational matrices inextricably interwoven with the affective lives of speaking beings, plays a significant part in generating the very feel of feeling. Consequently, in those previously discussed cases prompting Freud hesitantly to resort to the phrase "unconscious sense of guilt," it now could be maintained that the feelings constitutive of guilt feel like guilt as such and per se when they enjoy a "true connection" with their "proper representative [*eigentlichen Repräsentanz*]," whereas these "identical" feelings don't feel like guilt when decoupled from their (unconscious) ideational ur-origin and forced into "false connections" with other ideas (*Vorstellungen*). In the latter instance, guilt could be deemed to be unconscious not as an oxymoronic unfelt feeling, but instead as a feeling that is, as all feelings in human subjects potentially can be, misfelt (to repeat Freud's phrasing, "perceived but misconstrued")—and this insofar as the feel of this feeling is inflected by misleading associative displacements along the strands of the psyche's webs of ideational contents. In fact, Freud says as much approximately a page later, toward the end of this section of "The Unconscious," proposing that "the development of affect can . . . proceed from this conscious substitute [*bewußten Ersatz*], and the nature of that substitute determines the qualitative character of the affect."[20] (The "conscious substitute [*bewußten Ersatz*]" is related to the earlier-invoked "other idea [*anderen Vorstellung*].")

And yet, no sooner does Freud open up these possibilities for coherently conceptualizing unconscious affects than he quickly shuts down these promising metapsychological avenues, promptly reverting to a theory according to which an unconscious affect is, strictly speaking, a contradiction in terms. He stipulates at length:

> If we restore the true connection [*richtigen Zusammenhang*], we call the original affective impulse an "unconscious" one. Yet its affect was never unconscious; all that had happened was that its *idea [Vorstellung]* had undergone repression. In general, the use of the terms "unconscious affect" [*unbewußter Affekt*] and "unconscious emotion" [*unbewußtes Gefühl*] has reference to the vicissitudes undergone, in consequence of repression, by the quantitative factor in the instinctual impulse. We know that three such vicissitudes are possible: either the affect remains, wholly or in part, as it is; or it is transformed into a qualitatively different quota of affect [*einen qualitativ anderen Affektbetrag*], above all into anxiety; or it is suppressed [*unterdrückt*], i.e. it is prevented from developing at all. . . . We know, too, that to suppress the development of affect is the true aim of repression and that its work is incomplete if this aim is not achieved. In every instance where repression has succeeded in inhibiting the development of affects, we term those affects (which we restore when we undo the work of repression) "unconscious." Thus it cannot be denied that the use of the term in question is consistent; but in comparison with unconscious ideas there is the important difference that unconscious ideas continue to exist after repression as actual structures [*reale Bildung*] in the system *Ucs.*, whereas all that corresponds in that system to unconscious affects is a potential beginning which is prevented from developing.[21]

There is much to be unpacked in this passage, an unpacking that will occupy me in the next several paragraphs. Beginning with relatively simple, broad brushstrokes, the story Freud tells here is that what he really means by the phrase "unconscious affect" is a virtual potential-to-feel, rather than an actually felt feeling somehow not registered at the level of conscious awareness (something implicitly dismissed as self-contradictory). This virtual potential-to-feel, as not-yet-felt feeling cut off and strangulated (i.e., "suppressed" [*unterdrückt*]) by repression, is tied to certain "real formations" (*reale Bildung*) of repressed ideational representations (*Vorstellungen*) in the unconscious (what Lacan later calls "formations of the unconscious," as per the title of his fifth seminar of 1957–1958). The labor of analysis, in lifting the burdensome, heavy curtain of repression, allows these not-yet-felt affective potentials within the unconscious to become felt affective actualities in consciousness (a sort of variant on what is involved in the old idea of catharsis). Analytic therapy fleshes out emotional dead zones where appropriate feelings were previously lacking, in addition to filling in suspicious mnemic, conceptual, and symbolic-linguistic blanks within analysands' narratives. Moreover, Freud stresses that only ideas (*Vorstellungen*) truly can be repressed in the strict sense. Hence, affects are unconscious only as ideationally encoded non- or preaffective potentials for perhaps eventually coming to feel certain affects in connection with specific repressed *Vorstellungen* once those representatives are rendered conscious thanks to the lifting of repression.

But, even in the passage examined in freestanding isolation, things aren't so simple. Complications arise in relation to the senses in which to interpret and characterize the three psychical vicissitudes undergone by affective "quotas" as well as in relation to the distinction in this passage's background between affects as quantitative or economic variables (i.e., "the quantitative factor") and as qualitative or experiential phenomena. (As early as the *Project for a Scientific Psychology* [1895], the root source of so many enduring Freudian notions, Freud tries to formulate an explanatory quantitative reduction of the qualitative feel of affects.)[22] The term *affect* carries with it, especially in Freudian metapsychology, dangerous risks of several theoretically problematic equivocations, including a sloppy mixing together of quantitative and qualitative dimensions of description. Laplanche and Pontalis, among others, are careful to highlight the difference, evident in the preceding quotation from "The Unconscious," between the economic concept "quota of affect" (*Affektbetrag*) and affect (*Affekt*) as an experience with a given feeling-quality.[23] One of Freud's assumptions in 1915 on which his delineation of the three vicissitudes of affects rests is that there can be "quantitative" changes in libidinal, drive-level mechanisms or processes that fail to generate any corresponding conscious or felt qualities. (This assumption will be reexamined under the new illumination provided by the neurosciences, particularly Damasio's research.) Simply put, to be affected quantitatively isn't always, as one might presume, to be affected qualitatively. According to Freudian metapsychology, the phenomenology of affect (as *Affekt*) doesn't necessarily match up in any one-to-one manner with the economy of affect (as *Affektbetrag*)—and this by virtue of repressions bearing upon the libidinal economy.

Freud's three postrepression destinies of quotas of affect (*Affektbetrag*) lead to these quotas, as "the quantitative factor in the instinctual impulse," being felt (i.e., "the affect remains, wholly or in part, as it is"), misfelt (i.e., "it is transformed into a qualitatively different quota of affect [*einen qualitativ anderen Affektbetrag*], above all into anxiety"), or unfelt (i.e., "it is suppressed [*unterdrückt*], i.e. it is prevented from developing at all"). Sticking to the example of guilt, the first scenario refers to cases in which someone feels guilt without really understanding why he/she feels this way (as with the apparently irrational, excessive guilt typical of certain neurotics). The second scenario, of special interest to me, seemingly describes instances in which an underlying sense of culpability registers itself as a disturbing agitation not self-consciously felt as guilt per se. (Incidentally, maybe the excitement of being affected without knowing why tends to be spontaneously self-interpreted, under the constraints of repression, as anxiety because of the somatic excitations accompanying a range of affective feeling-states, including guilt, sexual arousal, and so on: on the next page of this paper, Freud characterizes anxiety as "the affect . . . for which all 'repressed' affects are exchanged.")[24] The third scenario is best construed as suggesting that someone's unconscious can harbor repressed memories or thoughts that, although charged with the potential power to give rise to guilty feelings if brought to light under the right circumstances, are prevented from actually stimulating a conscious sense of guilt (or any other palpable affective effect).

Additionally, a strange, troubling tension surfaces in the original German wording of the second of these three vicissitudes: Cutting against the grain of his metapsychological distinction between phenomenal *Affekt* and economic *Affektbetrag*, Freud imputes qualitative differences to different quantitative quotas of affect. Affects, as phenomena, can be qualitatively distinguished from one another by their distinctive feels. By contrast, how can quotas of affect, as pure economic quantities (not felt in themselves but only if and when they're translated into consciously registered experiences), differ from each other qualitatively? A strange short circuit between levels of metapsychological discourse appears to be operative here.

But, Freud has a few more noteworthy remarks to make in "The Unconscious." He continues: "Strictly speaking, then, and although no fault can be found with the linguistic usage, there are no unconscious affects as there are unconscious ideas. But there may very well be in the system *Ucs.* affective structures [*Affektbildungen*] which, like others, become conscious. The whole difference arises from the fact that ideas are cathexes [*Besetzungen*]—basically of memory-traces—whilst affects [*Affekte*] and emotions [*Gefühle*] correspond to processes of discharge, the final manifestations of which are perceived as feelings [*Empfindungen*]."[25] Many readers of Freud, particularly those of a Lacanian bent, tend to ignore what immediately follows and qualifies Freud's metapsychological statement claiming that "there are no unconscious affects"; significantly, Freud goes on to add "as there are unconscious ideas." In the two subsequent sentences, he struggles to clarify in what fashion it's indeed admissible to talk about affects being unconscious, albeit in a fashion other than that of designating the manner in which ideational representations subsist as unconscious. (In line with this Freudian addition, Green maintains that, for Freud, affects can be unconscious, although admittedly in modes different from unconscious representations.)[26] So, how are these clarifications to be comprehended, assuming the invalidity of simply concluding, particularly in the wake of a close reading of Freud's writing, that Freud categorically and without qualification rejects the very idea of unconscious affects?

The invocation of "affective structures" (*Affektbildungen*, which also could be translated as "affective formations," as in "formations of the unconscious") seemingly signals a falling-back upon the hypothesis according to which the phrase "unconscious affect" really refers not to affects as such (as experiential phenomena), but instead to constellations of repressed ideational representations with the potential, under the proper conditions, to give rise to certain affects within the sphere of conscious awareness. These repressed constellations within the unconscious are, strictly speaking, protoaffective rather than affective per se. In short, appealing to *Affektbildungen* would appear to enable Freud to square the notion of unconscious affect with his metapsychological postulate dictating that only ideas (*Vorstellungen*) can be truly unconscious in the precise technical sense. Read in this fashion, no serious threat looks to be posed by the passage quoted to the traditional Lacanian interpretation of Freud's metapsychology of affect, repeatedly and insistently alleged by Lacan and his adherents to be articulated by Freud with a decisive finality in 1915.

But, the following final sentence of the quoted passage indeed does problematize, if read closely and carefully, Lacan's persistent reliance upon "The Unconscious" to underwrite his generally sweeping denial of the existence of unconscious affects (a reliance that will be examined closely in the next chapter). With my putting aside for the time being the hidden nuances and subtleties contained in the term *cathexis* (*Besetzung*)—this term risks appearing simple and straightforward due to its ubiquity and familiarity in psychoanalytic discourse—it should be noticed that Freud resorts to using three separate but related words: *Affekte* (affects), *Gefühle* (emotions), and *Empfindungen* (feelings). Even if Freud himself, as an intentional authorial consciousness, isn't fully aware of the implications sheltering here in his sentences, these implications literally are there, on this very textual surface itself. Moreover, in light of this tripartite distinction in "The Unconscious," a retroactive payoff becomes visible in relation to the regular underscoring of Freud's German in the prior pages of this project (an underscoring that might have seemed, at least to some readers perhaps, to be pointless or even excessive in an irritatingly obsessional sort of scholarly style). Green likewise draws attention to this German terminological triad, although he doesn't go on, as I do, to develop in detail its precise systematic ramifications for a Freudian-Lacanian psychoanalysis interfaced with neurobiology.[27]

Freud manifestly draws a distinction, in 1915, between, on the one hand, affects and emotions and, on the other hand, feelings. The former (i.e., *Affekte* and *Gefühle*) are said to designate "processes of discharge" (presumably discharges driven by ideational *Affektbildungen* with their economic *Affektbeträge* [quotas of affect]), processes of which only a partial portion are consciously registered—and this insofar as Freud clearly states, regarding affects and emotions, that solely their "final manifestations . . . are perceived as feelings [*Empfindungen*]." The two extreme poles of, on one end, *Affektbildung* and *Affektbetrag* and, on another end, *Empfindung* map onto Freud's underlying metapsychological dichotomy between economic quantities (akin to structure) and experiential qualities (akin to energy) in a parallel, one-to-one correspondence. However, *Affekte* and *Gefühle* (or, what hereafter I will dub "*Affekte*-qua-*Gefühle*") are left hanging in a strange metapsychological limbo, a conceptual liminal space, between these two poles. *Affekt*-qua-*Gefühl* is neither *Affektbildung* or *Affektbetrag* nor *Empfindung*, neither the structural or ideational potential for being consciously affected through feeling nor the phenomenal or sensational being consciously affected through feeling.

Further support for thus demarcating these subdivisions in Freud's metapsychology of affect are readily to be found by casting a glance backward over the textual ground already covered in the preceding pages. First of all, what Freud circa 1915 indisputably would reject would be any suggestion that feelings-as-*Empfindungen* could be unconscious, since this would entail indefensibly positing self-contradictory feelings that are not felt. Secondly, if all *Empfindungen*, as sensed sentiments, are consciously registered "final manifestations" of psychical dynamics set in motion by underlying affective structures or formations, *Affekte*-qua-*Gefühle* directly are implied to be, as distinct from *Empfindungen*, un- or nonconscious (but, perhaps, in a manner different from the un- or nonconsciousness of ideational *Affektbildungen* and, especially, economic *Affektbeträge*). In fact, when Freud refers to "unconscious affects" or "unconscious emotions," both in the title of this third section of "The Unconscious" presently under discussion and elsewhere (before and after 1915), he consistently attaches the adjective *unconscious* to *Affekte* and *Gefühle*, not to *Empfindungen*. (There is one exception to this rule, maybe the proverbial exception that proves the rule, occurring in the second chapter of *The Ego and the Id*: therein, Freud stipulates that feelings [*Empfindungen*] are either conscious or unconscious, but never preconscious.)[28] More specifically, apropos the "unconscious sense of guilt" (guilt being the affect Freud [disproportionately] focuses on as possibly unconscious), the term Freud invariably employs is *Schuldgefühl*. Guilt is unconscious as an instance of *Gefühl*, not *Empfindung*. For now-obvious reasons, Freud avoids using the more common, quotidian German word *Schuldbewußtsein* (consciousness of guilt) to designate the sense of guilt bound up with conscience, save for mentioning it in the paper "Obsessive Actions and Religious Practices" (1907) to stress "the apparent contradiction in terms" involved in speculating about unconscious guilt as a literal "unconscious consciousness of guilt" (*unbewußten Schuldbewußtseins*).

In response to this pinpointing of *Affekt*-qua-*Gefühl* as distinct from both, on the one side, *Affektbildung* and *Affektbetrag* as the structural-economic-quantitative part of affective life and, on the other side, *Empfindung* as the phenomenal-experiential-qualitative part of this dimension of the psyche's being, one might say that such a move, rather than answering any questions about the metapsychology of affect, introduces new mysteries raising further unanswered questions. But, even if this is all that's been accomplished thus far, this is indeed an accomplishment. Freud's account of affect (or, more accurately, accounts), especially in his metapsychological writings from the era around 1915, has been treated by the vast majority of his successors of various stripes, both Lacanian and non-Lacanian, as an open-and-shut matter of established exegetical fact—namely, the alleged fact that Freud flatly and without caveats denies the existence of unconscious affects. What the preceding attentive examination of the details of Freud's texts shows, if nothing else, is that his metapsychology of affect is simultaneously less consistent and more complex than his commentators and heirs tend to acknowledge.

To take a non-Lacanian example from mainstream Anglo-American clinical analytic literature: Sydney Pulver, in two articles from the 1970s (one in the *International Journal of Psycho-Analysis* and the other in *Psychoanalytic Quarterly*), tackles head-on the lingering enigma of unconscious affect(s) bequeathed by Freud to his successors. Pulver's interlinked pieces are highly instructive in this context. One of the general weaknesses of English-speaking psychoanalytic traditions vis-à-vis Freud—there are exceptions to this generalization—is that these traditions misunderstand a number of Freud's key claims and concepts because of, in part, a failure to understand adequately his original

German statements (such misunderstandings aren't minor matters of exegetical nitpicking, but have major effects on the theory and practice of analysis). A core component of Lacan's "return to Freud" is the effort to address this Anglo-American weakness through an insistence on reading Freud to the letter, taking seriously the devils residing in the details of his writings (including those dwelling in Freud's German). But, this rigorous interpretive vigilance preached and usually practiced by Lacan proves to be lacking as regards Freud's reflections on affective life; although there are frequent extended meditations on the connotations and resonances of specific German words used by Freud, the related words *Affekt*, *Gefühl*, and *Empfindung* nowhere are cited in either the nine-hundred-page *Écrits* or the twenty-seven volumes of *le Séminaire*. Pulver, approaching the Freudian corpus and legacy through a very different set of analytic lenses than those worn by Lacan, nonetheless concurs that Freud bluntly and categorically denies the possibility of affects being unconscious. He then, unlike Lacan, sets about contesting this denial through proposing different ways in which affects can be, and frequently are, unconscious in psychoanalytically meaningful senses. But, a careful rereading of Freud's pronouncements on affects in relation to the unconscious reveals that many of Pulver's suggestions already are anticipated by Freud.

With some justification, Pulver blames what he views as Freud's untenable dismissal of the concept of unconscious affects on a metapsychologically lax taking-for-granted of the everyday, folk-psychological association between the notions of "feeling" and "experience," an association in which both notions connote awareness.[29] This rare instance of complacency on Freud's part, Pulver implies, leads him to overlook various ways in which affects can be kept outside of the restricted sphere of conscious awareness (Pulver provides several clinical illustrations of these ways). Pulver's main concern is to argue for a distinction between two basic categories relevant to conceptualizing nonconscious affective life: "unconscious affects" and "potential affects." He contrasts these categories thus: "*Unconscious affects* are those in which the affect is aroused and experienced, but kept from awareness through some defensive process. *Potential affects* are those affects which are particularly susceptible to arousal *but have not yet been aroused*."[30] In a sequel article entitled "Unconscious Versus Potential Affects," he further clarifies and refines this distinction: "Stated simply, *unconscious affects* exist in an activated or aroused state outside of awareness. They may be either preconscious or dynamically unconscious. They are 'activated' because they exist experientially in a dynamically active state; that is, they have an effect upon motor or psychic activity at the moment under consideration. *Potential affects*, on the other hand, may arise from a dispositional state in which the affect is not aroused and active, but is 'more ready than usual' to be so. . . . Unconscious affects, then, are items of mental *content*, whereas potential affects, strictly speaking, are not affects at all, but *structural* dispositions to produce affects."[31]

Pulver subsequently summarizes this as follows: "Affects of which the individual is unaware may exert their behavioral effect in two different modes, as *unconscious affects* or as *potential affects*. Unconscious affects are those which exist in an activated state outside of awareness. Potential affects are those which may arise from a dispositional state of the individual in which the affect is not aroused and active but is 'more ready than usual' to be so. Unconscious affects are items of mental content; as such, they are in the realm of subjective experience. Potential affects, on the other hand, are, strictly speaking, not affects at all but *structural dispositions* to produce affects and, as structures, they are not in the realm of subjective experience."[32]

One might rename what Pulver calls "unconscious affects" "nonconscious affects," since, as he specifies, such affects can be either preconscious (as "feeling tones" activated in the here and now but not attended to by self-conscious attention) or unconscious (as these same sort of tones defensively avoided by self-conscious attention).[33] What both of these types of nonconscious affects have in common is the occurrence of phenomenal states of being affected minus an accompanying explicit cognizance of these same states. In the terms of Freud's metapsychology, an affect registered by the perception-consciousness system is neglected, whether for defensive or nondefensive reasons, by the attentive awareness of (self-)consciousness. (In defensive instances, unconscious mechanisms are topographically situated between perception consciousness and consciousness proper, contra the standard, misleading depth-psychological imagery frequently foisted on Freud's thinking, situated internally and immanently within the very surface of consciousness.) Translating Pulver's concept-phrase "potential affects" back into Freudian parlance, one can say that this concept-phrase designates those constellations of repressed ideational representations with the potential to give rise to a corresponding affect or affects, namely, constellations of unconscious ideas (*Vorstellungen*) liable to provoke particular feeling-states under specific conditions.

What evidence is there for either of Pulver's two categories of affects? He specifies that: "The evidence we are looking for to support the existence of unconscious affects consists of situations in which the individual shows physiological, ideational and motor behaviour usually associated with a central feeling state, in which he indicates a lack of awareness of that feeling state, and in which he is incapable of reporting such awareness after an ordinary effort of attention."[34] This criterion concerning evidence speaking in favor of there being unconscious affects ought to be reminiscent of the "as if" phenomena Freud alludes to, in "Obsessive Actions and Religious Practices," in connection with the possibility of the existence of an unconscious sense of guilt in certain neurotic analysands. For his part, Pulver, among other examples, highlights reaction-formations (as in, for instance, feeling fondness as a way of avoiding feeling anger, the latter thereby remaining an unconscious affect in a peculiar fashion) and behavioral tactics of unknowingly avoiding circumstances and situations apt to arouse defended-against (potential) affects.[35]

From his reflections on this topic, Pulver concludes that, in addition to clinical observations and data testifying to the existence of unconscious affects, nothing testifies against the legitimacy and accuracy of positing sides of affective life outside of the limited scope of the conscious ego's (self-)awareness[36] (save for what Pulver diagnoses as Freud's uncritical, mistaken acceptance of the everyday, ordinary-language lumping-together of affects and consciousness). However, after having passed through the preceding examinations of Freud's pronouncements bearing upon unconscious affects, Pulver's proposals seem familiar. Apart from Pulver overlooking all of those occasions when Freud entertains the hypothesis that actually activated affects indeed can be unconscious in Pulver's sense of "unconscious affects"—one need only point to the recurrent invocations of *Schuldgefühl* in Freud's writings—he also ignores what Freud terms "affective structure" (*Affektbildung*). Pulver's category of "potential affect" designates, despite his not acknowledging this, the same thing as Freud's affective structure. But, the merit of Pulver's articles resides in their helping to pull together a less cloudy vision of nonconscious affects than the one floating around in fragments scattered throughout Freud's oeuvre. Pulver brings into sharper relief a picture of unconscious affect(s) arguably implicit and latent in Freud's texts.

Moreover, a statement made by Pulver productively serves as a bridge to the examination of Lacan's treatment of affects to ensue in the next chapter: "'pure feelings' do not exist in nature. . . . Rather, affects from the very beginning of psychic life are linked with perceptual, cognitive and motor processes."[37] While this assertion is true, this same truth can be grasped and put to work in strikingly different ways. On the one hand, it can serve as a base axiom for projects (including this one) seeking to enrich, extend, and deepen, in conjunction with contemporary philosophical and neuroscientific resources, Freud's less-than-fully-elaborated metapsychology of unconscious affects. On the other hand, it can serve as a justification for downplaying affects as secondary, residual by-products of processes fundamentally governed by the dynamics of structures comprising ideational representations. This latter path is the one Lacan tends to follow. It is to his handling of affect that I turn now.

II.

FROM SIGNIFIERS TO *JOUIS-SENS*

LACAN'S *SENTI-MENTS* AND *AFFECTUATIONS*

As the Lacanian analyst and scholar Bruce Fink correctly observes, Freud is far from consistent in his theorization of affect.[1] Yet another illustration of this Freudian inconsistency, apart from the shifts and vacillations already highlighted, is to be found in the metapsychological paper on "The Unconscious," a mere two paragraphs after the invocations of affect (*Affekt*), emotion (*Gefühl*), feeling (*Empfindung*), and affective structure (*Affektbildung*) examined in chapter 10: the distinction between affect and feeling, in which the latter designates qualitative phenomena that must be felt consciously in order to be, looks to be revoked to the extent that Freud soon proceeds to relapse, at the end of the third section of this paper from 1915, into again conflating affects with felt feelings registered by the awareness of consciousness ("in actuality . . . the affect does not as a rule arise till the break-through to a new representation in the system *Cs.* has been successfully achieved [*der wirkliche Vorgang... ist in der Regel, daß ein Affekt so lange nicht zu stande kommt, bis nicht der Durchbruch zu einer neuen Vertretung im System* Bw *gelungen ist*]"[2]). What absolutely must be acknowledged is that Freud is indeed genuinely and entirely inconsistent apropos a metapsychology of affect, erratically oscillating in indecision between various speculations regarding the existence and nature of unconscious affects in particular. Lacan, perhaps strongly motivated in this instance by what could be deemed (in his own parlance) a "passion for ignorance"[3] (perhaps a passion for ignorance about passion), tends not to admit even this much; as will be seen soon, he repeatedly insists with vehemence that Freud unflinchingly bars affective phenomena from the unconscious qua the proper object of psychoanalysis as a discipline. By contrast, Fink at least concedes that Freud wasn't of one mind on this issue, especially concerning the topic of guilt.[4] However, Fink's concession is tempered by a very Lacanian qualification to the effect that, despite his superficial changes of mind concerning affective life, Freud's metapsychological apparatus is, at a deeper and ultimate theoretical level, consistent in ruling out *a priori* the existence of unconscious affects.[5] And, following closely in Lacan's footsteps, Fink likewise ignores the letter of Freud's original German texts by conflating as synonymous affect (*Affekt*) and feeling (*Empfindung*) so as to sustain the claim that affects are felt feelings and, hence, cannot be unconscious strictly speaking.[6]

Most other Lacanians simply pass over in silence those numerous textual occasions in which Freud mobilizes the hypotheses that (certain) affects can be and, in actuality, are unconscious. These followers of Lacan present an utterly false portrait of a Freud steadfastly unwavering in his dismissal of the notion of unconscious affect as a muddleheaded contradiction in terms inadmissible to correct psychoanalytic reason. Although somewhat superficially faithful to the letter of Lacan's text, such Lacanians flagrantly flout its spirit, failing to "return to Freud" by not, like Lacan before them, reading Freud's oeuvre as closely and carefully as possible; they are content to accept the Freudian corpus as digested for them by Lacan. Recalling the fact that, in relation to the topic of the psyche's affective side, Lacan uncharacteristically makes no references whatsoever to the German words *Affekt*, *Gefühl*, *Empfindung*, and *Affektbildung* as these words operate literally in Freud's texts, one might risk asserting that Lacan violates the spirit of his own endeavor when discussing the Freudian metapsychology of affect. One only can guess why this breakdown befalls Lacan. Why does he turn a blind exegetical eye, typically so sharp and discerning, to everything Freud says about affective life in addition to, and in a way that is often at odds with, the far-from-unqualified denial of unconscious affects connected to the claim that solely ideational representations (ideas as *Vorstellungen*, to be identified by Lacan as "signifiers") can become unconscious through repression?

And yet, like Freud, Lacan too isn't thoroughly consistent in the manners in which he addresses affect in psychoanalysis. Although his wavering and hesitations on this matter are more muted and less explicitly at the fore than in Freud's work, they are audible to an appropriately attuned interpretive ear. Especially in his tenth and seventeenth seminars (on *Anxiety* [1962–1963] and *The Other Side of Psychoanalysis* [1969–1970]), Lacan does more than just underscore the nonexistence of unconscious affects for a psychoanalysis grounded upon properly Freudian concepts. But, before turning to focus primarily on these two seminars, I must foreground the nuances and subtleties of Lacan's own contributions to a yet-to-be-systematized Freudian-Lacanian metapsychology of affect, which requires establishing a background picture of his general, overarching account of affects. This is best accomplished via a condensed chronological tour through the seminars, with topical detours into corresponding *écrits* and other pieces.

In the first seminar (*Freud's Papers on Technique* [1953–1954]), Lacan argues against distinguishing between the affective and the intellectual such that the former becomes an ineffability beyond the latter. He states his staunch rejection of "the notorious opposition between the intellectual and the affective—as if the affective were a sort of colouration, a kind of ineffable quality which must be sought out in itself, independently of the eviscerated skin which the purely intellectual realisation of a subject's relationship would consist in. This conception, which urges analysis down strange paths, is puerile. The slightest peculiar, even strange, feeling that the subject professes to in the text of the session is taken to be a spectacular success. That is what follows from this fundamental misunderstanding."[7] Particularly during the first decade of *le Séminaire*, the primary audience to whom Lacan addresses himself consists of practicing analysts. Discussions of clinical work in Anglo-American analytic circles, both in Lacan's time and nowadays, indeed frequently do give the impression that prompting patients on the couch to produce verbalizations of feelings in the here and now of the session is the principle concern of analysis; when listening to analysts of the stripe Lacan has in mind in this context, it sounds as though therapeutic progress is measured mainly by the degree to which an analysand is willing and able to struggle to voice affects as he/she is being affected by them between the four walls of the analyst's consulting room. In short, this is to treat upsurges of emotion irrupting into patients' forty-five-minute monologues as analytic pay dirt, as self-evident ends in themselves requiring no further explanation or justification (i.e., a spectacular success).[8] Although this is an aggressively exaggerated caricature, it informs Lacan's remarks here. He warns those analysts listening to him not to go down this "puerile path" in their practices.

However, Lacan isn't saying that affects are irrelevant to or of no interest in analytic practice. He's reacting to what he sees as an indefensible and misguided elevation of affective life into the one and only alpha-and-omega of analysis. What he actually claims, with good reason, and which has been steadily and increasingly vindicated since the 1950s, is that neither the intellectual nor the affective (or, in more contemporary vocabulary borrowed from neuroscientific discourse, the cognitive and the emotional) are independent of each other, with each standing separately on its own. Not only, contra other analytic orientations guilty of fetishizing the appearance of affects within the scene of analytic sessions, are affects inextricably intertwined with ideas (as thoughts, memories, words, concepts, and the like), but ideas, as incarnated in living speech, are permeated with something other than themselves, affected by nonideational forces and factors[9] (as indicated in the quoted passage when Lacan speaks of "the eviscerated skin which the purely intellectual realisation of a subject's relationship would consist in").

Lacan's point can be made by paraphrasing Kant: Affects without ideas are blind (the dynamic movement of the affective or emotional is shaped and steered by the intellectual or cognitive), while ideas without affects are empty (the structured kinetics of the intellectual or cognitive are driven along by juice flowing from the affective or emotional). Of course, given the tendencies and trends within psychoanalysis Lacan is combating at this time, his comments immediately following the ones in the quotation a couple of paragraphs earlier highlight one side of this two-sided coin, namely, the dependence of the affective on the intellectual: "The affective is not like a special density which would escape an intellectual accounting. It is not to be found in a mythical beyond of the production of the symbol which would precede the discursive formulation. Only this can allow us from the start, I won't say to locate, but to apprehend what the full realisation of speech consists in."[10] This is of a piece with Lacan's denunciation, in his "Rome Discourse" from 1953 ("The Function and Field of Speech and Language in Psychoanalysis"), of an "illusion" plaguing analysts and their practices, one "which impels us to seek the subject's reality beyond the wall of language."[11] (Fink also points out this connection between the mirage of language being a barrier between those who use it and certain conceptions of affect.)[12] In other words, analysts shouldn't erroneously strive somehow to gain access to a reservoir of feelings and emotions sheltering behind the manifest façade of analysands' utterances. It's not as though there really is a transcendent Elsewhere of ineffable qualitative phenomena subsisting in a pure state of extralinguistic immediacy outside of the strictures of the linguistic latticework woven session after session by the patient's speech. When dealing with speaking beings—analysis deals with nothing but—any affects inevitably will be immanent and impure in a way that is tied up with constellations and configurations of ideational representations (i.e., Freudian *Vorstellungen* as Lacanian signifiers). At least as regards these particular observations made in 1954 bearing on affects in analysis, Lacan's position seems to be that the affective or emotional and the intellectual or cognitive are mutually entangled, although, to counterbalance what he considers to be misguided deviations from Freudian orthodoxy, he slants his stress in the direction of underscoring the intellectual or cognitive mediation of the affective or emotional.

In the ensuing years, this slanted stress seems to lose its status as strictly a tactical counterbalance against prevailing clinical analytic developments, with Lacan coming to contend that signifier-ideas have absolute, unqualified metapsychological priority over affects. That is to say, as is particularly evident between 1958 and 1962 (in the sixth, seventh, and ninth seminars specifically), Lacan tilts the balance in the complex ideational-affective rapport decisively in favor of ideational structures, maintaining that these are the driving, determining variables in relation to affective (epi)phenomena. This rapport, deprived of a dialectic of bidirectional, reciprocal influences between its poles, now appears to be organized by a unidirectional line of influence originating from one side alone, namely, in signifiers and their interrelationships. In a session of the sixth seminar (*Desire and Its Interpretation* [1958–1959]), Lacan, basing himself on what he takes to be Freud's metapsychological exclusion of affects from the unconscious (as oxymoronic unfelt feelings) in 1915, claims that affects are only ever displaced within consciousness relative to chains of signifiers as concatenations of ideational drive representatives, some of which can be and are repressed. Stated differently, whereas *Vorstellungen* as signifiers are able to become parts of the unconscious through being dragged, via the gravitational pull of material or meaningful associations, into the orbit of branching formations of the unconscious, affects, as felt qualitative phenomena, must remain within the sphere of conscious experience. In line with what Freud posits in another paper from 1915 on metapsychology (the essay "Repression"),[13] Lacan views repression as bringing about false connections similar to red herrings; more precisely, Lacan thinks the Freudian position here is to assert that affects, after repression does its job and disrupts the true connection of these affects with their original ideational partners, drift within the sphere of conscious awareness in which they remain and form false connections through getting (re)attached to other signifiers.[14] As Roberto Harari, in his examination of Lacan's tenth seminar on anxiety, puts it, "there are *no unconscious affects but, rather, affects drift*."[15] Both Harari and, in certain contexts, Fink express agreement with this aspect of Lacan's reading of Freud articulated in 1958.[16] In this same session of the sixth seminar, Lacan also underscores Freud's reservations when speaking of unconscious affects, emotions, and feelings (three terms Lacan lumps together on this occasion). With a calculated weighting of exegetical emphasis, he thereby aims at supporting the thesis that, for Freudian metapsychology, such talk can amount, when all is said and done, only to incoherent, contradictory formulations without real referents.[17]

The seventh and ninth seminars continue along the same lines. In the seventh seminar (*The Ethics of Psychoanalysis* [1959–1960]), Lacan denounces "the confused nature of the recourse to affectivity" so prevalent in strains of psychoanalysis basing themselves on what he alleges to be "crude" non-Freudian psychologies—although he's careful to add, "Of course, it is not a matter of denying the importance of affects."[18] In the ninth seminar (*Identification* [1961–1962]), responding to a presentation by his student Piera Aulagnier in which she appeals to an unbridgeable abyss separating affective phenomena from their linguistic translations (i.e., to something akin to the earlier-denounced image of the "wall of language"), Lacan denies that affects enjoy an immediate existence independent from the mediation of words. On the contrary, even in affective life, signifiers (as ideas, symbols, thoughts, and the like) are purported to be the primary driving forces at work in the psyche. Lacan encapsulates his criticisms with a play on words, a homophony audible in French: insisting on affects as somehow primary (*primaire*) is tantamount to simplemindedness (*primarité*).[19] Instead, affects, in Lacanian psychoanalysis, are secondary, namely, residual by-products secreted and pushed to and fro by the kinetic relations between networks of signifiers. Harari maintains that the true "Lacanian conception" of affects is that which "*postulates affect as one effect of the signifier.*"[20] Soler likewise bluntly states, "affect is effect."[21]

Although, starting the following academic year (1962–1963), Lacan significantly refines and enriches his metapsychology of affect, it isn't as though this poorer, less refined treatment of affects as mere aftereffects of the interactions of ideational representations falls entirely by the wayside. For instance, in the text of the published version of Lacan's appearance on television from 1973, he reiterates his earlier opinions on affect. Complaining about "the story of my supposed neglect of affect," a narrative by then quite popular and widespread in the poststructuralist intellectual climate of Paris in the wake of May 1968, Lacan indignantly retorts: "I just want an answer on this point: does an affect have to do with the body? A discharge of adrenalin—is that body or not? It upsets its functions, true. But what is there in it that makes it come from the soul? What it discharges is thought."[22] The word *thought* here functions as a synonym for ideational representations as signifiers, as chains of multiple linguistic-symbolic constituents. The affected body is affected by words and ideas; even though the effect might be somatic, the cause is not. Lacan adds: "All I've done is rerelease what Freud states in an article of 1915 on repression, and in others that return to this subject, namely that affect is displaced. How to appreciate this displacement, if not so the basis of the subject, which is presupposed by the fact that it has no better means of occurring than through representation?"[23]

From the vantage point reached through the preceding examination of the literal details of Freud's writings relevant to the debated enigma or problem of unconscious affects, Lacan's professions of modesty are in danger of ringing false: even in his papers on metapsychology from 1915, Freud, as seen, doesn't limit himself to saying solely that affects are invariably conscious experiential qualia displaced relative to the shifting ground of webs of representational contents—and this in addition to those numerous other places in the Freudian corpus, both before and after 1915, where affect is discussed in ways relevant to the issues at stake here, places neglected by Lacan's highly selective and partial rendition of Freud's metapsychology of affect. In struggling against the excessive overemphases on affectivity, embodiment, and energetics promoted by a range of figures and orientations (non-Lacanian analysts, disenchanted ex- or post-Lacanians, existential phenomenologists, feminist theorists, and so on), Lacan sometimes succumbs to an equally excessive counteremphasis on the foundational, fundamental primacy of "representation" in psychical life.

Along the same lines and echoing remarks made in the seventh seminar, Lacan, in the twenty-third seminar (*Le sinthome* [1975–1976]), sidelines the topic of affect as too bound up with vulgar, unsophisticated psychologies based on the "confused image we have of our own body"[24] (i.e., mirages mired in the Lacanian register of the Imaginary). In a late piece from 1980, Lacan contrasts the indestructible fixity of desire with the "instability" (*mouvance*) of affects, an instability symptomatic of their status as volatile fluctuating displacements within consciousness buffeted by the achronological machinations of the unconscious formations configuring desire in its strict Lacanian sense[25] (the latter, not the former, thus being identified as what is really of interest in analysis). Once again, at the very end of his itinerary, Lacan insists that intellectual or cognitive structures, and not affective or emotional phenomena, are what psychoanalysis is occupied with insofar as the unconscious, as constituted by repression and related mechanisms, is the central object of analytic theory and practice.

Before directing sustained critical attention toward the tenth and seventeenth seminars, in which determining the status of affect in Lacan's thinking is a trickier task, mention must be made of a peculiar German term employed by Freud and singled out as being of crucial importance by Lacan: *Vorstellungsrepräsentanz* (a compound word whose translation, as soon will become evident, raises questions and presents difficulties not without implications for analysis both theoretical and practical—hence, its translation will be delayed temporarily in this discussion). Lacan's glosses on this word's significance, as used by Freud, often accompany his pronouncements regarding the place of affect in the Freudian framework.[26] In the third section on "Unconscious Emotions" in the metapsychological paper "The Unconscious" (1915)—as is now obvious, these three pages of text lie at the very heart of the controversies into which I have waded—the *Repräsentanz* represented by the *Vorstellung* isn't a representation that is an idea distinct or separate from an affect, but instead an affectively charged (i.e., "cathected," in Freudian locution) ideational node. To be more specific and exact, a *Repräsentanz* is, in this context, a psychical drive representative that is a mental idea (representing a drive's linked aim [*Ziel*] and object [*Objekt*]) invested by somatic drive energy that is the affecting body (consisting of a drive's source [*Quelle*] and pressure [*Drang*]). Such cathexes are the precise points at which soma and psyche (and, by extension, affects and ideas) overlap in the manner Freud indicates in his contemporaneous paper on "Drives and Their Vicissitudes."[27] *Vorstellungen* are ideational representations that represent representations-as-*Repräsentanzen* once these *Repräsentanzen* have been submitted to the vicissitudes of defensive maneuvers rendering them unconscious (à la the patterns of "repression proper" in connection with "primal repression," as described by Freud in his metapsychological paper on "Repression.")[28] As Freud words it in "The Unconscious" apropos the concept of an "affective or emotional impulse" (*Affekt- oder Gefühlsregung*), "Owing to the repression of its proper representative [*eigentlichen Repräsentanz*] it has been forced to become connected with another idea [*anderen Vorstellung*], and is now regarded by consciousness as the manifestation of that idea."[29] The violent cutting of repression tears away affects or emotions from their own primordial and initial accompanying representatives (*Repräsentanzen*). Thereafter, they move in, along, and about "other ideas" as *Vorstellungen* associated, however loosely and indirectly, with their original *Repräsentanzen*.

Incidentally, Fink, on a couple of occasions, indicates that Lacan identifies the *Vorstellung* as a primordially repressed Real (i.e., a pre-Symbolic "x" inscribed in the psyche as a protosignifier) and the *Repräsentanz* as the

Symbolic delegate of the thus repressed, unconscious *Vorstellung* (i.e., the signifier signifying that which is primordially repressed).[30] However, the preceding sentence from "The Unconscious" (quoted in the previous paragraph) indicates that this reverses Freud's metapsychological usage of these two German words. Moreover, in Freud's contemporaneous metapsychological paper on "Repression" (a text Lacan refers to apropos Freud's use of the compound word *Vorstellungsrepräsentanz*), the German makes clear that Freud identifies the ideational representatives of drives (*Triebrepräsentanzen*) that are submitted to repression (both "primal" and secondary or "proper" repression [*Urverdrängung* and *Verdrängung*]) as *Repräsentanzen*, not *Vorstellungen*.[31] Contra Fink (and, perhaps, Lacan himself), the Freudian usage will be respected throughout the rest of the ensuing discussion.[32]

This Lacanian (mis)reading of Freud aside, an upshot of the preceding to bear in mind in what follows is that affective elements (intimately related to the drives of the libidinal economy) are infused into these ideational representations right from the start. One cannot speak, at least while wearing the cloak of Freud's authority, of intra-representational relations between *Repräsentanzen* and *Vorstellungen* as unfolding prior to and independently of drive-derived affective investments being infused into the ur-*Repräsentanzen* constituting the primordial nuclei (i.e., the primally repressed) of the defensively eclipsed unconscious. In Freud's name, one might (as does Green)[33] venture positing as an axiom that a *Repräsentanz* is a strange locus of convergence in which energy and structure are indistinctly mixed together from the beginning. Rather than theorizing as if affective energies and ideational structures originally are separate and distinct, only subsequently to be brought together over the course of passing time in unstable admixtures through ontogenetic processes, maybe this metapsychological perspective needs to be inverted: the neat-and-clean distinction between energy and structure, between affect and idea, is a secondary abstraction generated by both the temporally elongated blossoming of the psyche itself (a blossoming made possible in part by repressions) and the psychoanalytic theorization of this same emergence. In short, one might speculate that energetic affects and structural ideas, separated from each other as isolated psychical constituents, are fallouts distilled, through repression and related dynamics, from more primordial psychical units that are neither/both affective energies nor/and ideational structures.

A paragraph in Lacan's *écrit* "In Memory of Ernest Jones: On His Theory of Symbolism" (1959) summarizes the basic gist of what he sees as entailed by the Freudian concept-term *Vorstellungsrepräsentanz*. As usual, when the topic of affect is at stake, Lacan appeals to Freud's papers on metapsychology from 1915 in particular:

> Freud's conception—developed and published in 1915 in the *Internationale Zeitschrift*, in the three articles on drives and their avatars, repression, and the unconscious—leaves no room for ambiguity on this point: it is the signifier that is repressed, there being no other meaning that can be given in these texts to the word *Vorstellungsrepräsentanz*. As for affects, Freud expressly formulates that they are not repressed; they can only be said to be repressed by indulgence. As simple *Ansätze* or appendices of the repressed, signals equivalent to hysterical fits [*accès*] established in the species, Freud articulates that affects are simply displaced, as is evidenced by the fundamental fact—and it can be seen that someone is an analyst if he realizes this fact—by which the subject is bound to "understand" his affects all the more the less they are really justified.[34]

Nearly everything Lacan pronounces apropos *Vorstellungsrepräsentanzen* in Freudian metapsychology over the course of seminars ranging from 1958 through 1971 is contained in this passage. Before turning to the issues involved in translating Freud's German word into both English and (French) Lacanese—these issues will be gotten at through examining relevant moments in *le Séminaire* running from the sixth through the eighteenth seminars—a few remarks on this quotation are in order. First of all, Lacan clearly asserts that his Saussure-inspired notion of the signifier is synonymous with Freud's *Vorstellungsrepräsentanz*.[35] (As I already indicated, and as I will maintain subsequently, this alleged terminological equivalence is debatable.) Secondly, the implied delegitimization of any theses regarding unconscious affects looks to be in danger of resting on the erroneous assumption that repression is the sole defense mechanism by virtue of which psychical things are barred from explicit conscious self-awareness. (As Lacan well knows, for the later Freud especially, there are a number of defense mechanisms besides repression—and this apart from the fact that what is meant by "repression" [*Verdrängung*] in Freud's texts is far from simple and straightforward in the way hinted at by Lacan here.) Third, in tandem with emphasizing the displacement of affects within the sphere of consciousness following repression, Lacan indicates that these mere "signals"—in a session of the seventh seminar, he again contrasts affects as signals with *Vorstellungsrepräsentanzen* as signifiers[36]—are fixed, natural attributes of the human animal (i.e., "signals . . . established in the species"). That is to say, emotions and feelings themselves don't distinguish speaking beings from other living beings. Rather, only the web-like network systems of ideational nodes into which affects are routed, and within which they are shuttled about through drifting displacements, mark the denaturalized human psyche as distinct from other animals' nature-governed minds. Put differently, affective phenomena on their own, as signals, are purportedly no different in kind from the stereotyped repertoire of invariant reactions characteristic of any animal species. Finally, Lacan, presuming that affects remain conscious in the wake of repression (albeit thereafter reattached to other representations-as-signifiers in what Freud deems "false connections"), insists that a properly analytic stance vis-à-vis affects is to call into question the pseudoexplanatory rationalizations people construct in response to seemingly excessive displaced sentiments whose "true" ideational bases have been rendered unconscious.

In the sixth seminar, Lacan reiterates much of this apropos the Freudian *Vorstellungsrepräsentanz*.[37] The following academic year, he returns to discussing this term several times. Lacan starts with the first half of this compound German word, namely, the word *Vorstellung* (usually rendered in English by Freud's translators as "idea"; thus, *Vorstellungsrepräsentanz* could be translated into English as "representative of an idea" or "representative of an ideational representation"). Lacan situates these ideas "between perception and consciousness,"[38] thus suggesting, along accepted and established Freudian lines, that *Vorstellungen*, although they are ideational representations registered by the psychical apparatus, aren't necessarily registered in the mode of being attended to by the awareness of directed conscious attention. However, when it comes to the unconscious, Lacan is careful to clarify that its fabric is woven not of *Vorstellungen* as freestanding, atomic units of mental content, but instead of differentially codetermining, cross-resonating relations between multiple representations. This is taken as further justification for his psychoanalytic recourse to a modified Saussurian theory of the signifier à la structural linguistics, a theory including the stipulation that signifiers as such exist only in sets of two or more signifiers.[39] (A signifier without another signifier isn't a signifier to begin with; for there to be an S1, there must be, at a minimum, an S2.) This, he claims, is the significance of Freud's mention of *Vorstellungen* in connection with *Repräsentanzen* in his paper on "The Unconscious." The concept-term *Vorstellungsrepräsentanz* "turns *Vorstellung* into an associative and combinatory element. In that way the world of *Vorstellung* is already organized according to the possibilities of the signifier as such."[40] For Freudian psychoanalysis as conceptualized by Lacan, everything in psychical life (affects included) is "flocculated" through the sieve-like matrices of interlinked signifiers, with these signifiers mutually shaping and influencing one another in complex dynamics defying description in the languages proffered by any sort of psychological atomism of primitive, irreducible mental contents.[41] (In the contemporaneous talk "*Discours aux catholiques*," he relates the Freudian *Vorstellungsrepräsentanz* to a "principle of permutation" in which the possibility of displacements and substitutions is the rule.)[42] Lacan reads *Vorstellung* and *Repräsentanz* both as equivalent to what he refers to under the rubric of the signifier, with one signifier (the S1 *Vorstellung*—really, Freud's *Repräsentanz*) represented by another signifier (the S2 *Repräsentanz*—really, Freud's *Vorstellung*).

This becomes even clearer a few years later. Jacques-Alain Miller entitles the opening subsection of the session from June 3, 1964, of Lacan's deservedly celebrated eleventh seminar "The Question of the *Vorstellungsrepräsentanz*." Lacan gets his lecture underway by again stressing the importance of this term in Freud's discourse.[43] He ties it to the Freudian metapsychological account of repression, including this account's purported denial and dismissal of the possibility of affects being rendered unconscious.[44] Moreover, auditors are reminded of the correct Lacanian translation of *Vorstellungsrepräsentanz*: not "the representative representation (*le représentant représentatif*)"[45] but instead "*the representative (le représentant)*—I translated literally—*of the representation (de la représentation)*."[46] Or, as he quickly proceeds to formulate it, "The *Vorstellungsrepräsentanz* is the *representative representative (le représentant représentatif*), let us say."[47]

Lacan's point, here and elsewhere,[48] is that a *Vorstellungsrepräsentanz* is not the psychoanalytic name for a single, special piece of ideational content in the psychical apparatus. It isn't as though a *Vorstellungsrepräsentanz* is one individual item of representational material. Rather, according to Lacan, it designates the co-determining rapport between two (or more) ideational representations wherein one representation (the repressed S_1) is represented by another representation (the nonrepressed S_2, different from, but associationally linked in a chain with, the repressed S_1).[49] In this vein, he goes on to claim, "The *Vorstellungsrepräsentanz* is the binary signifier"[50] (and this in the context of elaborations concerning the now-famous Lacanian conception of "alienation," elaborations too elaborate to deal with at the moment). In the next session, this is restated: "this *Vorstellungsrepräsentanz* . . . is . . . the signifying S_2 of the dyad."[51] A few years later, in the fifteenth seminar, the *Vorstellungsrepräsentanz*, as the "representative of representation" (*représentant de la représentation*), is similarly linked to the notion of a "combinatorial" (*combinatoire*).[52] In the sixteenth seminar, he warns against equivocating between the terms "represen-tative" (*représentant*) and "representation" (*représentation*).[53] These terms are distinct from one another insofar as representation is a function coming into operation between two or more representatives. (In terms of the psychoana-lytic *Vorstellungsrepräsentanz* involved with repression, this interval is the con-nection between, on the one hand, the repressed S_1 *Repräsentanz* and, on the other hand, the nonrepressed S_2 *Vorstellung* as both that which contributes to triggering retroactively the repression of the S_1 *Repräsentanz* and, at the same time, the associative or signifying return of this same repressed.) Hence, the function of representation isn't reducible to one given representative as an iso-lated, self-defined atomic unit constituting a single element of discrete content lodged within the psychical apparatus.[54]

What Lacan means when he claims that the *Vorstellungsrepräsentanz*, accu-rately translated and understood, is the "representative of the representation" is the following:[55] In the aftermath of repression constituting the unconscious in the strict psychoanalytic sense (with the unconscious being the proper object of psychoanalysis as a discipline), certain repressed signifiers (remembering that, for Lacan, only ideas or representations qua signifiers can be subjected to the fate of repression) are represented by other, nonrepressed signifiers associ-ated in various ways with those that are repressed. In the restricted, circum-scribed domains of self-consciousness and the ego, the Lacanian "subject of the unconscious" manages to make itself heard and felt (or, perhaps, misheard and misfelt) through the S_1-S_2 signifying chains that Lacan equates with Freud's *Vorstellungsrepräsentanzen*, with these chains bearing witness to significant "effects of truth" (*effets de vérité*)[56] having to do with the repressed. (This also helps to explain why Lacan maintains that "repression and the return of the repressed are the same thing.")[57] These claims about the place of *Vorstellung-srepräsentanzen* in the vicissitudes of repression are reiterated in subsequent seminars after 1964 too.[58]

What, if anything, is problematic in Lacan's glosses on Freud's *Vorstellung-srepräsentanz*? Arguably, difficulties arise as soon as Lacan (again in the June 3 session of the eleventh seminar) proceeds further to flesh out the sense in which he uses the word "representation" with respect to Freudian metapsychology:

> We mean by representatives what we understand when we use the phrase, for
> example, the representative of France. What do diplomats do when they
> address one another? They simply exercise, in relation to one another, that
> function of being pure representatives and, above all, their own signification

must not intervene. When diplomats are addressing one another, they are supposed to represent something whose signification, while constantly changing, is, beyond their own persons, France, Britain, etc. In the very exchange of views, each must record only what the other transmits in his pure function as signifier, he must not take into account what the other is, *qua* presence, as a man who is likable to a greater or lesser degree. Inter-psychology is an impurity in this exchange.[59]

He continues: "The term *Repräsentanz* is to be taken in this sense. The signifier has to be understood in this way, it is at the opposite pole from signification. Signification, on the other hand, comes into play in the *Vorstellung*."[60]

There are (at least) two ways to read this invocation of the figure of the diplomat: one, so to speak, more diplomatic (i.e., charitable) than the other. The less charitable reading, for which there is support here and elsewhere in Lacan's oeuvre, is that Lacan completely neglects the fact that, according to Freud, the repressed portions of *Vorstellungsrepräsentanz* configurations or constellations are not "pure" (à la the "pure function as signifier") qua functionally independent of affective and libidinal investments. In fact, for Freud and much of psychoanalysis after him, intrapsychical defense mechanisms, repression included, are motivated and driven by the recurrently pressing demands of affect-regulation within the psychical apparatus (primarily fending off and tamping down unpleasurable negative affects). Additionally, for Freud in particular, the repressed drive representatives (*Triebrepräsentanzen*) constituting the nuclei of the unconscious are saturated with cathexes (*Besetzungen*), with the potent "energies" of emotions and impulses. Such electrified representatives, laden and twitching with turbulent passions, are anything but bloodless diplomatic functionaries, cool, calm, and collected representatives (*Repräsentanzen*) able to conduct negotiations with other representatives (*Vorstellungen*) in a reasonable, sober-minded manner.

The more charitable reading of Lacan's invocation in 1964 of the figure of the diplomat in specifying the meaning of "representative" at work in Freudian psychoanalysis involves further elucidating what lies behind this figure. Lacan is sensible enough to realize that the flesh-and-blood human beings charged with the status of being diplomatic representatives are, as all too human, influenced by their particular interests, motives, reactions, tastes, and the like (i.e., their peculiar "psychologies"). And yet, as diplomatic representatives, they can and do conduct their business with others in ways that put to the side and disregard these idiosyncrasies of theirs as irrelevant to the matters at stake in their negotiations. But, the states these representatives represent frequently are far from being as dispassionate as their diplomats. In 1915, Freud, responding to the outbreak of the First World War, is quick to note, with a sigh of discouragement he proceeds to analyze, just how emotionally discombobulated and irrationally stirred up whole countries can become, even the most "civilized" of nations;[61] the essay "Thoughts for the Times on War and Death" is from the same period as the papers on metapsychology upon which Lacan relies in his downplaying of the importance of affect in psychoanalysis. And, to render Lacan's reading of Freud's metapsychology of affect even more suspect, Freud's war-inspired reflections emphasize the top-to-bottom dominance of affects in the mental life of humanity, in relation to which the intellect is quite frail and feeble.[62]

Considering this fact about the relation between diplomats and the nation-states they represent, a sympathetic and productive way to read Lacan here (in the eleventh seminar) is to interpret the processes unfolding at the level of *Vorstellungsrepräsentanzen* (qua representational or signifying materials) as set in motion by something other than such Symbolic "stuff." Starting in the seventh seminar, the Lacanian register of the Real consistently plays the part of that which drives the kinetic concatenations of signifiers without itself being reducible to or delineable within the order of the signifier. However, once set in motion, these representational or signifying materials help shape subsequent psychical-subjective trajectories in fashions not entirely determined by their originary non-Symbolic catalysts (just as diplomats are dispatched at the behest of their country's whims, although, once caught up in the intricacies of negotiations, these representatives can and do contribute an effective influence of their own on events). As regards a metapsychology of affective life, this would mean that fusions of energy and structure (i.e., *Repräsentanzen*, as analogous to nation-states qua combinations of collective will, with all its passions and sentiments, and sociosymbolic edifices) mobilize and push along signifier-like representational networks (i.e., *Vorstellungen*, as analogous to diplomatic representatives of nation-states licensed to speak on their behalf), with these networks taking on a relative autonomy of their own that comes to exercise a reciprocal, countervailing influence over that which propels them forward (or, sometimes, drags them backward).[63]

Fink rightly observes that the concept of representation in Freudian-Lacanian theory is very much in need of further clarification.[64] As I will argue at regular intervals in what follows, such much-needed clarifications lead to revisions of or deviations from Lacan's signifier-centered version of Freud's metapsychology of affect and repression. But, in the meantime, certain things should be articulated apropos Lacan's more nuanced pronouncements concerning affective life, pronouncements located in the tenth and seventeenth seminars in particular. The first session of the tenth seminar, a seminar devoted to the topic of anxiety, closes with Lacan rapidly enumerating a series of points bearing upon the psychoanalysis of affects. (Considering that this seminar's treatment of anxiety has been gone over at length by others, my focus will be highly selective and partial.) To begin with, here and in the next session, Lacan insists that anxiety is indeed an affect.[65] Few people, whether analysts or not, would disagree with this seemingly banal observation. But, Lacan proceeds to clarify his relationship to affect as a psychoanalytic thinker: "Those who follow the movements of affinity or of aversion of my discourse, frequently letting themselves be taken in by appearances, undoubtedly think that I am less interested in affects than in anything else. This is absurd. I have tried on occasion to say what affect is not. It is not being [*l'être*] given in its immediacy, nor is it the subject in some brute, raw form. It is not, in any case, protopathic. My occasional remarks on affect mean nothing other than this."[66] He adds: "what I have said of affect is that it is not repressed. Freud says this just like me. It is unfastened [*désarrimé*]; it goes with the drift. One finds it displaced, mad, inverted, metabolized, but it is not repressed. What are repressed are the signifiers that moor it."[67]

Lacan's comments betray a palpable awareness of charges indicting him for negligence with respect to affects, accusations with damning force in many clinical psychoanalytic circles. (Several years later, starting in the late 1960s, various so-called poststructuralists in France, including many nonclinicians, started to noisily repeat this long-standing refrain of complaint about Lacanian theory, which continues today.) At the very start of the tenth seminar, he lays the foundations for what becomes a repeated line of defensive self-exculpation: I, Lacan, devoted a whole year of my seminar to the topic of anxiety; therefore, I am not guilty of neglecting affect, as I'm so often accused of doing.[68] Of course, critics might be tempted to respond by pointing out that one academic year out of twenty-seven (not even including the mountain of other texts) isn't all that much time for a psychoanalyst to spend addressing affects. (Even if the titles of Lacan's seminars indicate that, for instance, the analytically crucial topic of transference too is the focus of only one academic year, this is misleading; to stick with this example, transference, unlike affect, is repeatedly treated at length by Lacan across the full span of his teachings.) Lacan himself admits that his "remarks on affect" are "occasional." What's more, as he goes on to say in the closing moments of this inaugural session of the tenth seminar, he has no plans to elaborate a "general theory of affects" (at least not prior to an exploration of anxiety as one specific affect of momentous significance for psychoanalysis), an elaboration derided as a nonpsychoanalytic endeavor for mere psychologists.[69]

Anyhow, in the passages from the tenth seminar quoted earlier, Lacan also, as is manifest, repeats his mantra according to which Freud flatly denies the existence of repressed (i.e., unconscious) affects. (This mantra ignores the fact that Freud, as seen, tacitly distinguishes between, on the one hand, feelings [*Empfindungen*] and, on the other hand, affects [*Affekte*] and emotions [*Gefühle*]; additionally, as shown, he vacillates considerably on the issue of whether affects or emotions can be unconscious.) Again, in the wake of repression, affects are said to undergo only detachment from their original ideational partners (i.e., Freud's ideas or Lacan's signifiers) to which they are coupled initially; subsequent to this, they meander off and end up reattached to other ideational partners further away down the winding, branching tendrils of enchained representations. Curiously, Lacan, instead of declaring that what he states regarding affect echoes Freud, announces the reverse: what Freud states regarding affect echoes him ("Freud says this just like me" [*Cela, Freud le dit comme moi*], and not "I say this just like Freud"). Perhaps, whether consciously or not, Lacan is signaling, through this odd reversal of positions between himself and Freud, an awareness that the Freud he presents in his teachings as regards affect is one retroactively modified and custom-tailored to the needs, constraints, and requirements of a specifically Lacanian framework.

But, although none of the above is new relative to Lacan's basic metapsychology of affect as sketched in earlier contexts, he does utter something very important, something pregnant with crucial implications: affect "is not being [*l'être*] given in its immediacy, nor is it the subject in some brute, raw form." As ought to be crystal clear by now, I agree with Lacan on this key point. That is to say, there's agreement here that affects, at least those affecting the sort of subjectivity of concern in analysis (i.e., the human qua speaking being [*parlêtre*]), are anything but primitive phenomena of a self-evident nature calling for no further analysis or explanation. Affects are not ground-zero, rock-bottom experiences incapable of additional decomposition; they are not *Gestalt*-like, indissolubly unified mental states of an irreducible sort. As per the very etymology of the word, to "analyze" affects (as an analyst) is to dissolve them into their multiple constituents. Along these lines, Harari, in his commentary on Lacan's tenth seminar, helpfully highlights what's entailed by Lacan emphasizing, in fidelity to Freud, anxiety's position as a "signal":[70] "The mere fact of pointing this out implies considering it as *something referring to another order*. Thus, it is not a self- or auto-referential phenomenon but, on the contrary, has a condition of retransmission to another field. *Anxiety does not represent itself*."[71] However, on this reading, if anxiety is emblematic of affects in general, then the "other order" in relation to which this affect is a residual phenomenal manifestation (i.e., a signal) is none other than Lacan's "symbolic order." Affect is thereby once more reduced to the role of a secondary by-product of the intellectualizing machinations of "pure" signifiers. But, what if it's possible for certain affects to "represent" different affects? Or, what if the complex, nonatomic organizations of subjects' affects involve components that aren't strictly of either an affective or signifying status? These are hypotheses yet to be entertained whose consequences await being pursued.

In 1970, during the seventeenth seminar, Lacan refers back to the tenth seminar. Speaking of the latter, he observes: "Someone whose intentions I don't need to describe is doing an entire report, to be published in two days time, so as to denounce in a note the fact that I put affect in the background, that I ignore it. It's a mistake to think I neglect affects—as if everyone's behavior was not enough to affect me. My entire seminar that year was, on the contrary, structured around anxiety, insofar as it is the central affect, the one around which everything is organized. Since I was able to introduce anxiety as the fundamental affect, it was a good thing all the same that already, for a good length of time, I had not been neglecting affects."[72] Immediately after using the seminar on anxiety to exonerate himself, Lacan continues: "I have simply given its full importance, in the determinism of *die Verneinung* [negation], to what Freud has explicitly stated, that it's not affect that is repressed. Freud has recourse to this famous *Repräsentanz* which I translate as *représentant de la représentation*, and which others, and moreover not without some basis, persist in calling *représentant-représentatif*, which absolutely does not mean the same thing. In one case the representative is not a representation, in the other case the representative is just one representation among others. These translations are radically different from one another. My translation implies that affect, through the fact of displacement, is effectively displaced, unidentified, broken off from its roots—it eludes us."[73] Lacan's reference to "*die Verneinung*" sounds like an invocation of the concept of negation à la Freud, and not a citation of the paper of the same title from 1925. That is to say, he seems to be asserting that he indeed pays attention to affects, albeit in a negative mode emphasizing what affects are not: not repressed, not unconscious, not irreducible, not primitive, not self-explanatory, and so on. If he talks about them as a psychoanalyst, it tends to be under the sign of negation. Furthermore, Fink's previously noted reading of the Lacanian translation of Freud's *Vorstellungsrepräsentanz* appears to be supported here; in these particular remarks, Lacan too evidently reads backward the positioning of *Repräsentanzen* and *Vorstellungen* relative to each other in the core texts of Freudian metapsychology. Perhaps a contributing factor to the confusion evinced by Lacan and Fink with respect to Freud's original German writings is the distinction between "primal repression" (*Urverdrängung*) and "repression proper" (*eigentliche Verdrängung*) in the paper on "Repression." More precisely, in primal repression, a *Repräsentanz* qua *Triebrepräsentanz* is condemned to unconsciousness, thereafter to be represented in the psyche by other ideas qua *Vorstellungen*. Some of these *Vorstellungen* of the primally repressed *Triebrepräsentanz*, if the former become too closely associated with the latter, can succumb to (secondary) repression as repression proper.[74] But, once repression proper, as secondary in relation to primal repression, is up and running—by this point, a whole web-like network of ideational representations is established in the psychical apparatus—one could speak of certain representatives (signifiers as *Vorstellungen*) being represented by other representatives (signifiers as *Repräsentanzen*).

The alternative translation of the Freudian *Vorstellungsrepräsentanz* that Lacan mentions seems to be that of his two protégés Jean Laplanche and Serge Leclaire. In their famous paper "The Unconscious: A Psychoanalytic Study" (given in 1960 at the Bonneval colloquium, the same venue in which Lacan orally delivers his *écrit*, rewritten in 1964, "Position of the Unconscious"), Laplanche and Leclaire discuss this vexing compound German word. They indeed translate it as "*représentant représentatif*."[75] In the third chapter of this text, Leclaire explains: "It is emphasized that the drive, properly speaking, has no place in mental life. Repression does not bear on it, it is neither conscious nor unconscious and it enters into the circuit of mental life only through the mediation of the '*(Vorstellungs-)Repräsentanz*.' This is a rather unusual term of which it must be immediately said that in Freud's usage, it is often found in divided form as one of its two components. We will translate this composite expression by 'ideational representative' and we shall inquire into the nature of this mediation, through which the drive enters into (one could even say 'is captured by') mental life."[76] Laplanche and Pontalis, in their psychoanalytic dictionary, echo this interpretive translation and definition proffered by Leclaire.[77] Therein, Laplanche and Pontalis explain: "'Representative' renders '*Repräsentanz*,' . . . a German term of Latin origin which

should be understood as implying *delegation*. . . . '*Vorstellung*' is a philosophical term whose traditional English equivalent is 'idea.' '*Vorstellungsrepräsentanz*' means a delegate (in this instance, a delegate of the instinct) in the
sphere of ideas; it should be stressed that according to Freud's conception it
is the idea that represents the instinct, not the idea itself that is represented
by something else—Freud is quite explicit about this."[78] In the passages from
his seventeenth seminar quoted in the preceding paragraph, what appears
to concern Lacan about the way his students Laplanche, Leclaire, and Pontalis translate and define Freud's *Vorstellungsrepräsentanz* is that their rendition of this compound German word implies that the affective forces of
libidinal life are adequately represented by the ideational inscriptions (as
Lacan's signifiers) forming the signifying networks of the structured psychical apparatus. Although he grants that his students' perspective on this
issue of interpreting Freud's texts is hardly unjustified ("not without some
basis"), Lacan feels that, when it comes to the (non)relation between affects
and signifiers in the speaking subjectivity of interest to psychoanalysis, it's
inappropriate to imply that affects are accurately represented (i.e., depicted,
mirrored, reflected, transferred, translated, and so on) by signifiers as ideational representations—hence, Lacan's emphasis that, in his own translation
and definition of this Freudian term, "the representative is not a representation" (and, as he proceeds to clarify apropos this point, "My translation
implies that affect, through the fact of displacement, is effectively displaced,
unidentified, broken off from its roots—it eludes us"). As Lacan presents this
disagreement in which he's embroiled, Laplanche et al. hint at the hypothesis that fundamental affective phenomena connected with the driven psyche
can be and are distilled into more or less faithful representational delegates,
whereas he insists upon the disjunctive break creating a discrepancy or gap
between affects and their nonrepresentative "representations" (maybe akin
to renegade diplomats). According to this presentation, Laplanche and
company posit a synthesizing rapport that is harmonious enough between
affects and their signifier-like delegates; Lacan, by contrast, maintains that
(to paraphrase one of his most [in]famous one-liners) *il n'y a pas de rapport
représentatif entre l'affect et le signifiant*. The Lacanian metapsychology of
affect stresses, among other things, the estrangement of the *parlêtre* from its
affects. Rather than remaining self-evident, self-transparent experiences, the
affective waters are, at certain levels, hopelessly muddied from the viewpoint
of the speaking subject struggling to relate to them. For signifier-mediated
subjectivity, the feel of its feelings ceases to be something immediately clear

and unambiguous. Or, as Green, even in his post-Lacanianism, expresses this, "The human condition is affective alienation."[79]

In the seventeenth seminar where the last passage quoted from this text leaves off, Lacan remarks, "This is what is essential in repression. It's not that the affect is suppressed, it's that it is displaced and unrecognizable."[80] To be more precise, there arguably are two senses of displacement operative here (parallel to the two types of repression, primal and secondary or proper): first, the shuttling of an affect from one signifier-like ideational representation to another (a displacement of affect corresponding to secondary or proper repression); and second, the split between an affect and its nonrepresentative "representations" introduced with the originary advent of the mediation of signifiers (this mediation amounts to a primal repression of affects through irreversibly displacing them into the foreign territories of symbolic orders). Consequently, not only can affects become "unrecognizable" (*méconnaissable*) through being transferred from one ideational-representational constellation onto another (à la such common analytic examples as the displacement of emotional responses linked to one significant other onto a different person who is somehow brought into associational connection with the significant other); the foundational gap between affects and signifiers means that, to greater or lesser extents, the subject's knowledge (*connaissance* as much as *savoir*) of its affective life in general is problematized through the unavoidable distorting intervention of the signifying systems shaping speaking subjectivity. These statements are made by Lacan during a question-and-answer session entitled "Interview on the Steps of the Pantheon" (May 13, 1970). Right after this discussion of the representation (or lack thereof) of affect, Lacan is asked an unrecorded question about "the relations between existentialism and structuralism." All he says in response is this: "Yes, it's as if existential thought was the only guarantee of a recourse to affects."[81] This one-sentence reply is worth highlighting if only because it serves as yet another indication that Lacan doesn't conceive of himself as seeking to eliminate any and every reference to the affective in psychoanalysis (as he is sometimes accused of doing). He doesn't perceive his Saussure-inspired rereading of Freud as entailing the reductive elimination of everything other than the signifier systems of Symbolic big Others.

At the start of the immediately following session of the seventeenth seminar (May 20, 1970), the topic of affect resurfaces. Lacan's succinct statements here with respect to this topic are rather inscrutable, at least at first glance. To begin with, he comments that "thought is not a category. I would almost say it is an affect. Although, this is not to say that it is at its most fundamental under the aspect of affect."[82] This easily could be read in several fashions. However, Lacan undoubtedly intends in this context to call into question what is often assumed to be a firm, sharp distinction between the cognitive-structural and the emotional-energetic (but, as the last sentence of this quotation indicates, he nonetheless doesn't deny some sort of distinction between the intellectual and the affective). He then proceeds to declare: "There is only one affect—this constitutes a certain position, a new one to be introduced into the world, which, I am saying, is to be referred to what I am giving you a schema of, transcribed onto the blackboard, when I speak of the psychoanalytic discourse."[83] Lacan goes on to note that there are those, such as some student radicals who reproached him when he appeared at Vincennes in 1969, who would protest that Lacan's mathemes in dry white chalk against a black background (such as his formulas for the four discourses forming the focus of his annual seminar in 1969–1970) are bloodless, sterile academic constructs with no bearing whatsoever on anything truly "real" (qua concrete, palpable, tangible, and so on).[84] Lacan retorts, "That's where the error is."[85] On the contrary, "if there is any chance of grasping something called the real, it is nowhere other than on the blackboard."[86] Resonating with prior reflections on the dialectical entanglement of the concrete and the abstract in both Hegelian and Marxist reflections on the nature of reality (not to mention with the history of mathematical models in the modern natural sciences from the seventeenth century through the present), Lacan denounces the naïve appeal to any concreteness unmediated by abstractions. Human social and subjective reality is permeated and saturated by formal structures and dynamics irreducible to what is simplistically imagined to be raw, positive facts on the ground. Hence, only a theoretical grasp of these abstractions, abstractions that do indeed "march in the streets" in the guise of socialized subjects, has a chance of getting a handle on a real(ity) that is so much more than a mere aggregate of dumb, idiotic, concrete givens.[87] It ought to be observed that Lacan makes this point on the heels of talking about affect, thus insinuating that affects are not to be thought of (as some in psychoanalysis do) as elements of a brute, preexistent psychical concreteness already there before either the analysand on the couch speaks (or even becomes a speaking subject in the first place) or the analyst clinically interprets or metapsychologically theorizes.

Lacan quickly returns to his assertion of there being solely a single affect. Again invoking the "psychoanalytic discourse" (i.e., the discourse of the analyst, as distinct from the other three discourses delineated in the seventeenth seminar, those of the master, university, and hysteric), he maintains that "in effect, from the perspective of this discourse, there is only one affect, which is, namely, the product of the speaking being's capture in a discourse, where this discourse determines its status as object."[88] A series of steps are necessary to spell out the reasoning behind Lacan's assertion. First of all, one must remember that, according to the Lacanian theory of the four discourses, the analyst's discourse has the effect of "hystericizing" the analysand.[89] In other words, through the peculiar social bond that is an analysis, a language-organized situation in which someone occupies the position of an analyst in relation to another speaking being, he/she who speaks under the imperative to associate freely (i.e., the analysand) is led to lose the certainty of being equal to his/her discourse, of meaning what he/she says and saying what he/she means. Such a loss of self-assured certainty is inseparable from what is involved in any genuine confrontation with the unconscious. Along with this, the analysand comes to wonder whether he/she is equivalent to his/her previously established coordinates of identification, coordinates embedded in sociosymbolic milieus (i.e., avatars and emblems of identity embraced by the analysand as constitutive of his/her ego-level "self"). Hystericization occurs when the *parlêtre* on the couch is hurled into a vortex of doubts through coming to be uncertain about being comfortably and consciously in charge of his/her discourse and everything discourse entails for an entity whose very identity depends on it. From a Lacanian perspective, one of the analyst's primary aims in an analysis, to be achieved through various means, is to derail the analysand's supposed mastery of speech and meaning, to disrupt the discourse of the master as the (illusory) mastery of discourse.[90] In reference to the brief quotation at the start of this paragraph, the thus-hystericized subject becomes riveted to questions about what sort of "object" he/she is, first and foremost, for both intersubjective others (i.e., incarnate alter egos, embodied partners actual and imagined, and so on) and transsubjective Others (i.e., the symbolic order, the anonymous "They," institutions and societies, and so on), as well as for him-/herself in terms of self-objectifications: "Who or what am I for you and others?"; "Am I really the 'x' (man, woman, husband, wife, son, daughter, authority, professional) I have taken myself to be?"

In short, the position Lacan labels the discourse of the hysteric, unlike that of the master, is essentially characterized by uncertainty. However, what, if anything, does all of this have to do with the topic of affect? There are several connections. To begin with, another possible line of questioning speaking subjects hystericized through analyses inevitably will be prompted to pursue on a number of occasions is: "How do I truly feel?" "Do I honestly feel the way that I feel that I feel?" Not only is the figure of the master certain of being equivalent to what he/she says and how he/she identifies and is identified sociosymbolically; the *parlêtre* pretending to occupy a position of masterful agency (in Lacan's discourse theory, agency itself, in any of the four discourses, is invariably a "semblance" [*semblant*] beneath which lies the obfuscated "truth" [*vérité*] of this agent-position)[91] is also certain of how he/she feels: "I know exactly how I feel"; "When I feel 'x,' that's how I really feel." Hystericization undermines confident sureness as regards affects just as much as regards anything else— and this insofar as, within the subjective structures of speaking beings, affective phenomena, like everything else, are inextricably intertwined with socio-symbolic mediators.[92] Moreover, in an effective analysis worthy of the name, doubts arise about the seeming obviousness and trustworthiness of feelings.[93] The analyst can and should guide the analysand to realizations that affects aren't always directly related to what they appear to be related to in conscious experience (thanks to displacement, transference, and so on) and that given feelings can work to conceal other emotions and their associated thoughts (such as, to take one common example, affection or love masking aggression or hate and vice versa). Soler claims that "affects have for the affected the force of immediate evidence, of a pseudo-evidence."[94] Although this is generally true for nearly everybody, including analysands in earlier stages of their analyses, a good analysis dispels this illusory immediacy qua self-evidence, bringing to light its "pseudo" status.

Lacan's neologisms *senti-ment* (a neologism linking sentiments to lying)[95] and *affectuation* (a neologism linking affects to affecting qua putting on a false display)[96] both point to the analytic thesis that, as Žižek bluntly and straight-forwardly puts it, "emotions lie."[97] But, whereas Lacanians often explicitly assert or implicitly assume that the unconscious "truths" masked by the "lies" of conscious emotions (as felt feelings [*Empfindungen*]) are nonaffective entities (i.e., signifiers, structures, and so on), the preceding parsings of Lacan's inade-quately elaborated metapsychology of affect indicate that behind the façade of misleading felt feelings might be other, misfelt feelings (rather than phenom-ena of a fundamentally nonaffective nature). As will be seen later (chapters 12 and 13), the breakthroughs of contemporary research in affective neuroscience are indispensable for any effort to clarify and develop further what is suggested in this context with regard to human emotional life.

In his seminar in 1971–1972 on *Le savoir du psychanalyste*, Lacan intro-duces the neologism *lalangue*.[98] This neologism is formed through collapsing the space between the definite article and the noun in the French *la langue* (which could be translated as "the tongue" or "the natural language"). One could say that a nonsense word is created through skipping over the spacing so crucial to the syntactical and grammatical structures of recognizably meaningful (uses of) natural languages. Moreover, the sound of the word *lalangue* recalls, through its first two repeating sounds (*lala*), the murmurings of infants before mastering their "mother tongue" (*la langue maternelle*) as a transparent medium of socially comprehensible communication. An infant's babbling, prior to his/her acquisition of and accession to *la langue* as a system of signifying signs employed in exchanges of ideas, frequently involves playing with phonemic elements of his/her auditory milieu as meaningless materials to be enjoyed for the sensations they produce in the libidinally charged orifices of the mouth (when vocalized) or the ears (when heard). The nonsense neologism *lalangue* is coined by Lacan to designate, among other things, the nonsense uttered by babbling infants joyfully and idiotically reveling in the bodily pleasures of pure, senseless sounds.[99]

But, in line with Freud's crucial psychoanalytic thesis according to which ontogenetic development doesn't entail the effacing, superseding replacement of previous "stages" by subsequent ones—the earlier subsists side by side with the later in the temporally emergent organizations of the psychical apparatus—Lacan's *lalangue* lingers on in the linguistic productions of more mature speaking subjects[100] (albeit in forms pruned and modified by being folded into successive sheaths of *la langue*). In his final seminars of the mid-to-late 1970s, it becomes apparent that Lacan accords *lalangue* an absolutely central place in clinical analysis. From Freud to the present, one of the few statements able to elicit near-universal assent from among the diverse array of psychoanalytic traditions and orientations—the psychoanalytic field as a (non) whole is marked by disagreement and bickering among its various constituents and parties—is the claim that the practice of analysis ultimately is based on the "fundamental rule" requiring of analysands that they freely associate. The very acoustic or graphic materiality of the language with(in) which patients on the couch freely associate inevitably results in the derailment of consciously intended meanings through the sounds and images of asignificant language matter generating consciously unintended slips, homophonies, equivocations, and so on. When language, as *la langue*, does this, it momentarily operates as *lalangue*.[101] These unintended productions of the analysand reveal the, so to speak, private language of his/her unconscious. Like the nonsense-murmuring infant, the unconscious plays with the mother tongue heedless of whether or not the products of this playful process "make sense." The opening session of

Lacan's twenty-fifth seminar (*Le moment de conclure* [1977–1978]) is entitled *Une practique de bavardage*; analysis, based as it is on free association, is "a babbling practice."[102] The analysand is asked to "babble," to lie there in the consulting room and mutter on for a time, vocalizing whatever happens to cross his/her mind with as little concern as possible for whether what comes out of his/her mouth is meaningful, significant, or even readily comprehensible to him-/herself or the listening analyst. One of the results of this activity is the surfacing of residual elements of the idiosyncratic-yet-interpretable *lalangue* spoken by the speaking subject's unconscious.[103] These elements are keys to unlocking and decoding the unconscious.[104]

On a more general metapsychological plane, Lacan's contrast between *lalangue* and *la langue* can be aligned precisely with Freud's distinction between primary and secondary processes, respectively.[105] Freud depicts secondary process conscious cognition as a specific style of chaining together interlinked ideational contents. Whereas this style of cognition is unfree insofar as it is restricted by concerns about whether the connections it makes between ideational contents are logical or meaningful according to shared conventions, primary process mentation disregards such concerns and the accompanying restrictions they dictate. This other style of thinking, a comparatively less restricted style characteristic of the unconscious as revealed by dreams, jokes, slips of the tongue, literary and musical engagements with language, and free associations, forges links between *Vorstellungen* in unconventional fashions, sometimes exhibiting a surprising degree of creativity and inventiveness. Likewise, for Lacan, *la langue* (as akin to Freudian secondary processes) establishes rules and boundaries fixing the slippery, runny overflowing of surplus meanings and nonsense supported by the materiality of *lalangue* (as akin to Freudian primary processes), a materiality underpinning and mixed in with any and every instance of language qua *la langue*.[106]

To take an additional Lacanian step, one could argue that *lalangue* lingers on in *la langue* as *jouis-sens* (another, related neologism introduced in the seminar running parallel to *Le savoir du psychanalyste* [in which the neologism *lalangue* is coined], the nineteenth seminar entitled " . . . *ou pire*" [1971–1972]).[107] The best possible translation into English of this French neologism, which is homophonous with *jouissance* (enjoyment), is "enjoy-meant."[108] The link between the two neologisms *lalangue* and *jouis-sens* is evident in Lacan's televised interview of 1973. Therein, soon after discussing *lalangue* as closely related to what Freud designates when referring to primary process unconscious thinking, Lacan observes: "What Freud discovers in the unconscious—here

I've only been able to invite you to take a look at his writings to see if I speak truly—is something utterly different from realizing that broadly speaking one can give a sexual meaning to everything one knows, for the reason that knowing has always been open to the famous metaphor (the side of meaning Jung exploited). It is the real that permits the effective unknotting of what makes the symptom hold together, namely a knot of signifiers. Where here knotting and unknotting are not metaphors, but are really to be taken as those knots that in fact are built up through developing chains of the signifying material."[109] He immediately adds: "For these chains are not of meaning but of enjoy-meant [*jouis-sens*] which you can write as you wish, as is implied by the punning that constitutes the law of the signifier."[110]

Jouis-sens is *jouissance* entwined with and mediated by language not as *la langue* (i.e., an intersubjective and transsubjective system of meaningful signs, as signifiers stitched to signifieds, employed in exchanges between conscious communicators), but as *lalangue* (i.e., the not-yet-meaningful or meaningless signifiers-apart-from-signifieds whose acoustic and graphic materialities facilitate associative enchainings of psychical contents in excess of the circumscribed sphere of shared, consensus-reality "sense"). Echoing his recurrent insistence that he doesn't employ the word *material* metaphorically when referring to the acoustic and graphic elements of symbolic orders,[111] Lacan here indicates that the symptomatic formations of concern to analysis consist of literal "knots of signifiers," namely, bundles of auditory and visual traces inscribed in the psychical apparatus and associatively woven together, via primary process patterns (as "the law of the signifier" insofar as the pure signifier is substantial rather than significant), into tangles of interconnected relations producing certain effects in the speaking being. Moreover, as will be explored further subsequently, the concept-term *jouis-sens* suggests an interest on Lacan's part in problematizing and complicating the crude, simplistic, black-and-white distinction between, as it were, energy (as libidinal or affective forces related to the body [*jouis*]), on the one hand, and structure (as representational or ideational factors related to the subject [*sens*]), on the other hand. Following this suggestion alluded to by Lacan's neologism, it might be feasible to outline a neuro-psychoanalytic account of affective life, bringing together the odd couple of empirical studies of the emotional brain and Lacanian metapsychological theory, a coupling from which both partners, it is hoped, will benefit in terms of increased accuracy and sophistication.

The preceding discussion of *lalangue* à la Lacan sets the stage for productively examining a moment in the famous twentieth seminar where *lalangue* is said to generate affective repercussions. At the (self-)conscious level of language use, a level neglecting the material signifier in its focus on the meaningful sign (with the former treated as nothing more than a transparent medium for intended significations), the *parlêtre* remains largely oblivious to its own unknown knowledge in the form of a speaking unconscious entangled with the *jouissance*-saturated meanderings of *lalangue* as something "in *la langue* more than *la langue* itself." Lacan explains: "The unconscious evinces knowledge that, for the most part, escapes the speaking being. That being provides the occasion to realize just how far the effects of llanguage go, in that it presents all sorts of affects that remain enigmatic. Those affects are what result from the presence of llanguage insofar as it articulates things by way of knowledge (*de savoir*) that go much further than what the speaking being sustains (*supporte*) by way of enunciated knowledge."[112] Fink translates *lalangue* as "llanguage." Lacan continues: "Language is, no doubt, made up of llanguage. It is knowledge's hare-brained lucubration (*élucubration*) about llanguage. But the unconscious is knowledge, a knowing how to do things (*savoir-faire*) with llanguage. And what we know how to do with llanguage goes well beyond what we can account for under the heading of language."[113] This is promptly brought back to bear on the topic of affect: "Llanguage affects us first of all by everything it brings with it by way of effects that are affects. If we can say that the unconscious is structured like a language, it is in the sense that the effects of llanguage, already there qua knowledge, go well beyond anything the being who speaks is capable of enunciating."[114]

From the perspective of secondary process conscious cognition, fixated as it is on the recognizably logical and meaningful dimensions of *la langue*, the (apparently) illogical and meaningless "false connections" between multiple pieces of psychical content made by the primary process styles of thinking, styles of thinking characteristic of an unconscious that thinks in and through *lalangue*, usually go unnoticed. But, these consciously unnoticed associative cross resonances of a *lalangue* mixed in with *la langue* spoken by the *parlêtre* are not without their effects for all that. Among other consequences, these chains and knots of sounds and images generate affective reverberations.[115] When someone experiences his/her affects as mysterious or puzzling (i.e., "enigmatic"), as apparently without rhyme or reason, Freudian-Lacanian psychoanalysis hypothesizes that there is indeed, nonetheless, a rhyme or reason at play (sometimes even a literal rhyme). However, standard (nonanalytic) protocols of narration and explanation, governed by the semantic and syntactic restrictions imposed by normal, ordinary uses of natural language as a communicative conveyor of sensible significations, are unable to discern and comprehend the seemingly irrational and nonsensical free associations between *Vorstellungen* responsible for catalyzing certain emotions and feelings. As a result, such emotions and feelings thus catalyzed cannot but manifest themselves as strange and inexplicable to "rational" conscious cognition.

For Lacan, enigmatic affects aren't the exception—they're the rule. That is to say, instead of treating emotions and feelings as typically transparent and self-evident phenomena, with perplexing affective experiences being relatively infrequent anomalies or pathological aberrations, Lacan considers most consciously felt affects to be unreliable, dissembling indicators of things other than themselves—and this even when the awareness registering these experiences doesn't experience them as such (many emotions and feelings regarded as straightforwardly unenigmatic by self-consciousness might not be what it takes them to be). As noted earlier, he neologistically designates affective phenomena as a matter of *senti-ment* and *affectuation*. Additionally, his well-known characterization of anxiety as the one affect that doesn't deceive obviously indicates that all other affects are, at least potentially if not actually, deceptive.[116] Similarly, a less well-known aside by Lacan, in the eighteenth seminar (*D'un discours qui ne serait pas du semblant* [1971]), mentions hate as "the only lucid sentiment" (*le seul sentiment lucide*).[117] Hence, by implication, all other sentiments are *senti-ments*, namely, dark and cloudy sensations that always can be doubted as to whether they mean what they seem to mean, whether they, so to speak, tell the truth about themselves. Apart from anxiety and hate, affects, in the Lacanian view, are generally misleading and opaque. And, the preceding also implies that anxiety can be nondeceptive yet nonlucid (as in superficially mysterious anxiety of the free-floating or phobic types, which, in either case, reliably signals the presence or proximity of elements and entities central to the desiring unconscious) and that hate can be lucid yet deceptive (when one vividly feels intense hatred, one undoubtedly really feels hatred as such, although this might be transferentially displaced from one object onto another or be the flip side of passionate love). Anyhow, if, as Lacan tacitly alleges, all other affects are both deceptive and nonlucid, this entails that they can and should be placed under a cloud of suspicions: "Do I truly feel 'x?'"; "Do I truly feel 'x' in relation to 'y?'"; "Is feeling 'x' related to 'z' rather than 'y?'"; "Does feeling 'x' hide or code for different feelings?" and so on. Furthermore, if, according to Lacan, the *jouis-sens* of *lalangue* is responsible for enigmatic affects, then, despite Lacan's prevailing tendency to posit nonaffective signifier-structures as the unconscious truths distorted by the phenomenal lies of conscious emotions, behind the façades of feelings might be defensively occluded psychical factors having as much to do with the passions of the enjoying body (*jouis*) as with the calculations of symbolic constellations (*sens*).

It is time to return to a sentence from the seventeenth seminar quoted quite a while ago: "In effect, from the perspective of this discourse, there is only one affect, which is, namely, the product of the speaking being's capture in a discourse, where this discourse determines its status as object."[118] Again, "this discourse" refers to the discourse of the analyst depicted during this particular period of Lacan's teachings. Additionally, it must be recalled that the analyst's discourse strives to interrupt the discourse of the master (as the mastery of discourse, namely, the semblance of intentional conscious control over speech, meaning, and so on) and, in so doing, to hystericize he/she who formerly spoke from a posturing position of masterful agency. As I've argued here, such hystericization amounts not only to someone becoming uncomfortably skeptical about whether he/she is what he/she took him-/herself to be at the level of sociosymbolic identities (i.e., egos and selves mediated by the images and words of surrounding intersubjective and transsubjective environments), but also to losing any firm, stable certainties at the level of his/her affective life. Through this loss, feelings are deprived of a previously taken-for-granted reflexive self-identity in which one can be sure that one's feelings really feel the way that they apparently feel (i.e., in which there are no non-self-identical affective phenomena in the form of unfelt or misfelt feelings). However, two features of this quotation from 1970, features related to each other, have yet to be adequately explicated: first, the issue of there being "only one affect" for Lacanian psychoanalysis and, second, exactly what is involved with the *parlêtre*'s "status as object" in this context.

For anyone familiar with Lacan's discussions of affects, the assertion of there being solely a single affect is a familiar one: Based, in part, on specific observations made by Freud, he maintains that anxiety alone is the key affective phenomenon of concern for psychoanalysis.[119] Elsewhere in the seventeenth seminar, Lacan describes anxiety as "the central affect, the one around which everything is organized," as "the fundamental affect."[120] The Freudian-Lacanian justifications for this thesis are too numerous and complex to go into at present. What's more, it will be necessary in what follows eventually to turn to the task of articulating conceptual definitions of affects, emotions, and feelings as related-but-distinct metapsychological categories. For now, suffice it to say that, as Lacan sees it, anxiety (the "one affect") is intimately linked to "the speaking being's capture in a discourse, where this discourse determines its status as object." To cut a long story short, the objectification of the *parlêtre* mentioned on this occasion is tantamount to the hystericization described earlier. Anxiety arises from various uncertainties that themselves can become sources of tangible disturbances exclusively for a being whose relations with itself (via intrasubjective self-objectification) and others (via inter- or trans-subjective objectification) are routed through and modulated by ensembles of sociosymbolic configurations (i.e., "discourses"). Thanks to discourses and everything they bring with them, the subject "captured" by the signifier can come anxiously to ask what it is, as an object (especially an object of desire), for both others and itself; and, also thanks to immersion in the worlds of signifiers, such inquiring subjectivity never will alight upon definitive, final answers to its questions granting unshakeable certainty.[121] If anxiety is not only the one-and-only affect for psychoanalysis but also the sole affect that doesn't deceive, then all other affects (as emotions and feelings) can become causes for anxiety (as an affect proper) insofar as their deceptiveness, a deceptiveness engendered by their sociosymbolic mediation, invariably allows for casting them into doubt. As a sociosymbolic being (i.e., a *parlêtre*), one always can wonder warily, in a gesture of self-objectification, whether one honestly feels what one seemingly feels (in addition to whether others honestly feel what they indicate they feel). What could be more anxiety-inducing than feeling that one cannot trust one's feelings, that one's heart and soul might tell half-truths or utter falsehoods?

To borrow the title of one of Laplanche's books (*La révolution copernici-enne inachevée*), there is another "unfinished" aspect to the Copernican revolution of psychoanalysis. As I've observed already (in chapter 8), Lacan, apropos Freud's references to Copernicus, emphasizes the analytic dissolution of the illusion of knowledge's inherent reflexivity that is transparent to itself; the (subject of the) unconscious subverts the notion of the self-conscious subject that supposedly, when it knows, necessarily knows that it knows. In the Lacanian account, what remains unfinished in the Freudian Copernican revolution is the thinking-through of the full extent of the subversion of knowing subjectivity brought about by the psychoanalytic discovery of the unconscious as a knowledge that doesn't know itself, a subversion partially obfuscated by Freud's manner of interpreting his own invocation of Copernicus. (As explained previously, the pain of the blow to humanity's self-image by the earth's celestial decentering is mitigated and compensated for by narcissistic pride at having achieved knowledge of this decentering.) Along these lines, Lacan positions himself with respect to Freud as extending to their consequent logical ends certain crucial revolutionary trajectories that, although not followed through to their ultimate conclusions by his predecessor, manifestly originate in the foundations provided by this predecessor's work. Lacan's "return to Freud" could be depicted as an analytic-dialectical retrieval and deployment of the "unknown knowns" of the Freudian oeuvre (as Heidegger would phrase it, Lacan "thinks the unthought" of Freud). Whereas Lacan's finishing of unfinished Freudian business generally focuses on thinking and knowing, with the thinking that doesn't think that it thinks and the knowing that doesn't know that it knows both being dynamics and structures of a fundamentally conceptual-intellectual-linguistic-representational nature, my finishing of unfinished Lacanian business focuses on feeling as being not transparent to itself. Additionally, unlike the many critical readings of Lacan that see nothing in his teachings doing real justice to things not of a conceptual-intellectual-linguistic-representational nature, I acknowledge that, although underemphasized and in need of further elaboration, a number of resources indeed are to be found in the Lacanian corpus for the development of a richer, more subtle metapsychology of affective life that is able to be interfaced productively with the findings of the contemporary neuroscience of the emotional brain. Even though Lacan repeatedly denies the existence of unconscious affects, considering the very phrase "unconscious affects" to be self-contradictory (as Freud too sometimes does), his scattered reflections on affects nonetheless hint that subjects can be "strangers to themselves" at the level of feeling as well as at the levels (not unrelated to feeling) of thinking and knowing. But, a "return to Lacan" modeled on Lacan's return to Freud is required if these resources and hints are to be extracted and extrapolated in new directions that are neither simply Lacanian nor non-Lacanian.

12.

EMOTIONAL LIFE AFTER LACAN

FROM PSYCHOANALYSIS
TO THE NEUROSCIENCES

Among those readers of Lacan not inclined immediately to denounce his version of psychoanalysis as entirely devoid of any serious and sustained treatment of affective life—Lacanian psychoanalysis is all too frequently caricatured as a disembodied, formalist structuralism neglecting everything apart from static symbolic-linguistic systems—much attention has been paid to his tenth seminar. As noted, Lacan himself appeals to this particular seminar, with its focus on anxiety, as exculpatory evidence against accusations that he mishandles or ignores affects (accusations coming from a number of quarters: phenomenologies, poststructuralisms, deconstructionisms, feminisms, non-Lacanian psychoanalytic orientations, and so on). Various exegetes sympathetic to Lacan, taking their lead from this appeal, attempt to derive a broader Lacanian metapsychology of affect from his discussions of anxiety in 1962–1963.

But, one already might ask at this point: given the undeniable existence of numerous phenomena that are identifiable as "affective," how can a mere one-academic-year-out-of-twenty-seven examination of anxiety alone be presented as an adequately thorough psychoanalytic theorization of affects? Preemptively anticipating one likely Lacanian response among others to this question, one might pose another query that seems appropriate: what justifies asserting that anxiety is the single, sole affect recognized as such by psychoanalysis, when so many other affects appear to be important and relevant in both clinical and theoretical psychoanalysis? For Lacan, if becoming a speaking being (the precise sort of being who ends up babbling on analysts' couches) entails, as one of many consequences, estrangement from one's emotions and feelings as self-evident, self-transparent conscious experiences—in other words, as a *parlêtre*, one is deprived of the guarantee of certainty that, when one feels a feeling, one feels that one feels this feeling as such—then anxiety is the uniquely human affect. Why? Only human beings become subjects qua speaking beings ($); and, one of the results of such subjectification is, by virtue of the mediation of signifiers, a loss of any (pre)supposed immediacy at the level of affective experience. The subject's ensuing uncertainties about its emotions and feelings, uncertainties deliberately aggravated and intensified in analysands by the analytic process, generate any number of sensations that can span the negative emotional-sensational spectrum, ranging from subtle, low-burn discomfort to acute, all-consuming angst, from being vaguely ill at ease to being frantic with panic (the latter state sometimes precipitating rash behaviors of the sort referred to by all analytic orientations as instances of "acting-out").[1] Every point along this range arguably involves anxiety, itself arguably distinct from any similar states of sensation (such as fear) apparently common to both humans and animals.

Thus, on this interpretation, Lacan isn't saying that anxiety is the one-and-only emotion or feeling of interest and pertinence to psychoanalysis. Rather, his partially outlined metapsychology of affective life proposes a tacit distinction between, on the one hand, affect and, on the other hand, emotion and feeling (one ought to recall the earlier unearthing and extensions of the *Affekt-Gefühl-Empfindung* triad buried in Freud's original German texts and, somewhat surprisingly, passed over without remark by Lacan). Hence, countless emotions and feelings could be taken into account by a Lacanian analysis. But, with respect to these passions and sentiments, if analytic attention should be paid principally to those moments when doubts of various sorts can and do arise regarding conscious emotions and feelings, then anxiety, as the affective accompaniment of such doubts, is indeed, as Lacan contends, the "central" and "fundamental" affect, at least as far as analyses of the unconscious dimensions of speaking beings qua split subjects of signifiers are concerned.

However, to be perfectly exact before proceeding further, the Lacan of the tenth seminar doesn't claim, as these previous articulations are at risk of suggesting, that doubts (as intellectual causes) give rise to anxiety (as an affective effect). Quite the contrary: one of Lacan's theses on anxiety, stated during the year of *le Séminaire* devoted to it, is that "anxiety is the cause of doubt."[2] Anxiety is a "pre-sentiment," "that which is before the birth of a sentiment,"[3] namely, a vague premonition of the bursting-forth of new, unexpected affective or libidinal intensities indicative of that which has been unconscious. These statements are made with reference to phenomena familiar in the clinical treatment of obsessional neurosis: When anxiety arises in obsessionals—and, for Lacan, this agitating presentiment doesn't deceive insofar as it can be trusted as a signal that objects closely associated with unconscious desires are lurking somewhere in the contextual vicinity—they try to fend it off, tamp it down, and fool themselves about it. Obsessional neurotics attempt this mainly through intellectualizations and rationalizations taking the form of a proliferation of hesitant, tentative self-interpretations creating feelings of uncertainty (i.e., doubt) about feelings. How they feel is thereby buried in a hodgepodge haystack of conflicting, incompatible speculations. As Lacan puts it, "Doubt . . . is made for nothing else but combating anxiety, and this precisely by its lures."[4] When this type of neurotic anxiety surfaces as an advance indication that defended-against emotions and desires are threatening to irrupt into the scene of consciousness, a verbal swarm of confusing pseudoexplanations is conjured up to create deceptions allowing for skepticism as to whether any affective disturbance really is occurring. This skepticism struggles to sustain the illusion that nothing deviating from the narrow parameters of what the obsessional deems normal and manageable actually is in danger of transpiring.

So, do Lacan's stipulations in 1962 to the effect that affective anxiety is the cause of intellectual doubt, as glossed in the previous paragraph, invalidate preceding discussions here in which it's hypothesized that the doubt-anxiety relation can operate in the opposite causal direction too? The answer is a definite "No!" for several reasons. First of all, at a very basic and broad level, one might simply (and not without justification) disagree with Lacan about the dynamics of interaction between the affective and the intellectual, dynamics he tends not to delineate in a sufficiently dialectical fashion. The approach adopted by me in this project is most certainly not one governed by a mindless, rigid presumption that Lacan is infallible. Second, whether Lacan's indications regarding the role of doubt specifically in obsessional neurotic defenses against anxiety generally apply across the board to any and every psychical subject in an overarching metapsychological model is quite questionable. As should be apparent from my prior citations of other assertions made by Lacan in the course of my arguing for the view that anxiety is related to a hystericization particularly vis-à-vis emotions, passions, sentiments, and the like, there is plenty of evidence to suggest that Lacan elsewhere admits the existence of an anxiety generated by doubts about the feel of feelings, worries about the specters of misfelt feelings (if not unfelt feelings). Third, the preceding analysis of affective hystericization relies primarily on seminars given by Lacan beginning at the end of the 1960s, several years after the seminar on *l'angoisse* in which obsessional doubt is said to be triggered by anxiety (instead of vice versa). Debates undoubtedly could be had about whether and to what extent Lacan's comments on affects starting in the seventeenth seminar are consistent with those situated in earlier contexts (such as the tenth seminar). Fourth and finally, as regards doubt, Lacan talks about it along different lines the following year, in his famous eleventh seminar on *The Four Fundamental Concepts of Psycho-Analysis* (as well as on a number of other occasions too). In addition to the doubts of obsessional neurotics, one might wonder about the functions and significance of doubt in nonobsessional analysand-subjects; one also might wonder about doubts on the side of the listening analyst apart from those on the side of the speaking analysand. All I need to point out in the current setting is that Lacan's multifaceted character-izations of doubt subsequent to the tenth seminar are far from pigeonholing it as nothing more than a defense against anxiety mounted exclusively by obses-sional neurotics in analysis.[5]

As seen, my excavation of the rudiments of a Lacan-inspired metapsychol-ogy of affects—this metapsychology of affects is both centered on the thesis that, like knowing and thinking according to psychoanalysis, feeling also is non-self-reflexive and a theoretical framework potentially compatible with the neurosciences—derives many of its findings from the seventeenth semi-nar. And, as I mentioned a while ago (in chapter 8), this seminar recently has attracted a lot of attention from Lacanians interested in exploring Lacan's dis-course on affect and, in so doing, providing additional testimony to the effect that Lacan isn't guilty, as regularly and recurrently charged by a chorus of crit-ics, of an unpardonable silence on this psychoanalytically unavoidable subject matter. However, these contemporary Lacanian scholars don't address those parts of the seventeenth seminar scrutinized earlier here; instead, they share an exclusive preoccupation with a few passing observations Lacan utters about shame at the opening and closing moments of the final seminar session (June 17, 1970) of this academic year.[6] Jacques-Alain Miller and others argue that, in surrounding collective atmospheres infused with the lingering scents of Paris's May '68 and everything of which this convulsive outburst was a symptom, Lacan sees fit to make his audience aware of the historically unprecedented shamelessness so widespread in the crass, materialistic world of consumerist mass-media late capitalism[7] (a vulgar, exhibitionistic shamelessness on display among some of the provocative agitators in the audience when Lacan spoke at

Vincennes in 1969).[8] The lines of inquiry drawn by these interesting and suggestive sociocultural readings of shame in Lacanian psychoanalysis, critically summarized by me elsewhere,[9] will not be directly pursued further in what follows. Instead, my reflections will zero in on the implications of Lacan's few scant-but-allusive comments on the topic of shame for a psychoanalytic theory of affective life whose relevance isn't confined to a postmodern era of cheap plastic toys and television reality shows. As with his renowned recasting of the superego in the twentieth seminar,[10] Lacan's perspectives on shame are situated in two registers simultaneously: one more historical and contextual, the other more structural and transcontextual (i.e., metapsychological).

Joan Copjec is among those notable Lacanian scholars who highlight Lacan's calls for a bit more shame at the last meeting of the seventeenth seminar. In particular, her essay "May '68, The Emotional Month" is a careful, sophisticated historical contextualization of this academic year, an academic year situated in an unsettled cultural and political climate palpably perturbed by the aftershocks of France's mass uprisings of students and workers alike. Copjec's meticulous, thoughtful exploration of Lacanian shame gets well and truly underway thus: "In response to May '68, a very emotional month, he ends his seminar, his long warning against the rampant and misguided emotionalism of the university students, with an impassioned plea for a display of shame. Curb your impudence, your shamelessness, he exhorts, cautioning: you should be ashamed! What effrontery! What a provocation is this seminar! But then: what are we to make of it? Because the reference to shame appears so abruptly only in the final session and without elaboration, this is not an easy question to answer."[11] Like other recent readers of Lacan's appeals to shame in 1970, Copjec seems to adopt an angle of exegetical approach privileging the sociohistorical motivations behind and resonance of these appeals. And yet, Copjec's ensuing efforts to answer her opening question regarding shame ("what are we to make of it?") reveal a convergence of interests between her endeavors in this essay and the project I'm pursuing here. In both cases, the seventeenth seminar, admittedly situated as it is in such intensely determinative cultural and institutional circumstances, is interpreted as saying things about affect that go well beyond the limits of its proximity to the event of May '68. Of course, Lacan does intervene in manners intended to address those of his auditors gripped by the passions of their specific time and place; these interventions indeed speak to a peculiar late-capitalist *Zeitgeist* differing in important respects from the era enveloping Freud. But, apropos affects and their delineation in psychoanalysis (not to mention a number of other topics too), the Lacan of

1969–1970 remains just as committed as always to carrying forward faithfully Freud's theoretical framework as he simultaneously becomes, in this academic year especially, concerned with revising and refining Freudian metapsychology by putting this conceptual apparatus into a dialectical rapport with the evident facts of new widespread phenomena unknown to and unforeseen by Freud.[12] Again, a transcontextual metapsychology of affects can and should appropriate resources from the Lacan of this event-conditioned context of post–May '68 Paris.

However, despite some overlap at the level of aims and approaches, I part company from Copjec with respect to two key matters: the question of unconscious affect in general and the understanding of the significance of the words *affect* and *shame* in Lacan's texts in particular. To begin with the first of these differences, Copjec reiterates several times the Lacanian assertion, supposedly resting on firm Freudian foundations, that, in terms of being repressed, "affect never is."[13] Invoking "Freud's critical assertion that only ideas are ever repressed," she maintains: "Affect remains on the surface. This does not mean that repression has no effect on affect [*jouissance*]; it means, rather, that this effect is something other than the removal of affect from consciousness. The specific effect of repression on affect is displacement. Affect is *always* displaced, or: always out of place."[14] Copjec takes Lacan's word that affects, according to Freud, cannot succumb to the psychical vicissitude of repression insofar as they are feelings. This is problematic for several reasons: Not only does this claim ignore the different terms Freud employs when discussing affective life (i.e., *Affekt*, *Gefühl*, and *Empfindung*), but it also wrongly alleges that Freud consistently and categorically denies the existence of emotional phenomena below the superficial threshold of explicit conscious awareness. As shown previously, there are a plethora of instances, starting as early as 1907, in which Freud ponders the possibility of unconscious affect. But, what's more, the place in which Freud purportedly issues the decisive decree stating that affects can only ever be displaced within consciousness instead of repressed into unconsciousness—the place in question, regularly cited by Lacan and those sympathetic to his views on this point, is the third section ("Unconscious Emotions") of the metapsychological paper on "The Unconscious" (1915)—is far from decisive. As revealed by my earlier detailed examination of Freud's German, Freud wavers in relation to this topic even within the span of this single three-page section. And, as will be seen shortly, what his hesitations and oscillations therein (ignored by Lacan and Copjec, as well as many others) reveal has consequences for the Lacanian handling of shame as an affect.

Another limitation to Copjec's reading of Lacan's seventeenth seminar is its relative neglect of the nuances and subtleties of the remarks regarding affect (remarks unpacked at length in chapter 11) in all but the final session of that academic year. Like a handful of other Lacanians, she devotes most of her attention to shame as it appears in that year's last meeting. However, like Alenka Zupančič,[15] Copjec rightly observes that this annual seminar involves, among other things, Lacan reworking his long-standing black-and-white dichotomy between the signifier (as the intellectual-representational) and *jouissance* (as the affective-libidinal).[16] *Jouis-sens*, with its muddied shades of gray, begins to crystallize at this moment. And yet, none of this leads to questioning skeptically the old story, erroneously imputed to the authority of Freud, about affects as nothing more than mobile lumps in the carpet of consciousness set in motion by being pushed about (i.e., displaced) as a secondary result of the effects of defense mechanisms (repression first and foremost) operating exclusively on ideational and mnemic materials. Although both Freud and Lacan sometimes articulate conceptions of affects along these lines, a comprehensive survey of their various and varying pronouncements bearing upon matters of passions renders such a clear-cut, straightforward depiction of affect in Freudian-Lacanian psychoanalysis (as never repressed, as always displaced) suspect. Furthermore, when this survey takes into account the precise German and French phrasings of these pronouncements, the picture gets even more complex.

Sometimes sounding audibly frustrated and contemptuous, Lacan tirelessly pleads with his audience to acquaint themselves with Freud's texts in their original tongue, insisting that fundamental conceptual understandings and misunderstandings hinge on whether or not one gains adequate access to the syntax and semantics of the German language in which the founding documents of psychoanalysis are written. The devil resides in the details not only in the clinical setting of the analyst's consulting room. Although Lacan's neglect of the translation and interpretation difficulties posed by the German words Freud employs in his discussions of affective life is a notably rare and uncharacteristic exception to the former's own rule—this exception indeed proves the rule insofar as these strangely neglected German concept-terms arguably come back to haunt Lacan's own analytic understanding and handling of affects—a return to Lacan interested in affect must scrutinize the French used by the "French Freud." When it comes to affect-language of all sorts, the distinctions between connotations of words for affective phenomena in various natural languages are crucial to observe for at least two reasons: first, different natural languages splice up and organize fluid emotional spectrums differently; second, these differing linguistic renditions of shaded affective hues are not without real and direct repercussions for the affective lives of the speaking beings whose visceral emotions and feelings are mediated by the very languages that they speak. In fact, particularly when it comes to an English-language exegesis of a French-language discourse on shame, this sensitivity to linguistic precision is especially crucial.

Copjec contends that Lacan's talk of shame in 1970 is far from unprecedented in his teachings, citing, among other references, his famous seventh seminar of a decade prior.[17] This is where certain problems begin to arise. The French word translated as "shame" at the end of the seventeenth seminar is *honte*,[18] and this final session of that academic year is one of only three occasions on which Lacan speaks, briefly and in passing, of *honte* in *le Séminaire* (the other two occur in seminars eight and eleven,[19] with Copjec citing the latter but not the former). A different French word, *pudeur* (also translated as "shame"), is used by Lacan in the majority of those contexts referenced or alluded to by Copjec as precursors of his post–May '68 revival of shame. But, how do *honte* and *pudeur* differ from each other? Moreover, what difference does recognizing this English-elided terminological distinction make? Why is this important, particularly as regards a psychoanalytic metapsychology of affect?

The contrast between *honte* and *pudeur* consists in the former word referring to an affect as a felt feeling (i.e., as a consciously registered sensation tangibly experienced) and the latter word referring to a predisposition toward being capable of feeling certain feelings. Simply put: "*Honte* is shame as an excruciatingly uncomfortable, embarrassed feeling actually felt (as in 'I feel ashamed right now'). By contrast, *pudeur* is the potential capacity for or susceptibility to experiencing *honte*, a capacity/susceptibility that, in the form of the ethico-moral self-restraints of what is sometimes called 'modesty' or 'tact,' keeps one from crossing lines or transgressing those boundaries that would produce an actually felt upsurge of negative affect (as in, apropos a person lacking this tactful modesty, 'Have you no shame?')."[20] Interestingly, this French semantic difference can be correlated with Freud's previously traced German distinction between *Empfindung* (feeling) and *Affektbildung* (affective structure or formation): *Honte* designates a felt feeling qua *Empfindung*, whereas *pudeur* designates a potential to feel qua *Affektbildung* (rather than a feeling felt in actuality); indeed, German allows for a distinction between *Scham* and *Schamgefühl* (as per the title of a book by Max Scheler) corresponding to that between *pudeur* and *honte*, respectively. Accordingly, *honte*, as an *Empfindung*, is a conscious experience involving a specific set of sensations; by contrast, *pudeur*, as an *Affektbildung*, involves chains of ideational representations that can be either conscious or unconscious (as in the Freudian superego, a conscience not all of which is conscious). To say that *honte* and *pudeur* both mean "shame" in the same sense and are both words for an "affect" in the same sense would be inaccurate and misleading.

In fact, if one identifies *pudeur* qua *Affektbildung* as an affect, then, contra the Lacanian line adhered to by Copjec, one concedes the existence of unconscious affects, unless one is willing to contradict Freud's well-supported and explanatorily invaluable contention that much of the superego, itself responsible for intrapsychically enforcing modest, tactful restraint (*pudeur*), is unconscious. In her analyses of shame in Lacan's teachings, Copjec's lovely, polished English, usually so deft and illuminating, reveals a tendency to conflate the two senses of shame as *honte* and *pudeur*. While addressing shame (as *honte*) in the seventeenth seminar, she claims this to be a continuation of preceding Lacanian reflections on shame (generally as *pudeur*), proceeding to present all of these scattered instances in Lacan's seminars as occasions on which Lacan tackles the problem of affect (with no mention made of crucial distinctions such as those between *Empfindung* and *Affektbildung*, actual and potential affects, and so on).[21]

Admittedly, Lacan, once in a while permitting himself a more relaxed relationship to his native French tongue, sometimes lapses into an indistinction between *honte* and *pudeur* allowed for in nontechnical quotidian speech. In the sixth seminar, when describing the blush of a miser provoked by another's gaze glimpsing the unveiled secret treasure of one of his hoarded "intimate objects," Lacan employs *pudeur* as synonymous with *honte* to designate the felt feeling of embarrassment.[22] In the eighth seminar, *honte* and *pudeur* are used in close proximity to each other.[23] However, these few aberrant and casual equivocations between *honte* and *pudeur* aside (not to mention the rare references to *honte* alone in the eleventh and seventeenth seminars), the rest of Lacan's interlinked, cross-resonating remarks on "shame" (*pudeur*) implicitly but clearly pertain not to shame as an affect (i.e., *honte* qua *Empfindung*, an excruciating, burning affective state of consciousness), but to affective structures or formations (*Affektbildungen*) enforcing a limiting restraint, in the forms of modesty and tact (whether consciously or unconsciously respected), through the potential to produce the feelings of embarrassment, humiliation, and so on.

Starting in the fifth seminar and the contemporaneous *écrit* "The Signification of the Phallus," Lacan repeatedly summons the "demon of shame"

(*le démon de la Pudeur*).[24] This invocation occurs with reference to the picture of "the terrified woman" from the frescos of the Villa of the Mysteries
at Pompeii (the image-scene depicting this recoiling female figure adorns
the cover of the French edition of Lacan's *Télévision* published in 1973).[25]
Lacan interprets this painted ancient woman, at the threshold of a *katabasis*-
type passage, as horrified precisely by the sudden unveiling of the phallus;
she is said to embody the shame qua modesty (i.e., *pudeur*) that is integrally
complicit in sustaining the apparent potency of this symbolic entity through
refusing to tear aside the layers of cloth beneath which it normally remains
hidden.[26] Among other things, the Lacanian phallus signifies a potent whole-
ness and vital fullness ("by virtue of its turgidity . . . the image of the vital
flow as it is transmitted in generation") both inaccessible and unattainable
for speaking subjects; as such, this illusory *x* effectively functions as a lure
solely when its presence is hinted at indirectly through screens and disguises
("it can play its role only when veiled").[27] According to the general Lacanian
logic of the curtain or veil, coverings sustain the sense that there is something
being covered, a substantial thing concealed behind the barrier of a façade.
Through this effect, curtains or veils, such as those covering phallic entities,
even can create the illusion of something where there is nothing.[28] Alluring
avatars and promises of phallic power and completion retain their seductive
aura solely insofar as respectful restraint (again, *pudeur*) stays the hand that
might otherwise, in aiming to seize such phalli directly, inadvertently tear
away masks hiding nothing, thus disrupting the masquerade by calling its
bluff (and ending up empty-handed in the process). Immodestly and tact-
lessly tossing aside the crowns of kings and the gavels of judges reveals the
near nothingness of mere mortals, of miserable, fragile animal bodies. Those
who are shameless (*sans pudeur, sans vergogne*), like children who have yet to
know shame, are prone to blurt out such disturbing truths as that the phallic emperor is naked, that emperor-phallus is nothing more than a sagging,
wrinkled bit of spent flesh (and not, as it appears when veiled, an eternally
erect font of an indestructible life force). Like both Freud's "little Hans" and
his curious young fetishist-to-be, those who peer behind the ornamental coverings of clothes see—oh! horror of horrors—gaping absence where eager
anticipation expected full, protruding presence. When the limits maintained
by *pudeur* are disrespected and violated, *honte* and disgust tend to arise.[29]
These affects (as felt feelings, as *Empfindungen*) are symptomatic of subjectivity itself as constituted partially on the basis of restraining barriers and borders,[30] of limiting constraints of which *pudeur* qua *Affektbildung* (sometimes

conscious, sometimes unconscious) is an instance ("the dimension of shame, a dimension that is proper only to the subject as such").[31]

The seventh seminar, turned to by Copjec in her commentary on shame à la Lacan,[32] enriches and extends these observations regarding *pudeur*. Lacan's contemplations therein bearing on beauty play a key role in this vein: "The true barrier that holds the subject back in front of the unspeakable field of radical desire that is the field of absolute destruction, of destruction beyond putrefaction, is properly speaking the aesthetic phenomenon where it is identified with the experience of beauty—beauty in all its shining radiance, beauty that has been called the splendor of truth. It is obviously because truth is not pretty to look at that beauty is, if not its splendor, then at least its envelope."[33] In terms of Lacan's preceding discussions of *pudeur* apropos the phallus, the ugly truth concealed by material and not-so-material veils is (symbolic) castration, the fact that there is nothing equal to the phallic façade, nothing measuring up to this impossible standard. The curtains covering this bitter, distasteful deficiency can use the ruses of aesthetic appeal, of decorative adornments, to hide or dress up any small, hairy disappointments, whoever or whatever they may be. Later on in the seventh seminar, Lacan links the "limit" of beauty as the barrier, curtain, envelope, or veil of truth to the specter of death:[34] "I wanted to show you how the function of the signifier in permitting the subject's access to his relationship to death might be made more concrete than is possible through a connotation. That is why I have tried to have you recognize it in our recent meetings in an aesthetic form, namely, that of the beautiful—it being precisely the function of the beautiful to reveal to us the site of man's relationship to his own death, and to reveal it to us only in a blinding flash."[35]

Coming quickly on the heels of his commentary on Sophocles's *Antigone*, one example of a "blinding flash" of beauty Lacan undoubtedly has in mind here is the fascinating dramatic-tragic figure of "Antigone in her unbearable splendor."[36] Another example that may be suitable in this context is the depiction of Christ as a fetishized martyr associated with certain styles of Catholicism in particular, a depiction lingering with obscene, *jouissance*-laden relish over every detail of his wounded bare body. In both cases, an aesthetic sublation or sublimation of suffering unto death covers over doomed-to-rot sexed skin in the gleaming sheen of art's mercifully distracting, cathartic pleasures.

Lacan proceeds to draw parallels between beauty and shame. He begins this by noting: "I should like to introduce here, as a parallel to the function of the beautiful, another function. I have named it on a number of occasions without emphasizing it particularly, but it seems to me essential to refer to it here. It is with your permission what I shall call Αἰδώς or, in other words, a sense of shame. The omission of this barrier, which prevents the direct experience of that which is to be found at the center of sexual union, seems to me to be at the origin of all kinds of questions that cannot be answered."[37] The shame at stake here is again *pudeur*.[38] At first, one might think that, for Lacan, shame is to sex what beauty is to death: just as beauty shields the mortal subject from the blunt, unmitigated experiential effects (or affects) of facing the ugly truth of its own unglorious mortality with no fantasmatic embellishments and illusions, so too is shame something that "prevents the direct experience of that which is to be found at the center of sexual union" (or, as Lacan later puts it, *pudeur* as a modest restraint shields one from the truth that "*il n'y a pas de rapport sexuel.*")[39] But, additional remarks in both the seventh seminar and subsequent contexts indicate that Lacan, in good Freudian fashion, refuses to partition sex and death as two cleanly distinct topics, thus problematizing the neat separation of when they are correlated to shame and beauty, respectively.

Soon after comparing beauty and shame as parallel defensive "functions"—both serve in protective capacities relative to painful facts[40]—Lacan asks, "Do the fantasm of the phallus and the beauty of the human image find their legitimate place at the same level?"[41] Arguably, this is a rhetorical question, the answer to which is "Yes." Why? For Freudian-Lacanian psychoanalysis, sex and death are mutually entangled in multiple manners. In connection with this, the aesthetics of phallic sexuality require repressing from view, through the artful manipulation of veils of various sorts, an underbelly of time-ravaged, putrescent flesh spitting out spluttering trickles of smelly discharges. Even when two sexual partners face each other in their apparent nakedness, a nakedness which really isn't so naked thanks to the interplay of fantasmatic projections between them,[42] each must unknowingly coat both bodies there in layers of fantasies making possible the effect or affect of sexiness. The masquerades of such fantasy-supported sexuality wrap titillating films of spectral images and meanings around a repulsively rotten core of senseless filth, of idiotic, pointless enjoyment driven along by the raw facticity of a sexuality coupled with mortality.[43] In later seminars, Lacan indeed speaks of *pudeur* vis-à-vis the anxieties and horrors of the faceless Real of death-tinged sexuality.[44]

If Lacanian *pudeur* (over and above *honte* qua *Empfindung*, the felt feeling of shame as embarrassment, humiliation, and so on) is qualified as something affective, then the truly subtle dimensions of Lacan's underdeveloped, largely tacit metapsychology of affect present a much more intricate picture than is commonly assumed by the majority of his readers. In other words, this would mean that Lacan doesn't simply and flatly deny categorically the existence of anything affective at unconscious levels; in this hypothetical instance, he wouldn't reduce affective phenomena to the status of residual, epiphenomenal conscious by-products of unconscious formations solely comprising nonaffective structures of pure signifiers. Again, if *pudeur* is affective, then the Lacanian unconscious is not without affect. But, this remains quite vague insofar as it raises a series of yet-to-be-answered questions, questions Lacan himself doesn't explicitly address: Is the distinction between *honte* and *pudeur* to be lined up in a way that corresponds to the distinction between actual and potential affects, respectively? Can *honte* or *pudeur* be misfelt, that is, consciously registered and reflexively interpreted as affective hues other than themselves? Similarly but differently, can *honte* or *pudeur* be enlisted in intra-affective defensive maneuvers in which one consciously feels ashamed or modest so as to avoid feeling other possible feelings instead, in which case these defended-against other (potential) feelings would be, in a certain sense, unconscious? The most effective and productive way to handle these difficulties bequeathed to contemporary thought by Freud and Lacan is to interface their metapsychologies with the neurosciences.

Some of Žižek's recent work constructs a very useful and unconventional bridge between Lacanian psychoanalytic theory and neuroscientific accounts of emotional life and affective selfhood or subjectivity. Interestingly, there is evidence that Žižek admits the existence of unconscious affects, a controversial admission in psychoanalysis generally and Lacanianism especially. On at least one occasion, he speaks of guilt, in faithful Freudian fashion, as "ultimately unconscious."[45] In this context, he even indicates two modes in which guilt can be unconscious: (1) "the subject is unaware of his or her guilt" (i.e., an unfelt feeling), and (2) "he or she, while experiencing the pressure of guilt, is unaware of what he or she is guilty of" (i.e., an enigmatic, free-floating feeling).[46] The latter mode arguably also could be (or morph into) a misfelt feeling: in the absence of an explicit cognizance of culpability apropos a misdeed relative to a certain rule, the feeling that might otherwise be self-interpretively felt as guilt is consciously registered as some other affective tonality (such as anxiety, nervousness, vague discomfort, or even physical illness).

Žižek's book *The Parallax View* (published in 2006) contains detailed engagements with the sciences of the brain. Among other figures in this set of disciplines, he turns his attention to Damasio in particular, specifically the latter's neuroscience-based theories of emotional matters elaborated primarily in the book *The Feeling of What Happens* (published in 1999). Before turning to what Žižek has to say regarding Damasio, a few introductory remarks obviously should be made about the ideas and positions of the latter. To begin with, Damasio is generally sympathetic to psychoanalysis and particularly sympathetic to the neuro-psychoanalytic movement in Anglo-American clinical analytic circles; for instance, he sits on the Neuroscience Editorial Advisory Board of the journal *Neuro-Psychoanalysis*, of which Solms is one of the founding editors.[47] Damasio (and, in fact, neuroscience as a whole) fundamentally accepts an unconscious along the lines of that described by analytic metapsychology.[48] What's more, whereas the notion of unconscious affect remains controversial in certain sectors of psychoanalysis—for many Lacanians, the phrase "unconscious affect" is oxymoronic—Damasio (and, as will be seen, many of his fellow researchers investigating the emotional brain) posits the reality of affective phenomena below the threshold of self-awareness.[49] Like Freud, he even acknowledges the ostensibly unavoidable awkwardness of proposing that there are feelings that aren't felt as such: "Someone may suggest that perhaps we should have another word for 'feelings that are not conscious,' but there isn't one."[50]

In the three shadows cast by Freud, Lacan, and Žižek, the current discussion, with its selective focus, will be limited to touching upon Damasio's fashion of distinguishing between "emotions" and "feelings" (as well as between nonconscious and conscious feelings). Properly understanding this Damasian distinction requires initially noting that Damasio insists, as I've done here too, on the essentially mediated nature of human beings' affective lives, on the ineliminable modulation (even constitution) of passions and sentiments by intellectual, linguistic, and representational configurations.[51] To put it in the language of the neuroscience trinity of cognition, emotion, and motivation, the emotional brain cannot be separated from the cognitive brain[52] (not to mention the motivational brain, whose facets also are of great importance to psychoanalysis, with its reliance on a theory of drives).

For Damasio, emotions are, by his definition, nonconscious phenomena, rather than, as in quotidian parlance, felt feelings. To be more precise, Damasian emotions are physiological processes visible to third-party observers; feelings, by contrast, are private, first-person phenomena.[53] He thus aligns emotions with the publicly accessible body and feelings with the publicly inaccessible mind.[54] However, Damasio is far from resting content with an indefensibly simplistic opposition between a nonconscious body of physiological emotions and a conscious mind of psychological feelings. This becomes clear in Damasio's delineation of a three-stage diachronic sequence running from nonconscious emotions to potential and actual conscious feelings (with emotions having temporal priority over feelings):[55] "I separate three stages of processing along a continuum: *a state of emotion*, which can be triggered and executed nonconsciously; *a state of feeling*, which can be represented nonconsciously; and *a state of feeling made conscious*, i.e., known to the organism having both emotion and feeling."[56]

The second of these three stages is where Damasio is perhaps at his most psychoanalytic. On his account, the human brain is a compulsive, reflexive self-modeler, constantly generating map-like depictions of the states of the subject's body, its world of objects, and the ongoing interactions between these two enmeshed poles (with consciousness being an outgrowth of these self-mapping dynamics).[57] The conceptions and pictures thus formed can be, in Damasio's view, either conscious or nonconscious.[58] He's entirely open about his reliance on the (originally Freudian) assertion according to which the large domain of mental life that isn't conscious contains not only motivational energies and impulses (as per the pseudo-Freudian notion of the unconscious as the dark depths of a writhing, primordial animal id), but also cognitive images and representations (something Lacan adamantly insists upon again and again in his "return to Freud"): "Images may be conscious or unconscious. It should be noted, however, that not all the images the brain constructs are made conscious. There are simply too many images being generated and too much competition for the relatively small window of mind in which images can be made conscious—the window, that is, in which images are accompanied by a sense that we are apprehending them and that, as a consequence, are properly attended. In other words, metaphorically speaking, there is indeed a subterranean underneath the conscious mind and there are many levels to that subterranean."[59] With the preceding details in mind, a better appreciation of the nuances and potentials of Damasio's fine-grained distinctions concerning affective life is now possible. Damasio states: "This perspective on emotion, feeling, and knowing is unorthodox. First, I am suggesting that there is no central feeling state before the respective emotion occurs, that expression (emotion) precedes feeling. Second, I am suggesting that 'having a feeling' is not the same as 'knowing a feeling,' that reflection on feeling is yet another step up. Overall, this curious situation reminds me of E. M. Forster's words: 'How can I know what I think before I say it?'"[60]

Emotions are "expressions" in the sense of physiological processes manifested by the body (everything from heart rates and adrenalin releases to blushing and sweating). These bodily states then are cognitively mapped, translated into images and representations. Such maps of emotions, constructed by the spontaneous self-modeling activities of a brain that "is truly the body's captive audience,"[61] would be feelings in Damasio's parlance. However, he crucially stipulates that feelings thus defined are not automatically and necessarily conscious (i.e., consciously felt feelings, Freudian *Empfindungen*). As Damasio postulates, one can "have a feeling" (as a nonconscious or unconscious image or representation of an emotion qua physiological condition) without knowing it.[62] (Jean-Pierre Changeux, another neuroscientist, likewise observes that "the direct experience of feeling is readily distinguished from the knowledge that one has a feeling.")[63] And, perhaps there are two modes in which this gap between having and knowing can exist: on the one hand, the feeling is unattended to by first-person consciousness (i.e., it's an unfelt feeling), or, on the other hand, the feeling is interpreted by first-person consciousness (i.e., it's a misfelt feeling, examples of which might include the conscious registration of varieties of affective excitation as anxiety or of guilt as physical distress). At this point, it's tempting to establish one-to-one correspondences between the affective trinities of Freud and Damasio: *Affekt* (affect) is emotion (for psychoanalysis, this emotionally expressive body is already itself saturated by the denaturalizing influences of intertwined cognitive-ideational and motivational-libidinal dimensions); *Gefühl* (emotion) is feeling-had (which can be unconscious, as in unconscious guilt à la Freud [*unbewußte Schuldgefühl*]); and *Empfindung* (feeling) is feeling-known (which would be "feeling" in the everyday, nontechnical sense of the word).

Damasio's work on affective life should be of great interest for psychoanalysis, including even Lacanian theory. (Žižek once more, as in other respects too, is an admirable and rare exception, being one of the all-too-few Lacanians to address seriously the advances achieved by Damasio and the neurosciences as a whole; by contrast, Anglo-American neuro-psychoanalysis indeed has enthusiastically embraced affective neuroscience.) From a Freudian-Lacanian perspective, several features of the approach to parsing the affective phenomena selectively summarized immediately strike the eye. As in Freudian metapsychology, Damasio's intermediary realm of feelings-had, situated in a mediating capacity between nonconscious emotions and conscious feelings-known, consists of *Triebrepräsentanzen* (drive representatives), namely, the psychical inscriptions both structurally articulated and energetically charged that form the coordinates of the drives' aims (*Ziele*) and objects (*Objekte*). Along related Lacanian lines, one cannot help but think of *jouis-sens*, of the hybrid juxtapositions and unstable syntheses of (in Freud's terms) soma and psyche, of something neither strictly corporeal-libidinal nor subjective-meaningful.[64] Additionally, the line from Forster quoted by Damasio also elegantly encapsulates Lacan's take on an aspect of free association in the analytic process, a take in which the analysand, as a *parlêtre* voicing his/her thoughts and desires, comes to figure out what he/she really thinks and wants through the verbal labor of associational expression itself (rather than a take in which free association merely helps to reveal what already was present beforehand fully formed in the repressed recesses of the speaking subject's psyche).[65]

Before turning to Žižek's critical comments on Damasio, a quick examination of the latter's book *Looking for Spinoza*, published in 2003, promises to be helpful and relevant (in part because it further clarifies arguments and concepts first delineated in *The Feeling of What Happens*). Damasio's Spinozism is expressed via the assertion, taken straight from part 2 of the *Ethics* (especially propositions 13 and 23), that "*the human mind is the idea of the human body*."[66] For Damasio, an obvious extension of this, in connection with his distinction between emotions and feelings, is the proposition that "feelings . . . are mostly shadows of the external manner of emotions."[67] Again, emotions are "external" insofar as they are corporeal expressions made manifest as physiological phenomena potentially if not actually observable by third parties. Moreover, as indicated, they are, in and of themselves, nonconscious; they can be translated into consciously registered experiences in the guise of feelings, but they aren't automatically and necessarily thus registered. In this vein, Damasio observes—this observation obviously dovetails with assertions central to Freudian psychoanalysis—that pleasure and pain (as emotion-level bodily events) don't need the mediation of conscious experience to generate and guide behaviors.[68] He goes on to indicate that this independence relative to consciousness is enjoyed by emotions generally.[69]

Damasio, in line with the thesis that the mind consists of ideational reflections of the body, defines feelings (as mental, distinct from physical, emotions) as representations of body-states (i.e., the body's changing conditions and its ongoing interactions with entities and circumstances affecting it).[70] He proceeds to elaborate: "Feelings are perceptions, and I propose that the most necessary support for their perception occurs in the *brain's body maps*. These maps refer to parts of the body and states of the body. Some variation of pleasure or pain is a consistent content of the perception we call feeling."[71] He continues:

> Alongside the perception of the body there is the perception of thoughts with
> themes consonant with the emotion, and a perception of a certain mode of

thinking, a style of mental processing. How does this perception come about? It results from constructing metarepresentations of our own mental process, a high-level operation in which a part of the mind represents another part of the mind. This allows us to register the fact that our thoughts slow down or speed up as more or less attention is devoted to them; or the fact that thoughts depict objects and events at close range or at a distance. My hypothesis, then, presented in the form of a provisional definition, is that *a feeling is the perception of a certain state of the body along with the perception of a certain mode of thinking and of thoughts with certain themes*. Feelings emerge when the sheer accumulation of mapped details reaches a certain stage.[72]

As Damasio summarizes all of this a few pages later, "A feeling of emotion is an idea of the body when it is perturbed by the emoting process."[73] From a psychoanalytic angle, a number of details in these passages warrant commentary. As I suggested earlier, the pleasure-and-pain-infused "body maps," themselves not necessarily conscious but capable of becoming so in the trappings of the ideational-representational material of feelings, can be associated with Freudian drive representatives (composing configurations of libidinal aims and objects) and Lacanian *jouis-sens* (itself written in the fluid "language" of *lalangue*). These Damasian maps, continually drafted and updated by the perpetual self-modeling activity of the brain, are nec-essary-but-not-sufficient conditions for the experience of somatic emotions as psychical felt feelings: "an entity capable of feeling must be an organ-ism that not only has a body but also a means to represent that body inside itself."[74] What's more, this mapping process is the first step of a two-step translation process at the end of which emerge feelings-known (*Empfind-ungen*), affective phenomena consciously experienced. In addition to the initial step from emotions to maps as (proto)affective formations (a step in which representations of body parts and relations with exogenous objects must be integrated), a subsequent step from such maps to "metarepresenta-tions" (in which cognitive styles and contents must be linked and synthe-sized) is requisite for the genesis of a consciously felt feeling.[75] Although Damasio repeatedly acknowledges that something like the psychoanalytic unconscious plays a role in the vicissitudes of affective life,[76] his discussions of the trajectories of translation leading from emotions through feelings-had to feelings-known tend to pass over quickly and quietly features of this multistep movement with respect to which a Freudian-Lacanian metapsy-chology of affect has a lot to say.

The Lacanian rendition of the Freudian unconscious as a "superficial" (non) being at play in twists, turns, and gaps inscribed within the very surface of consciousness is worth recalling at this juncture. (As is well known, Lacan is adamantly opposed to the vulgar depiction of psychoanalysis as a hermeneutic depth psychology, an exploration of hidden pockets of profound meaning.)[77] To be more precise, the psychoanalytic unconscious (and not the vague non-analytic notion of the nonconscious) exists, in part, as events of interventions intervening between different components and operations along the line running from one end of Damasio's affective spectrum to the other, from nonconscious emotions to conscious feelings. In other words, the unconscious isn't itself a deep, obfuscated component or operation of the complex ensemble of affective machinery, but instead is something slipping into the intervals of spacing distinguishing emotions, feelings-had, and feelings-known. It even can and does affect the linkings internal to both feelings-had and feelings-known, that is, the linkings of body parts, states, and surrounding circumstances in Damasian feelings-had (i.e., first-order representations in the form of body maps mapping the far-from-elementary complexes that are emotions) as well as the linkings of cognitive modes and themes in Damasian feelings-known (i.e., second-order "metarepresentations" as reflective appreciations of affective experiences).

Put differently and more generally, the unconscious of intrapsychical defense mechanisms (i.e., the unconscious that is repressed, with "repression" to be taken here in its broadest possible analytic sense) is not reducible to any set of particular content-nodes in the networks of the psyche insofar as it kinetically slides between these nodes. Repression often bears on associative relations between pieces of psychical content. For example, in an analysis, an analysand might very well be able consciously to recollect every specific fragment of mnemic material involved in a given constellation underpinning a particular symptom. In such a case, what is repressed isn't one memory among others, but instead the web of associations woven between the memories constituting nodes in the network producing symptoms as its outgrowths. The relations between memories are repressed, rather than the memories themselves. The unconscious comes to light in such analytic circumstances as newly recognized connections between previously recognized contents.

Whereas Damasio speaks of organic "consonances" between the different layers and levels of his affective spectrum, a psychoanalytic approach, taking up his model, would prefer to emphasize dissonances. More precisely, by virtue of the psyche's defensive means of achieving a self-regulated homeostatic equilibrium in terms of affects, there inevitably are absences of translations or distorting mistranslations within and between emotions, feelings-had, and feelings-known (or, as Freud might put it, within and between *Affekte*, *Gefühle*, and *Empfindungen*). Additionally, this analytic metapsychological supplement to Damasio's theory rectifies what appears to be one of its shortcomings: Damasio seems to suggest entertaining the unconvincing hypothesis that a simple, straightforward quantitative factor is responsible for the qualitative shift from nonconscious affective mechanisms to felt affective qualia ("Feelings emerge when the sheer accumulation of mapped details reaches a certain stage"). By contrast, an analytic approach would speculate that much more than "sheer" quantity alone is at work here.

In several contexts, Damasio somewhat enigmatically refers to what he characterizes as "feelings of feelings."[78] At this point, an examination of Žižek's Lacanian criticisms of Damasio's account of affective life is appropriate and promises to be productive. Žižek devotes a certain amount of attention to a topic I did not delve into earlier, namely, the theory of the multiple degrees and strata of consciousness and selfhood in *The Feeling of What Happens* (in which Damasio sets out such conceptual categories as protoselfhood, core consciousness or selfhood, extended consciousness, autobiographical selfhood, and conscience).[79] On this score, Žižek's complaint is that reducing subjectivity to the two dimensions of embodied being (as protoselfhood and core consciousness or selfhood) and linguistic-representational identity (as extended consciousness, autobiographical selfhood, and conscience) leaves out the third dimension first isolated by Descartes in the figure of the *Cogito* (i.e., the subject proper as the emptiness of the negativity of $, Lacan's "barred subject"):[80]

Damasio's solution to the old enigma of the two sides of Self (Self *qua* the continuously changing stream of consciousness verses Self *qua* the permanent stable core of our subjectivity) misses the mark: "the seemingly changing self and the seemingly permanent self, although closely related, are not one entity but two"—the first being the Core Self, the second the autobiographical Self. There is no place here, however, for what we as speaking beings experience (or, rather, presuppose) as the empty core of our subjectivity: what am I? I am neither my body (I have a body, I never "am" my body directly, in spite of all the subtle phenomenological descriptions *à la* Merleau-Ponty that try to convince me to the contrary), nor the stable core of my autobiographical narratives that form my symbolic identity; what "I am" is the pure One of an empty Self which remains the same One throughout the constant change

of autobiographical narratives. This One is engendered by language: it is neither the Core Self nor the autobiographical Self, but what the Core Self is
transubstantiated (or, rather, desubstantialized) into when it is transposed
into language. This is what Kant has in mind when he distinguishes between
the "person" (the wealth of autobiographical content that provides substantial content to my Self) and the pure subject of transcendental apperception
which is just an empty point of self-relating.[81]

The entire philosophical framework informing this critique of Damasio cannot be exhaustively elucidated here insofar as this would require reconstructing
the entirety of the Žižekian theory of subjectivity, which is constructed at the
intersection of German idealism and Lacanian psychoanalysis (a reconstruc-
tion I carry out in my book *Žižek's Ontology: A Transcendental Materialist
Theory of Subjectivity*, published in 2008). But, what's crucial in this context
is Žižek's insistence, following Lacan, that Symbolic mediation (i.e., the passage of the substantial protosubject into the enveloping milieus of language
structures) creates a subject (i.e., the *Cogito*-like subject-as-$ central to Kan-
tian and post-Kantian German idealism) that thereafter escapes reduction to
either bodily nature (including Damasio's "Core Self") or linguistic culture
(including Damasio's "autobiographical Self"); this could be described as a
sort of immanent structural genesis of transstructural subjectivity.[82] Damasio
agrees with Žižek about the invalidity of reducing consciousness or selfhood
to language;[83] he even speculates that nonhuman animals have autobiographical selves, thereby clearly indicating that he doesn't consider this stratum of
selfhood to be entirely language-bound.[84] But, Damasio and Žižek certainly
seem to part company apropos the latter's Lacanian thesis that the corporeal
substance of the Damasian protoselves and core selves doesn't remain a purely
biological foundation over which is then subsequently laid utterly separate and
distinct higher-order mental scaffoldings. (Lurking in the broadest encompassing background is what would be a much more far-reaching, fundamental
debate about the extent to which sociosymbolic mediators penetrate and alter
the realities of the body.)

In *The Feeling of What Happens*, Damasio does concede that a certain
amount of dialectical interaction transpires between core consciousness or
selfhood and the additional tiers of different configurations of conscious-
ness/selfhood overlaid on top of it.[85] And yet, Žižek is quite right that Damasio nonetheless tends to stick persistently to the claim that an atomic center
of substantial biomaterial being utterly untouched by nonnatural influences

remains a pure, impermeable core ultimately grounding all other dimensions of mental life.[86] Against this claim, Žižek asserts that insertion into symbolico-linguistic matrices of mediation (or, in Lacanese, the submission of the protosubject S to "symbolic castration" by the big Other, thus producing the subject-as-$) "transubstantiates" and "desubstantializes" the Damasian hard kernel of bodily existence. However, Žižek's critique ignores Damasio's distinction between the protoself and the core self, conflating these two entities under the single heading of the "Core Self." For Damasio, the core self is a representational map of the protoself.[87] Nonetheless, in the spirit of Žižek's psychoanalytically inspired objection to Damasio, it would be justifiable to maintain that the advent of language use (especially the subjectifying acquisition of proficiency with proper names and personal pronouns) might "transubstantiate" the very means and results of the translation process leading from the protoself to the core self.

Put in combined Lacanian and Damasian vocabularies, an irreparable rift rendering all representational translation between the protoself as S and the core self as $ somewhat misrepresentative (à la Lacan's *méconnaissance*) may open like a gaping wound in organisms subjected to the cutting intervention of linguistic structures. This would be the initial, zero-level introduction into the corporeal reality of human animals of the dissonances and discrepancies that come to be characteristic of split speaking subjects through whose splits circulate unconscious dimensions. But, whereas Žižek sounds as though he flirts at this moment with a vaguely social-constructivist vision according to which the nature-based protoself-as-S is retroactively liquidated and replaced by the language-induced core-self-as-$ (now in the form of the Cartesian-Kantian-Hegelian-Lacanian void of self-relating negativity), what I am proposing presently is an alternative picture in which, to articulate this in Hegelian fashion, the distinction between S (as the protoself) and $ (as the core self) persists as a distinction internal to $ itself. That is to say, not only do chasms of varying widths crack open between the language-independent protoself as S and its (un)representational (mis)translations in and by the linguistically influenced core self as $, but a split within the core-self-as-$ mirrors this chasm, a split dividing the core self in two, into both a plastic avatar of substantial bodily being as well as a faceless blank of desubstantialized negativity. In other words, maybe there are two core selves dissonant with each other (in addition to the varyingly dissonant intervals between protoselves and core selves): a "full" core self and an "empty" core self (the latter being the *Cogito*-like void of interest to Žižek, something admittedly neglected by Damasio).

In *The Parallax View*, Žižek spells out some key implications of his critical reading of Damasio's portrait of consciousness or selfhood for this portrait's accompanying account of affective life. He begins: "Damasio's fundamental 'Althusserian' thesis is that 'there is no central feeling state before the respective emotion occurs, that expression (emotion) precedes feeling.' I am tempted to link this emotion which precedes feeling to the empty pure subject ($): emotions are already the subject's, but before subjectivization, before their transposition into the subjective experience of feeling. $ is thus the subjective correlative to emotions prior to feeling: it is only through feelings that I become the 'full' subject of lived self-experience. And it is this 'pure' subject which can no longer be contained within the frame of life-homeostasis, that is, whose functioning is no longer constrained by the biological machinery of life-regulation."[88] Žižek soon adds: "The chain of equivalences . . . imposes itself between the 'empty' *cogito* (the Cartesian subject, Kant's transcendental subject), the Hegelian topic of self-relating negativity, and the Freudian topic of the death drive. Is this 'pure' subject deprived of emotions? It is not as simple as that: its very detachment from immediate immersion in life-experience gives rise to new (not emotions or feelings, but, rather) affects: anxiety and horror. Anxiety as correlative to confronting the Void that forms the core of the subject; horror as the experience of disgusting life at its purest, 'undead' life."[89] What Damasio depicts as natural (i.e., the core self as the source of not-felt or not-yet-felt emotions) Žižek treats as radically antinatural, that is "no longer . . . contained within the frame of life-homeostasis, . . . no longer constrained by the biological machinery of life-regulation" (i.e., $, which is also the Lacanian subject of the unconscious, as itself a generator of affective phenomena). By arguing that "emotions are already the subject's," he signals his hypothesis that Damasio's protoself or core self (or, more accurately, selves) is thoroughly denaturalized *après-coup* by the intrusion of the signifiers of the symbolic order.

Of course, one might have reservations with respect to what sounds like a hyperbolic positing of a total and complete denaturalization without reserve or remainder. As regards the (human) "nature" underpinning subjectivity, I prefer to conceive of denaturalization as, at least in some circumstances, more of a sedimentary accumulation, a layering of heterogeneous montages of often conflicting dimensions running the gamut from the relatively "natural" (e.g., evolutionary tendencies rooted in archaic environmental contexts) to the relatively "nonnatural" (primarily sociohistorical factors and variables past and present). To misappropriate some of Žižek's language from *In Defense of Lost Causes*,[90] the whole problem is that "life 2.0" (i.e., the retroactive denaturalizer of life as such in and of itself) never succeeds fully at erasing and replacing what after the fact becomes "life 1.0" (i.e., naked, primitive life *an sich* once it has been retroactively affected by the genesis of life 2.0). At least in certain cases, the latter continues to operate in parallel with the former, with antagonisms and dysfunctions arising between them.

Human beings, in terms of where they stand between the natural and the nonnatural, could be described as creatures of temporal torsions. Parts of human beings lag behind in the time warp of evolutionary-genetic influences linked to long-past contexts, whereas other parts, which can and do come into conflict with these same evolutionary-genetic influences, take shape according to faster-moving historical temporalities. (Moreover, the latter are themselves outgrowths of evolution that have escaped control by evolutionary governance alone.)[91] Such beings are the products of incomplete, partial denaturalizations failing to eliminate without undigested leftovers the vestiges of things other than the sociosymbolically mediated structures and phenomena of human history both phylogenetic and ontogenetic. Of course, one should wholeheartedly agree with Žižek that "Nature does not exist" if "Nature" designates a balanced, harmonious One-All; this is another nonexistent big Other (as per Lacan's "*Le grand Autre n'existe pas*").[92] However, nature indeed does exist both as that which immanently allows for and generates the denaturalizations involved with subjectivity,[93] and as a bundle of anachronistic variables, within the substance of human being, out of joint with various and sundry aspects of more current historical-temporal milieus. Nature is a participant in this unbalanced ensemble of conflicting elements. So, to paraphrase Lacan's "there is no Other of the Other" (rather than his "the big Other does not exist"), I assert that there is no Nature of nature, although there is nature as fragmentary, self-sundering components caught up in the conflicts constitutive of the "human condition."[94]

Regardless of all this, Žižek's crucial move in the passages quoted three paragraphs earlier is his insightful proposal that the signifier-catalyzed explosion of the emptiness of $ out of the fullness of S, of (as per Hegel) subject proper out of substance, is not without significant repercussions in the spheres of affect. In fact, for Žižek, properly human-subjective affects are neither emotions nor feelings in Damasio's senses of these latter two terms. Damasio treats emotions as automatic physiological processes regulated by nonconscious bodily mechanisms, although he stipulates that the translation of emotions into consciously registered feelings allows for partial cognitive-intellectual mediation and modulation of embodied emotions.[95] By contrast, Žižek, for a number of

Freudian-Lacanian reasons, insists that the emoting body, insinuated by Damasio to rest on a natural or instinctual basis, is altered right down to its bare bones and raw flesh by its transformative insertion into the sociosymbolic matrices of the big Other. (First and foremost, the corporeal core self of Damasio is "transubstantiated" and "denaturalized" into the disembodied emptiness of Lacan's *Cogito*-like $, a void linked to such linguistic signifier-entities as proper names and personal pronouns.)[96] Žižek proceeds to refer to LeDoux, another major researcher in the field of affective neuroscience, best known for his empirical investigations of the role of the amygdala in generating fear, in extending his critique of Damasio:

> It would be interesting to conceive the very specificity of "being-human" as grounded in this gap between cognitive and emotional abilities: a human being in whom emotions were to catch up with cognitive abilities would no longer be human, but a cold monster deprived of human emotions. . . . Here we should supplement LeDoux with a more structural approach: it is not simply that our emotions lag behind our cognitive abilities, stuck at the primitive animal level; *this very gap itself functions as an "emotional" fact, giving rise to new, specifically human, emotions,* from anxiety (as opposed to mere fear) to (human) love and melancholy. Is it that LeDoux (and Damasio, on whom LeDoux relies here) misses this feature because of the fundamental weakness (or, rather, ambiguity) of the proto-Althusserian distinction between emotions and feelings? This distinction has a clear Pascalian twist (and it is a mystery that, in his extensive critique of "Descartes' error," Damasio does not evoke Pascal, Descartes's major critic): physical emotions do not display inner feelings but, on the contrary, generate them. However, there is something missing here: a gap between emotions *qua* biological-organic bodily gestures and emotions *qua* learned symbolic gestures following rules (like Pascal's kneeling and praying). Specifically "human" emotions (like anxiety) arise only when a human animal loses its emotional mooring in biological instincts, and this loss is supplemented by the symbolically regulated emotions *qua* man's "second nature."[97]

Indeed, LeDoux, like Damasio, sees neuroscience and psychoanalysis as far from incompatible. Moreover, like the Lacanian Žižek, he emphasizes the far-reaching "revolutionary" (rather than just "evolutionary," smooth, and gradual) ramifications for the human animal of its immersion in language, an immersion changing and reshaping brains and bodies.[98] (Damasio similarly speaks of "the biological revolution called culture.")[99] LeDoux even muses about the possible alterations of affective dynamics in human *parlêtres* driven by linguistic mediation.[100] But, how accurate and justified are Žižek's critical remarks regarding LeDoux's ideas about the relation between cognition and emotion in the human brain?

From a psychoanalytic perspective, perhaps one of the most important facts emphasized by LeDoux is that, as it might be expressed, the brain, although a bodily organ, is not organic in such a way that it is a piece of nature that is a harmonious and synthesized self-integrated system of balanced components in sync with each other.[101] In fact, LeDoux points to precisely the sort of phenomena that led Freud to posit the centrality in mental life of intrapsychical conflicts and Lacan to invoke again and again the figure of the split subject as evidence of the brain's hodgepodge, collage-like construction, a construction whose mismatched elements don't necessarily work well together.[102] Along these lines, in his study *The Emotional Brain*, he observes: "Although we often talk about the brain as if it has a function, the brain itself actually has no function. It is a collection of systems, sometimes called modules, each with different functions. There is no equation by which the combination of functions of all the different systems mixed together equals an additional function called brain function."[103] He goes on to add, "Evolution tends to act on the individual modules and their functions rather than the brain as a whole.... [B]y and large most evolutionary changes in the brain take place at the level of individual modules."[104] The brain, like the rest of the human body with which it's inseparably enmeshed, is a product not of Evolution with a capital E (itself yet another nonexistent Lacanian big Other), but of a plethora of different and distinct evolutionary circumstances and challenges spread out over a disparate number of times and places (as Damasio puts it, "Evolution is not the Great Chain of Being").[105] In this vein, Alain Badiou's denial of Nature as a monolithic cosmic One-All and parallel corresponding affirmation of the existence of a proliferation of natural multiplicities—"Nature has no sayable being. There are only *some* natural beings."[106]—can and should be applied to the natural-scientific notion of evolution. Moreover, these evolutionary pressures, not at all coordinated and unified with each other, act separately on a diverse array of independent systems and subsystems within the central nervous system. (Damasio notes that "the brain is a system of systems"[107] and highlights the mismatch between brain stem and cortex in the human nervous system, two [sub]systems of different evolutionary age forced to cooperate with each other.)[108] No top-down design plan governed the assembly process producing the peculiar lump of folded, meshwork matter that is the human brain. Its bottom-up genesis consists (inconsistently) of a chaotic vortex of accidents, chances, and contingencies. Consequently, the resulting product of such a process is, not surprisingly, prone to an incalculable number of internal antagonisms, tensions, and short circuits. Or, as the neuroscientist David J. Linden describes it, the human central nervous system is a "kludge": "The brain is . . . a kludge, . . . a design that is inefficient, inelegant, and unfathomable, but that nevertheless works"[109] and "at every turn, brain design has been a kludge, a workaround, a jumble, a pastiche."[110] Linden's book *The Accidental Mind*, published in 2007, repeatedly insists that the brain is inelegantly designed by a multitude of haphazard evolutionary tinkerings in which the newer is plopped on top of the comparatively older and, hence, is "poorly organized," "a cobbled-together mess."[111] (Incidentally, Linden devastatingly wields his kludge thesis against antievolution proponents of so-called intelligent design.)[112] In the year immediately after the publication of Linden's book, the psychologist Gary Marcus, in the book *Kludge*, analyzed a range of mental phenomena in light of the same basic thesis advanced by Linden.[113] Both Linden's and Marcus's positions are foreshadowed by, among other sources, François Jacob's *Science* article "Evolution and Tinkering" from 1977[114] (a quotation from which serves as one of the epigraphs to Marcus's book). One would have to be, as it were, utterly brainless not to see the importance of this neuroscientific picture of the material seat of subjectivity for a psychoanalytic metapsychology emphasizing the central structuring functions of conflicts in mental life.

Clearly consistent with his stress upon the nonexistence of the Brain with a capital B as "brain function" in the singular—echoing Badiou, there is, within each human being, no Brain, only some brains—is LeDoux's repeated and emphatic argument against the false impression that affective neuroscience can and does deal with emotional life in general or an ultimately homogenous emotion function in the brain (such as the so-called limbic system, something the objective reality of which is a bone of contention among neuroscientists).[115] So, not only is there no coherent brain function overall, but there is no emotion function overall either (and, with reference again to the trinity of cognition, emotion, and motivation, one might wonder, under the influence of psychoanalytic thinking, whether the same might be said for cognitive and motivational functions too). In his substantial survey *Affective Neuroscience*, Panksepp takes a further step along this same trajectory delineated by LeDoux (even though he and LeDoux disagree about the status of the notion of the limbic system).[116] Panksepp maintains that even particular individual emotions lack discrete corresponding "centers" in the physiological anatomy of the brain: "no single psychological concept fully describes the functions of any given brain area or circuit. There are no unambiguous 'centers' or loci for discrete emotions in the brain that do not massively interdigitate with other functions, even though certain key circuits are essential for certain emotions to be elaborated. Everything ultimately emerges from the interaction of many systems. For this reason, modern neuroscientists talk about interacting 'circuits,' 'networks,' and 'cell assemblies' rather than 'centers.'"[117]

Combining LeDoux's denial of a basic, general emotion function in the brain with Panksepp's denial of compartmentalized anatomical brain loci correlated in a one-to-one manner with various feeling states, one can postulate the following: even specific singular emotions are complex (or complexes), that is, nonatomic or nonelementary clusters of interconnections between multiple different systems and subsystems in the brain. What's more, it seems quite reasonable to suppose that all three dimensions of brain functioning (i.e., cognition, emotion, and motivation) come into play in affective phenomena. Panksepp says as much here. Moreover, elsewhere, he remarks that "it must be kept in mind that the brain is a massively interconnected organ whose every part can find an access pathway to any other part."[118] He subsequently links this fact to emotional phenomena, emphasizing that the brain's mind-bogglingly intricate internal interconnectedness makes it such that emotions are inextricably intertwined with nonemotional dimensions.[119] Additionally, both within and between these interacting functions, it also seems defensible to hypothesize that a plurality of separate strata of temporal layers deposited in the brain (deposits dating from natural-evolutionary times as well as nonnatural historical times) converge and clash throughout the neural interactions generating emotions, feelings, and the like.

The big picture that arises from all of this, if indeed such a picture can be drawn on the basis of the preceding, is one that LeDoux appears to endorse. This endorsement is expressed in a passage that Žižek undoubtedly has in mind when critically "supplementing" LeDoux's ideas in *The Parallax View*: "there is an imperfect set of connections between cognitive and emotional systems in the current stage of evolution of the human brain. This state of affairs is part of the price we pay for having newly evolved cognitive capacities that are not yet fully integrated into our brains. Although this is also a problem for other primates, it is particularly acute for humans, since the brain of our species, especially our cortex, was extensively rewired in the process of acquiring natural language functions."[120] Žižek's earlier-quoted comments on this passage rightly highlight how LeDoux views the discrepancies between cognition and emotion in the human central nervous system to be symptomatic of a negative imperfection, a deficiency or fault perhaps eventually to be remedied in the evolutionary future of humanity. Especially for a Lacanian, this lack (here a lack of coordination, harmonization, synthesis, and so on between different neurological functions) is positive as well as negative, a plus arising from a minus. And, like Lacan, LeDoux too identifies the cutting intervention of language as largely responsible for the severity of the cracks and fissures of desynchronization introduced into the human brain. Hence, Žižek, in consonance with a number of hypotheses recently put forward by various investigators into the brain,[121] speculates that in losing a presupposed prior evolutionarily integrated balance of neurological functions, people gain their very humanness, their denaturalized subjectivity with its peculiar, uniquely human affective potentials.

After formulating these observations in response to Damasio and LeDoux, Žižek proceeds to warn that one must mind "the gap that separates the brain sciences' unconscious from the Freudian Unconscious."[122] He argues that this gap is particularly palpable as regards the topic of emotions.[123] Other authors, such as Ansermet and Magistretti as well as Pommier, likewise caution against conflating the psychoanalytic unconscious with the unconscious often spoken of by those situated in the neurosciences, with the latter frequently referring to what analysis would identify as merely preconscious or nonconscious (rather than unconscious proper in the sense of being defensively occluded by such intrapsychical mechanisms as repression, disavowal, negation, rejection or foreclosure, and so on).[124] Interestingly, LeDoux himself issues the exact same warning: "Like Freud before them, cognitive scientists reject the view handed down from Descartes that mind and consciousness are the same. However, the cognitive unconscious is not the same as the Freudian or dynamic unconscious. The term cognitive unconscious merely implies that a lot of what the mind does goes on outside of consciousness, whereas the dynamic unconscious is a darker, more malevolent place where emotionally charged memories are shipped to do mental dirty work. To some extent, the dynamic unconscious can be conceived in terms of cognitive processes, but the term cognitive unconscious does not imply these dynamic operations."[125]

Damasio too is aware of and acknowledges these crucial differences.[126] Žižek and certain other psychoanalytically inclined interpreters of the neurosciences are quite justified in being concerned that many neuroscientists carelessly and indefensibly conflate Freud's unconscious with that of nonanalytic cognitive science. However, Damasio and LeDoux, the two neuroscientists mentioned by name in the section of *The Parallax View* under consideration in the present context, are notable exceptions to this tendency in the neuroscientific literature. What's more, although Žižek charges that Damasio problematically treats emotions (as distinct from feelings) as simply and straightforwardly natural in the sense of biologically hardwired—in his theory of the emotion-based self, Damasio indeed tends to speculate about a kernel of nature as the fixed foundation for additional later layers of higher-order nurture[127]—there are moments when Damasio appears to entertain the possibility of sociosymbolic mediation penetrating all the way down into the bedrock of even the most rudimentary bodily emotional ground of human being.[128]

The issue of neuroscientific naturalism (such as Damasio's, which is critiqued by Žižek) and its validity or invalidity vis-à-vis psychoanalysis will be returned to shortly. For the moment, four lines of thought in Damasio's defense apropos his alleged failure to account for the properly Freudian unconscious ought to be advanced. First, if the conclusions reached by my prior reexamination of the treatments of affective phenomena in Freud are correct, then the mutually exclusive contrast Žižek appeals to between an emotional unconscious and the Freudian unconscious is questionable, if not incorrect (for the same reasons that render problematic Lacan's dogmatic insistence that Freud flatly denies the existence of unconscious affects, an insistence upon which Žižek, at least in *The Parallax View*, evidently relies). Second, despite his general, prevailing emphasis upon the naturalness of the rudimentary emotional building blocks of the embodied human mind, Damasio (as I already have indicated) nonetheless occasionally allows for the possibility of cognitive (and, hence, cultural-linguistic) mediation and modulation even of physiological emotions, not just of psychologically parsed feelings. Third, Damasio's distinction between emotions and feelings, rather than threatening to reduce the unconscious to a roiling carnal sea of primitive impulses and passions (in a fashion counter to Freudian-Lacanian psychoanalysis), both dovetails with key features of Lacan's depiction of the unconscious and opens up new options for envisioning this set of mental dimensions central to psychoanalytic concerns.

As regards this third line of defense, Lacan continually combats the crude popular image of the unconscious as a dark, hidden depth, repeatedly maintaining (sometimes with recourse to topology, the mathematical science of surfaces) that the unconscious is, so to speak, profoundly superficial, situated right out in the open of the signifiers and structures within which subjects come to be and circulate.[129] Although Damasio, with respect to the topic of the unconscious, indeed often does focus on emotions as deep corporeal states of a naturally shaped body overlooked by conscious mental attention (i.e., as unfelt emotions), his distinction between emotions and feelings nonetheless implies a notion of the unconscious that is anything but complicit with the woefully unsophisticated picture thinking of old versions of depth psychology. The Damasian unconscious consists not so much of unfelt emotions bubbling away in the obscure, opaque depths of the flesh, but instead of the ensemble of intervening mechanisms and processes facilitating and interfering with the connections between emotions and feelings. In other words, Damasio's unconscious, like that of Lacan, is a thin, in-between function of gaps, the cause of discrepancies and splits between manifest features of the *parlêtre*. In this vein, it's important to recall that Damasio portrays emotions as public rather than private phenomena.[130] That is to say, emotional states, as corporeal events, are observable, at least in principle, by third parties, whether these third parties be scientists monitoring physiological changes in a human organism or nonscientific others taking stock of visible alterations expressed in and through the observed body of the person under consideration. (This is by contrast with feelings as mental events that, due to their first-person quality and corresponding experiential inaccessibility to other minds, can be "observed" only indirectly through linguistically conveyed reports.) So, an emotion à la Damasio, even if unfelt by the person whose body undergoes (un)said emotion, isn't associated by him with concealed depths. Quite the contrary: A Damasian emotion tends to be just as "out there" in the light of publicly visible day as the utterances spoken by the speaking subject. Along related lines, the Damasian unconscious subsists in the intervals between two types of manifestations: emotions as bodily conditions and thoughts as mental contents (which are potentially expressible in sociosymbolic terms, if not actually thus expressed). Thanks to these intervals as gaps between manifested emotions and their equally manifested translations, nontranslations, or mistranslations in ideationally inflected mediums—such intervals should be counted as constituting some of the "bars" barring the split subject ($) of Lacanian theory—emotions can be not only unfelt but also misfelt in any number of manners.

The fourth line of defense in favor of Damasio when faced with Žižek's criticisms requires circumnavigating back to the question of naturalism versus antinaturalism. The position I'm staking out here in response to this question could be succinctly encapsulated in Žižekian style as "Naturalism or antinaturalism? No, thanks—both are worse!"[131] Žižek closes the section of the fourth chapter of *The Parallax View* dealing with Damasio, a section entitled "Emotions Lie, or, Where Damasio Is Wrong," by insisting that

> we should bear in mind the basic anti-Darwinian lesson of psychoanalysis repeatedly emphasized by Lacan: man's radical and fundamental *dis*-adaptation, *mal*-adaptation, to his environs. At its most radical, "being-human" consists in an "uncoupling" from immersion in one's environs, in following a certain automatism which ignores the demands of adaptation—this is what the "death drive" ultimately amounts to. Psychoanalysis is not "deterministic" ("What I do is determined by unconscious processes"): the "death drive" as a self-sabotaging structure represents the minimum of freedom, of a behavior uncoupled from the utilitarian-survivalist attitude. The "death drive" means that the organism is no longer fully determined by its environs, that it "explodes/implodes" into a cycle of autonomous behavior.[132]

The invocation of the psychoanalytic notion of the death drive won't be treated in detail here; I've addressed Žižek's philosophical appropriation of the infamous Freudian *Todestrieb* at length elsewhere.[133] What I will address at present are the ways in which Žižek contrasts Damasio's naturalism with Lacan's antinaturalism. Both in the passage just quoted and others from the same portion of *The Parallax View*, one could read Žižek's remarks as referring to a partial, rather than a complete, denaturalization characteristic of human beings qua subjects (as indicated by the adverb "fully" in "the organism is no longer *fully* determined by its environs"). Interpreted in this manner, Žižek succeeds at resisting the temptation of an exaggerated pseudo-Lacanian antinaturalism insofar as he presupposes that the primitive emotions deposited within the base of humans' mammalian brains by archaic evolutionary conditions persist alongside sociosymbolic configurations and all the various subjectifying mediations they bring with them. Žižek's move here gestures at the notion of humans being creatures of incomplete, perpetually unfinished transformations, monstrous abortions of the failed sublations of a weak, anything-but-omnipotent dialectic incapable of digesting the animal bodies out of which it emerges without leaving behind remaining residual scraps. To resort to the lexicon of Marxism, this would be a dialectic of interminably "uneven development."

However, one also, perhaps less charitably, could construe Žižek as envisioning a total and thorough denaturalization befalling those living entities transubstantiated into $s by being taken up into the networks and webs of symbolic orders. In an essay entitled "From *objet a* to Subtraction," he indeed sounds as though he endorses an excessively extreme antinaturalism, hypothesizing a denaturalization without remainder that is brought about by the processes of subjectification affecting human beings (as he similarly sounds in the previously mentioned discussion of life 1.0 versus life 2.0 from *In Defense of Lost Causes*). In that essay, Žižek depicts "Freud's basic lesson" as the idea that "there is no 'human animal,' a human being is from its birth (and even before) torn out of the animal constraints, its instincts are 'denaturalized,' caught in the circularity of the (death-)drive, functioning 'beyond the pleasure principle.'"[134] Subsequently, in the same paragraph of this text, he suggests: "In a step further, one should even venture that there is no animal *tout court*, if by 'animal' we mean a living being fully fitting its environs: the lesson of Darwinism is that every harmonious balance in the exchange between an organism and its environs is a temporary fragile one, that it can explode at any moment; such a notion of animality as the balance disturbed by the human hubris is a human fantasy."[135]

Without contesting in the least the accuracy of this interpretation of Darwinian evolutionary theory, it ought to be noticed that Žižek appears partially to denaturalize nonhuman animals typically considered to be elements of "nature," which is imagined as a balanced harmony. (Žižek's larger body of philosophical work, especially in terms of his materialist ontology and corresponding theory of subjectivity, compels a radical rethinking of the protoconceptual pictures and metaphors constituting the images of nature informing standard varieties of naturalism.)[136] And although he partially denaturalizes nonhuman animals, he completely denaturalizes human animals, depicting such beings as always already "torn out of" their biological, instinctual animality. Although Damasio unambiguously evinces naturalist sympathies problematic from an orthodox Lacanian point of view, he and his like-minded brain researchers (such as LeDoux, Panksepp, and Keith Stanovich) don't subscribe to any sort of essentialist naturalism that unreservedly reduces cultural nurture to natural nature, the more-than-biomaterial subject to the physiology of the biological body in and of itself. In fact, in Damasio's defense, his multitiered model of the embodied self avoids the trap of the false dichotomy pitting antinaturalism against naturalism as an either-or choice (again, in Leninist-Stalinist phraseology, "both are worse!"). Sometimes Žižek himself elegantly navigates around this impasse. But, at select moments, he seems to force this false choice in elaborating his critical observations as regards, in particular, the neurosciences, evolutionary theory, and ecology.

Žižek points to a peculiarly human "*dis*-adaptation, *mal*-adaptation" as a fact that the neuroscientific perspectives of Damasio and LeDoux allegedly ignore or discount. However, as I will make evident in chapter 13 through a close reading of Panksepp's *Affective Neuroscience* in conjunction with further parsing of the proposals of Damasio and LeDoux, those aspects of neuroscience most relevant for forging a Freudian-Lacanian neuro-psychoanalysis are far from trafficking in the clumsy, unrefined oversimplifications of reductive strains of evolutionary psychology dogmatically insisting upon the ultimate centrality of "natural adaptation." (The non-Lacanian neuro-psychoanalysis of Solms and his collaborators will also be mentioned later in tandem with critical reflections on the engagements with the neurosciences elaborated by the Lacanian Pommier and the former Lacanian Green.) A specific combination of neuroscience and psychoanalysis requires critically amending and qualifying Žižek's Lacanian emphasis on the breadth and depth of human beings' identifying denaturalization: this denaturalization, as non- or antiadaptive relative to the presumed standards of deeply entrenched evolutionary rhythms and routines, is quite a bit less than absolute and all-pervasive.

The dis- or maladaptation of which Žižek speaks fails to break neatly and cleanly with older traces of "adaptation" as patterns of cognition and comportment laid down by much more archaic temporal strata of evolutionary history. A dis- or maladaptation as a sharp, absolute rupture with anything "natural" is, in a number of ways, far more adaptive than the partial and incomplete denaturalization that leaves humans stranded, as malformed Frankenstein-like jumbles of mismatched fragments thrown together over the course of unsynchronized sequences of aleatory events, halfway between nature and culture, between the lingering adaptations of evolutionary histories and those demanded by human histories past and present.[137] Additionally, when surfacing within the context of contemporary sociocultural circumstances, previously "adaptive" behaviors conditioned by ancient evolutionary pressures can be much more maladaptive than the thoughts and actions of subjects steered by the sociocultural mediators responsible for human disadaptation. Put differently, in the "inverted world" of human reality, dis- or maladaptation can be more adaptive than adaptation itself.

Related to this, the conflictuality of overriding interest to psychoanalysis (i.e., those conflicts analytic metapsychology portrays as tense fissures central to the structuration of psychical subjectivity) almost certainly includes conflicts between evolutionary nature (associated with adaptation) and nonevolutionary antinature (associated with dis- or maladaptation) as well as conflicts internal to the latter category. In *Civilization and Its Discontents*, Freud indicates that one of the root causes of this *Unbehagen* perpetually afflicting socialized humanity generation after generation is a defiant, rebellious constitutional base hardwired into the fundaments of "human nature" (the chief example of which is presumably innate instinctual quotas of id-level aggression and destructiveness).[138] "Civilization" (*Kultur*) can and does partially appropriate this base in a number of fashions to be turned to its own ends. But, whatever the extent of its partial successes, it repeatedly fails fully to tame and domesticate savage, resistant undercurrents whose archaic flows, however diluted by "civilizing" influences, continue to spill over into the present. Human subjectivity is constituted by neither nature nor antinature, but by the uneasy comingling and chaotic cross fertilizations between the poles of these two extremes, by the collisions of disparate temporal-structural layers sandwiched together so as to form multiple fault lines of tension. Nowhere are the consequences of humanity's abandonment to a limbo that is neither natural nor antinatural more apparent than in the peculiarities of human beings' emotional lives.

13.

AFFECTS ARE SIGNIFIERS

THE INFINITE JUDGMENT OF A LACANIAN
AFFECTIVE NEUROSCIENCE

Before turning to the task of elaborating a Freudian-Lacanian approach to the science of the emotional brain, a few general, preliminary remarks are in order. An irony acutely painful to partisans of psychoanalysis is that, over the course of the past several decades, Freud repeatedly has been pronounced dead and buried right at the moment when the life sciences are coming to confirm many of his core discoveries and insights, a moment of scientific vindication he anticipates starting with his earliest (proto)psychoanalytic writings.[1] The time of Freud's apparent defeat is precisely the time of his actual triumph. A little over a century ago, in the context of turn-of-the-century Europe, Freud was forced to argue fiercely against a deeply entrenched, widespread tendency to equate the mental with the conscious, a tendency responsible for some of the resistance to his central, fundamental ur-concept of the unconscious. Today, the assertion that not all of mental life is conscious is uncontroversial: every branch of nonpsychoanalytic psychology and neuroscience accepts as an empirically well-established truth the fact that the vast majority of mental life transpires below the threshold of explicit conscious awareness.[2] Nobody nowadays bickers about whether significant portions of the cognitive, emotional, and motivational processes of the brain or mind unfold in nonconscious ways. A number of eminent figures in the neurosciences have no problem whatsoever with acknowledging the existence of the psychoanalytic unconscious as a crucial, influential subsector of the broader category of the nonconscious. Additionally, there is an observation that ought to alleviate a typical Freudian-Lacanian worry aroused whenever anything having to do with the physical sciences is put forward as potentially relevant to psychoanalysis: contemporary neuroscientific research is far from pointing in the direction of a vulgar mechanistic materialism crudely reducing nurture to nature, the more than biological to pure biology alone. If anything, the neurosciences arguably are generating out of themselves a spontaneous dialectical materialism of a nonreductive sort in which the concepts and distinctions underpinning debates between already recognized varieties of naturalism and antinaturalism are being subverted and sublated in various fashions yet to be adequately appreciated.[3]

Reassuming a more precise angle of focus, Panksepp's *Affective Neuroscience*, a comprehensive overview of research into the emotional dimensions of both human and animal brains, provides a number of points of departure for the endeavor to entwine together the neurosciences, Freudian-Lacanian psychoanalysis, and the specific metapsychological perspectives on affective life outlined previously here. The fact that Panksepp refuses to limit his discussion of the emotional brain to human brains alone is based on his conviction that likely would ruffle more than a few Lacanian feathers: He insists that human and nonhuman mammals in particular share a great deal in common in terms of basic brain structures and functions, including emotional configurations and dynamics at various neural levels (especially at the most primitive levels of evolutionarily conserved neuroanatomy).[4] Panksepp hypothesizes that evolution has wired into the archaic base of the mammalian central nervous system a fixed set of seven rudimentary, elementary emotions and corresponding experiential tonalities. His taxonomy of the "major 'Blue-Ribbon, Grade A' emotional systems of the mammalian brain"[5] identifies four such systems, which are labeled "SEEKING" (stimulus-bound appetitive behavior and self-stimulation), "PANIC" (stimulus-bound distress vocalization and social attachment), "RAGE" (stimulus-bound biting and affective attack), and "FEAR" (stimulus-bound flight and escape behaviors).[6] Plus, there are, in mammals particularly, three additional systems, which are labeled "LUST," "CARE," and "PLAY".[7] These seven emotions and their accompanying tones of feeling are depicted as the primary colors of mammals' multihued affective lives.[8] (Solms and his coauthor Oliver Turnbull, in their sizable manifesto for a non-Lacanian neuropsychoanalysis *The Brain and the Inner World*, adopt Panksepp's hypothesis concerning "basic emotions").[9] Panksepp maintains that human beings are just as moved as nonhuman mammals by this set of foundational emotional elements. In this vein, Damasio, surveying a similar emotional landscape of primary affective phenomena, observes that the brain sculpted by evolution certainly looks as though it's much more prone to pain over pleasure: "There seem to be far more varieties of negative than positive emotions."[10] It would not be inappropriate to call to mind, in association with this, the factual detail that the early Freud, in *The Interpretation of Dreams*, originally christened the fundamental law of psychical life the "unpleasure principle" (later to be redesignated with the more familiar phrase "pleasure principle") so as to emphasize the avoidance of pain and suffering as the primary tendency of the psyche (instead of emphasizing the "positive" side of this principle, that is, the tendency to pursue ecstasy, gratification, joy, satisfaction, and so on).[11]

LeDoux, in his treatment of affective neuroscience, similarly proposes that "brain evolution is basically conservative."[12] LeDoux, like Panksepp, sees human affective life as resting on a base, shared with other mammals, of primitive emotional reactions and repertoires installed by ancient, long-gone evolutionary contexts and challenges. It should be noted once more that the "conservative" lingering-on of out-of-date neural machinery and programs is precisely part of what produces some of the tensions characteristic of the peculiarities distinguishing the unique "human condition" of such concern to psychoanalysis. As was stated in the earlier critical assessment of Žižek's reading of Damasio (in chapter 12), it would be mistaken to respond to the neuroscientific account of the persistence of evolutionarily archaic emotional systems hardwired into humans' brains with an antinaturalism, Lacanian or otherwise, which goes so far as to deny (at this juncture, quite untenably, not only theoretically but also empirically) that speaking subjects, thanks to the "castrating" intervention of symbolic orders, retain any significant links with their material or physical bodies as analyzed specifically by the natural sciences. (This response, often voiced by Lacanians and like-minded theorists, posits an always-already complete denaturalization as essential to the existence of subjectivity proper.) As partial rather than complete, the denaturalization that befalls those submitted to sociosymbolic subjectification splits human subjects between, as it were, nature and antinature, failing fully to liquidate the former retroactively and without remainder; the antagonisms and discrepancies between natural and antinatural residues embedded as strata and currents uneasily cohabitating within the psychical apparatus contribute to the splitting (*Spaltung*) central to the barred subject ($). Moreover, despite the understandable insistence of Panksepp and LeDoux on the reality of basic emotional systems in the brains of all mammals alike, neither of these researchers advance a naturalism according to which humans are nothing more than highly elaborate animal organisms whose sentiments and subjectivities can be entirely explained away through appeals to the secular god of Evolution with a capital E, an incarnation of Nature as really-existent big Other.

In light of my nascent version of neuro-psychoanalysis, LeDoux's work on the brain is appealing for several reasons. Apart from generally being sympathetic to psychoanalysis insofar as he both admits the existence of the analytic unconscious and highlights the significant role of language in the neuromental lives of human subjects, LeDoux claims again and again that, apropos affective phenomena, conscious awareness is the exception rather than the rule.[13] (Panksepp concurs,[14] likewise asserting, "Most of emotional processing, as of every other psychobehavioral process, is done at an unconscious level.")[15] And, in line with an established consensus in the neurosciences, LeDoux is adamant that a dialectic between genetic nature and epigenetic or nongenetic (with "nongenetic" encompassing behavioral and symbolic factors) nurture shapes emotional and other brain functions such that neither a simplistic biologism nor an equally unsophisticated social constructivism can offer remotely plausible explanations for affects (and many other things) in human beings.[16] (Eva Jablonka and Marion J. Lamb's four-dimensional analysis of evolution, taking into consideration genetic, epigenetic, behavioral, and symbolic dimensions, provides perhaps the best evolutionary-theoretic complement to this neuroscientific research and its results.[17] These two authors contend that "it is bad biology to think about the nervous system in isolation"[18] and that "the boundaries between the social sciences and biology are being broken down. People are aware that neither social nor biological evolution can be studied in isolation.")[19] The potentials of LeDoux's neuroscientific delineations of human emotional life for a Freudian-Lacanian neuro-psychoanalytic metapsychology of affect are manifest in the closing pages of his book *The Emotional Brain*: "Consciousness is neither the prerequisite to nor the same thing as the capacity to think and reason. An animal can solve lots of problems without being overtly conscious of what it is doing and why it is doing it. Obviously, consciousness elevates thinking to a new level, but it isn't the same thing as thinking."[20] After these statements echoing Freud's century-old gesture of decoupling thinking from consciousness—the psychoanalytic unconscious involves forms of thinking minus an accompanying reflexive self-awareness (i.e., "I think without thinking that I think")—LeDoux proceeds to discuss affective phenomena:

> Emotional feelings result when we become consciously aware that an emotion system of the brain is active. Any organism that has consciousness also

has feelings. However, feelings will be different in a brain that can classify the world linguistically and categorize experiences in words than in a brain that cannot. The difference between fear, anxiety, terror, apprehension, and the like would not be possible without language. At the same time, none of these words would have any point if it were not for the existence of an underlying emotion system that generates the brain states and bodily expressions to which these words apply. Emotions evolved not as conscious feelings, linguistically differentiated or otherwise, but as brain states and bodily responses. The brain states and bodily responses are the fundamental facts of an emotion, and the conscious feelings are the frills that have added icing to the emotional cake.[21]

According to LeDoux's dialectical model, the initial impetus and oomph under-lying affective life originates with and arises from evolutionarily primal and primary corporeal emotions of a fundamental and foundational nature (i.e., the emotions identified by Panksepp in his seven-category taxonomy). How-ever, in the exceptional animals that are human beings as *parlêtres*, the ener-getic, vital flows of these old mammalian juices run smack into language, being channeled through the mediating networks of the linguistic-representational structures constitutive of speaking subjectivities. Such structures then come to exert a reciprocal counterinfluence on these archaic influences, refracting, for instance, the effects of the FEAR and PANIC systems into a much more fine-grained spectrum of feelings (i.e., "fear, anxiety, terror, apprehension, and the like": Damasio, in *Descartes' Error*, similarly distinguishes between "pri-mary emotions" and "secondary emotions").[22] But, a pressing question must be posed at this juncture: do these thus refracted feelings react back on their emotional bases, dialectically transforming their corporeal causes or sources, and, if so, to what extent?

Despite elsewhere indicating that he indeed would at least admit and enter-tain the possibility of linguistic-representational nurture reflexively altering embodied emotional nature in a thoroughly dialectical fashion, LeDoux, at the very end of the last block quotation in the previous paragraph, seems to risk regressing back to a nondialectical position according to which alterations to affective life wrought by the nonnatural or not-entirely-natural dimen-sions determinative of humanity's distinguishing peculiarities are reduced to an ineffectual secondary status as mere window dressing arrayed around the fringes of a fixed, unchanged biomaterial ground ("the conscious feelings are the frills that have added icing to the emotional cake"). Once more, a brief reminder about the previous discussion of Žižek's perspective on these matters (in chapter 12) is appropriate. Two points are particularly topical here: First, this moment in LeDoux's reflections represents a naturalist tendency within even the most nonreductive neuroscientific materialisms (that of not only LeDoux but also Damasio)[23] that warrant the Lacan-inspired criticisms Žižek levels against Damasio and LeDoux (the prior defense of these latter two relies on other moments in their writings when they steer clear of nondialectical reductivism). Second, this same moment in the concluding pages of *The Emotional Brain* overlooks something *The Parallax View* rightly and insightfully highlights, namely, that the gap between the biological and the more-than-biological comes to function as itself an affective factor, rather than affective phenomena falling exclusively on one side or the other of this gap (i.e., as either emotions of a biological nature or feelings of a more-than-biological nurture). Maybe what makes an affect a specifically human experience (as distinct from the bodily emotions and psychological feelings evidently also undergone by nonhuman sentient mammals) is its bearing witness to humanity's status as stranded in an ontological limbo between nature and antinature, torn between split planes of existence irrupting out of the immanence of a self-sundering material Real.[24]

Returning to more empirical terrain and examining Panksepp's work in greater depth promises to be fruitful. Several times, he stresses that neuroplasticity holds for emotional systems as much as for other components of human neuroanatomy.[25] In relation to this, he (like both Damasio and LeDoux) grants that cognitive mediations and modulations, involving complex symbolic and linguistic representational constellations, play significant roles in coloring and inflecting affective phenomena in human life;[26] a two-way street of dialectical and reciprocal co-determination connects cognition and emotion for beings with highly developed cerebral cortices in addition to other, "lower" neural components left over from archaic evolutionary histories and shared with various other animal organisms.[27] Panksepp goes so far as to argue, as regards humans, that "one can never capture innate emotional dynamics in their pure form, except perhaps when they are aroused artificially by direct stimulation of brain areas where those operating systems are most concentrated."[28] Reiterating this argument later, he states:

> It is becoming increasingly clear that humans have as many instinctual operating systems in their brains as other mammals. However, in mature humans such instinctual processes may be difficult to observe because they are no longer expressed directly in adult behavior but instead are filtered and modified

by higher cognitive activity. Thus, in adult humans, many instincts manifest themselves only as subtle psychological tendencies, such as subjective feeling states, which provide internal guidance to behavior. The reason many scholars who know little about modern brain research are still willing to assert that human behavior is not controlled by instinctual processes is because many of our operating systems are in fact very "open" and hence very prone to be modified by the vast layers of cognitive and affective complexity that learning permits. Still, the failure of psychology to deal effectively with the nature of the many instinctual systems of human and animal brains remains one of the great failings of the discipline. The converse could be said for neuroscience.[29]

A number of comments are called for here. To begin with, in the second half of this quotation, Panksepp accurately and succinctly diagnoses the parallel short-comings of "psychology" (as associated with nurture-centric constructivism) and "neuroscience" (as associated with nature-centric biologism) with respect to the (partially obsolete) debate between naturalism and antinaturalism. In Panksepp's view, the plasticity of the human central nervous system, a plasticity affecting its emotional structures and dynamics, consists of the intertwining of inflexible "closed" and flexible "open" neural systems (i.e., on the one hand, those systems rigidly wired by genetics to produce relatively invariant patterns of cognition and comportment, and, on the other hand, those systems fluidly wired to be rewired by epigenetic or nongenetic accidents, contingencies, vari-ables, and so on).[30]

In response to Panksepp, someone with Hegelian or psychoanalytic leanings might be inclined to retort that the purportedly epistemological inaccessibil-ity of brute, raw instinctual emotions is not strictly and solely epistemological. Shouldn't Panksepp's spontaneous Kantianism, in which "pure" instinctual emotions are treated as thinkable-yet-unknowable noumenal things-in-them-selves that exist beyond the epistemologically accessible affective phenomena "filtered and modified by higher cognitive activity," be met with a Hegelian-ism speculating that this ostensible epistemological inaccessibility already directly discloses the "Thing itself," the ontological Real supposedly barred by subjective reflection? In other words, certain versions of Hegelian philoso-phy and Freudian-Lacanian psychoanalytic metapsychology would insist that the general absence of brute, raw instinctual emotions in the manifestations of specifically human existence is a testament to the thoroughgoing dialecti-cal digestion of the natural by the more-than-natural, rather than a reflection of a noumenal-phenomenal split between these two dimensions depicted as separate and distinct realms of a neatly partitioned, two-tiered reality, one inaccessible (i.e., the natural or biological), the other accessible (i.e., the more-than-natural/biological). Pommier, whose Lacanian glosses on the neurosciences I will address in more detail later, appears to adopt a stance along these lines, maintaining that "once the entry into speech has been accomplished, 'pure sensation' becomes that from which we exile ourselves."[31] He adds that conceding this necessitates abandoning the "myth of an original paradise, that of our improbable animality."[32]

Of course, to be perfectly honest and exact, portraying Panksepp as a spontaneous Kantian treating basic emotions (i.e., his seven "primary colors" of mammalian affective life) as akin to the notorious *Ding an sich* is far from fair. His denial of epistemological access to these emotional fundaments is not without qualification (in contrast with Kant's unqualified denial of access to the noumenal realm lying forever beyond "the limits of possible experience"). Panksepp posits that there are exceptional circumstances in which these primal constituents of human bodily being come to light in their undiluted immediacy. However, he stresses the artificiality of these circumstances; in addition to the experimental tools and techniques of the laboratory that he has in mind, one might also imagine, taking into account psychoanalytic and sociopolitical considerations, brutal ordeals and overwhelming traumas as excessive "limit experiences" violently unleashing unprocessed corporeal intensities pitilessly reducing those who suffer these experiences to the dehumanized state of naked animality, of convulsing, writhing flesh. This precise qualification noted by Panksepp signals an inversion that itself arguably is constitutive of the human condition: the reversal of the respective positions or roles of, so to speak, first and second natures (or Žižek's life 1.0 and life 2.0), a reversal in which the secondary becomes the primary and vice versa.

Such an inversion can be clarified further through reference to Giorgio Agamben's *Homo Sacer*. Therein, Agamben examines the distinction, rooted in the language of ancient Greece, between "*zoē*, which expressed the simple fact of living common to all living beings (animals, men, or gods), and *bios*, which indicated the form or way of living proper to an individual or a group."[33] Without getting bogged down in what would be, in the present context, a tangential exegesis of Agamben's genealogy of the distinction between *zoē* and *bios* in relation to structures of political sovereignty (a genealogy inspired by both Nietzsche and Foucault and particularly indebted to the latter's concept of "biopower"),[34] it suffices for now to draw attention to his contention that, in the always-already established individual and group forms or ways of life into which humans are thrown (i.e., *bios*), *zoē* as "bare life" is "produced" instead of being given.[35] As he puts it in *State of Exception*: "There are not *first* life as a natural biological given and anomie as the state of nature, and *then* their implication in law through the state of exception. On the contrary, the very possibility of distinguishing life and law, anomie and *nomos*, coincides with their articulation in the biopolitical machine. Bare life is a product of the machine and not something that preexists it."[36] In other words, in tandem with his rejection of standard, traditional "state of nature" narratives about humanity's transition from pre-sociohistorical *zoē* red in tooth and nail to the sociohistorical *bios* of the *polis* as established on the basis of a "social contract,"[37] Agamben proposes that humans are, at a default level, beings of *bios* (i.e., life organized and embellished by more-than-biological languages, institutions, practices, and so on) rather than creatures of *zoē*. Put differently, although the bare life that is *zoē* often is imagined as a first nature ontogenetically and phylogenetically preceding *bios* as the second nature of a nonbare life clothed by the artificial fabrications of language, society, and history, Agamben's remarks correctly point out that exceptional "artificial" means (for him, the means being actions taken by established sovereign power with respect to the subject-bodies it rules over) are necessary to strip away the default second-nature-become-first-nature that is *bios*. In the inverted world of human life, *zoē* is correspondingly a first-nature-become-secondary, an exception to the rule of *bios* that appears, in Agambenian parlance, exclusively in legal-political "states of exception" enacted in the names of unusual circumstances and alleged crises.[38]

To circumnavigate back to Panksepp and neuroscientific matters, a combination of Agamben's handling of the *zoē-bios* distinction with my position which is neither naturalist nor antinaturalist, a position centered on a hypothesized failed dialectic of incomplete denaturalization that is constitutive of human forms of subjectivity, enables the following to be said apropos a Lacan-influenced neuro-psychoanalytic metapsychology of affect: In human beings, the *zoē* of bare emotional life—this life doesn't disappear with the advent of the *bios* of feelings and the array of their accompanying conditions of possibility, but is only partially eclipsed and absorbed by the mediating matrices giving shape to *bios*—is fractured, like Damasio's core self, into unsublated brute, raw basic emotions (which manifest themselves solely in rare, extreme conditions) and sublated feelings as sociosymbolically translated emotions (or even, following Žižek, as affective states aroused by the gap between emotions and feelings). In Žižek's parlance, the life 1.0 of *zoē*, although inverted into the produced exception instead of the given rule in the never-finished denaturalizations brought about by subjectification, resists being taken up without remainder into the nonnatural or not-wholly-natural defiles of *bios* as life 2.0. The "updates" don't erase entirely the earlier versions, with bugs, glitches, and loopholes being generated by the unsynthesized layering of these materialized temporal-historical strata.

Panksepp is careful to stipulate that, despite their interpenetrating mutual entanglements, cognitive and emotional aspects of the human central nervous system nonetheless remain somewhat distinct and distinguishable.[39] One shouldn't sloppily lump them together into a muddy mess through an inelegantly quick-and-easy pseudodialectical approach that simply blurs the lines of conceptual demarcations in its haste to unite with what is imagined to be reality's subtle shades of grey. For Panksepp, the differences between cognition and emotion are at least as important to keep in view as the fact of their reciprocal, entwined relatedness insofar as these differences are the sites of palpable friction between conflicting components and tendencies of subjects' incompletely integrated, hodgepodge brains. He claims that, although the affective lives of human beings are substantially inflected by cognitive (i.e., cultural, ideational, linguistic, representational, social, symbolic, and so on) mediations, the compelling, gripping, potent pulsations of emotional phenomena issue forth from a comparatively ancient, primitive neural base.[40] Furthermore, he maintains that an imbalance obtains between cognition and emotion as unequal partners in mental life: "emotions and regulatory feelings have stronger effects on cognitions than the other way around."[41] In terms of the calibration constitutive of (neuro)plasticity between open flexibility and closed inflexibility, Panksepp stresses that a certain degree of genetic closure at the level of basic emotional systems (deposited in brains over the course of the old, slow-moving currents of evolutionary times) sets limiting boundaries for the bandwidths of possible epigenetic or nongenetic openness to denaturalizing alterations of affective spectrums (alterations unfolding at temporal rhythms and rates of comparatively much faster speeds than natural-qua-evolutionary times): "the ability of the human cortex to think and to fantasize, and thereby to pursue many unique paths of human cultural evolution, can dilute, mold, modify, and focus the dictates of these systems, but it cannot eliminate them."[42] (Damasio argues for a similar perspective.)[43]

To segue into a space of overlap between the neurosciences and Lacanian metapsychology, not only is the human brain a concrete, biomaterial point of condensation for the only partially compatible temporal tracks of nonhuman evolutionary phylogeny and human sociohistorical phylogeny, but, as psychoanalysis starting with Freud repeatedly contends, various streams and sedimentations of subjective ontogenesis generate out of themselves, as a cacophonous ensemble, disharmonies and clashes that are the conflicts around which psychical subjects are structured. As indicated in a much earlier discussion (in chapter 11), Lacan's distinction between *lalangue* and *la langue* is quite relevant in the context of the current analysis. Pommier says something odd that sounds less strange once one appreciates select details of Lacan's rich, multifaceted treatments of language: "neuroscientists forget . . . speech, . . . the support of which, far from being spiritual, is also material."[44] The oddness has to do with the fact that ample neuroscientific attention has been paid to language, at least in the Lacanian sense of *la langue*, which refers to the natural languages usually acquired by children and employed by linguistically competent members of given groups of language users. Pommier's insistence on the material dimension of "speech" (*la parole*) is crucial here: when it comes to both the spoken and the written, Freudian-Lacanian psychoanalytic metapsychology is at least as concerned with materiality as with meaning. The primary process mentation of *lalangue*, as a *jouis-sens* playing with phonemes and graphemes, flows through sounds and images in ways unconstrained by secondary process mentation's concerns to obey the constraining rules of a language's (as *une langue*) syntax and semantics so as to succeed at producing intersubjectively recognizable conventional significance. An analyst, in listening to an analysand's speech, should be as attentive to the murmurings of meaningless *lalangue* as to the meaningful utterances of *la langue* spoken by the (self-) conscious speaker on the couch. When Lacan draws attention to the material signifier (as being different from the sign), this is part of what's at stake at those moments.[45] This is one of the two fundamental aspects of language that Pommier sees the neurosciences overlooking (the other being the links between language and Otherness as understood in Lacanian theory, a topic to be taken up soon below).

As regards *lalangue* as distinct from *la langue*, Changeux, who Pommier cites in beginning to weave a neuro-psychoanalytic perspective on language,[46] indeed does touch upon infantile babbling in a neurological account of language acquisition.[47] One of Changeux's key theses is his assertion that "to learn is to eliminate."[48] He hypothesizes that the developing brain learns numerous things of various sorts through playing "cognitive games." These games involve the brain spontaneously generating "pre-representations," an activity that could be described as a process of actively fantasizing, imagining, or hallucinating at the surrounding world, creatively concocting "hypotheses" projected onto enveloping environs.[49] In terms of language learning specifically—it ought to be noted in passing that Changeux sympathetically refers to the Saussurian structural linguistics dear to Lacan and Lacanians in his reflections on language[50]—this means that infantile babbling is a type of game-playing in which a gurgling multitude of sounds automatically are experimented with by the young subject-to-be. Through interactions with the environment, especially the social milieus of language-using adult others, the infant is prompted to pare down the proliferating plethora of noises of its baby tongue (i.e., *lalangue*) so as to give voice to the narrower set of well-ordered phonemes recognized by the mother tongue (i.e., *la langue*) into which he/she is being inducted. (This is analogous to Kant's account, in his *Anthropology from a Pragmatic Point of View*, of how the externally dictated discipline of education and socialization transforms the excessive, unruly freedom of the human child as pre- or protorational into the tamed and domesticated autonomy of the adult rational subject.)[51] In other words, early childhood language acquisition isn't so much a matter of building up *une langue*; it's more a matter of tearing down and eliminating (or, more accurately, attempting to eliminate) the nonsensical meanderings and ramblings of *lalangue*, of the cognitive games *jouis-sens* plays with the vocal apparatus. *La langue* is part of what remains of *lalangue* after the contextually imposed trimming and snipping of "symbolic castration" by the transsubjective Other and intersubjective others of the linguistic universes into which the child is inserted has been undergone. However, psychoanalysis especially divulges veritable mountains of evidence that, sheltering within the *parlêtre* of *la langue*, vestiges of *lalangue* continue to manifest themselves, particularly in the forms familiar from the Freudian "psychopathology of everyday life," namely, dreams, jokes, parapraxes, slips of the tongue, and so on; the neuroscientific study of language would do well to consider more thoroughly such evidence and phenomena.

Apropos neurology, Changeux's theory of learning reflects what LeDoux characterizes as the "use it or lose it" doctrine of neural "selectionism." According to this doctrine, the initial "exuberance" of an infant's neural networks—there are more synaptic connections present in early stages of development than will be needed later by the more mature organism—is pruned down through "subtraction," through the exchanges between organism and environment determining which connections will be used (and, hence, will be kept) and which ones won't be used (and, hence, will be allowed to atrophy or completely wither away).[52] Changeux describes this selectionist process as "the epigenetic stabilization of common neural networks"[53] (i.e., a social dynamic mobilizing mirror neurons in which the language-supporting structures of the young child's brain are sculpted through pruning to be more or less sufficiently similar, for purposes of linguistic acculturation, to his/her older fluent socio-symbolic others).[54]

Pommier recapitulates everything summarized in the preceding para-graphs.[55] The Lacanian supplement he adds to the neuroscientific theories is an emphasis on the irreducible role of intersubjective and transsubjective variables (i.e., Imaginary others and Symbolic Others) in the genesis of sociosymbolic subjectivity in the immature subject-to-be. Pommier adamantly maintains that spontaneous endogenous developments within the physiological systems of the nascent *parlêtre* don't account for language acquisition and the subjectifi-cation it brings with it. That is to say, the eliminations and selections imposed on the child's neural networks—these eliminations and selections are pruning processes through which the wild thickets of *lalangue*'s *jouis-sens*-laden bab-blings (i.e., primary processes) are cut down (albeit, for psychoanalysis, not purged altogether without remainder) into the narrower confines of recogniz-ably meaningful forms of *une langue* (i.e., secondary processes)—are imposed thanks to the interactive interventions of significant (and signifying) others actively engaging with the child. For Pommier, "the signification of sounds depends on a sense given by an exterior authority: it breaks with the organicist model of auto-organization. This rupture with organizational self-sufficiency distinguishes itself from the muscular model. Organicism cannot render an account of neuronal modeling, since the only efficacious sonorities are those that signify something for the Other."[56] He quickly proceeds to link this with a more general theme emerging from the life sciences and philosophical inter-pretations of them: the plastic human brain in particular is genetically destined to be turned over to shaping vicissitudes far from entirely governed by evo-lutionary-genetic influences alone, and is naturally preprogrammed by genet-ics to be nonnaturally reprogrammed by epigenetics or nongenetics; in short, hardwired to be rewired.[57] As Pommier puts it regarding the Lacanian Other as the locus of epigenetic or nongenetic factors of a symbolico-linguistic sort, "It is henceforth innate that it wouldn't be innate";[58] or, as his fellow Lacanian neurosympathizers Ansermet and Magistretti articulate the same idea, it is "as though, when all is said and done, the individual were to appear genetically determined not to be genetically determined."[59]

To make one last fast-and-loose reference to Žižek's contrast between life 1.0 and life 2.0, an argument parallel to the one I laid out in chapter 12 apropos the layering of life 1.0 and life 2.0 that is neither natural nor antinatural (i.e., the critique of Žižek's critique of Damasio's alleged naturalism) can and should be made with regard to a Lacanian neuro-psychoanalytic recasting of the distinction between *lalangue* and *la langue*: just as life 1.0 isn't entirely erased after the fact of the genesis of life 2.0, *lalangue* (here analogous to life 1.0) likewise lingers on as indelible traces of primary process *jouis-sens* infused within and between the secondary process matrices of *la langue* (here analogous to life 2.0). Of course, such a claim is merely in good keeping with Freudian orthodoxy insofar as psychoanalysis, despite certain widespread misunderstandings, isn't a developmental psychology, at least not in any straightforward sense. More precisely, due to what Freud characterizes as the "timelessness" of the unconscious,[60] prior phases of ontogenetic development (i.e., past periods of psychical experience and structure) are not expunged and replaced by subsequent phases of development. Instead, the effects of the passage of time on the psyche involve the cumulative sedimentation of interacting layers, rather than successive demolitions of the old by the new (this point being illustrated by Freud with that image of the city of Rome in which all of the strata of its historical development are preserved side by side, sandwiched together).[61] But, what relevance does this have for a Freudian-Lacanian neuro-psychoanalysis of affective life?

The sociosymbolically subjectified *parlêtre* comes to consist (inconsistently) of, so to speak, a sort of Tower of Babel cobbled together out of a jumble mixing together flows and assemblages of both "immature" *lalangue* (which, as suffused with *jouis-sens*, is neither strictly affective-energetic nor signifying-structural) and "mature" *la langue*. Additionally, the affect-languages of the latter (i.e., the words and phrases of natural languages designating emotions and feelings) are notoriously ambiguous and vague. In fact, one of the most familiar ways in which people arrive at a palpable awareness of the limits of language is when they wrestle with the clumsy, clunky inadequacy of their mother tongue in trying to express linguistically the subtle nuances and fine-grained shades of fluid affective phenomena. The combination of affectively influential (yet consciously difficult-to-recognize) associations at the level of *lalangue* with the superimposed level of the inelegant affect-languages of *la langue* makes for a confusing and dizzyingly disorienting intrapsychical and subjective cacophony of tongues, a multivoiced soliloquy that sometimes loudly clamors and sometimes softly murmurs. Consequently, knowing how, what, and why one feels what one feels can be nearly impossible in certain instances. With this in mind, it now will be productive to circumnavigate back to the neurosciences of the emotional brain.

Pansepp mentions the complications that considerations of language introduce into the heart of affective neuroscience. From his perspective, the key problem here is one of constructing an accurate taxonomy of affects: how should primary and secondary emotions, various feeling states, and related phenomena be classified, and with what linguistic labels?[62] Pansepp directly evinces the concern that the affect-vocabularies of natural languages are too equivocal and imprecise to furnish affective neuroscience with concept-terms of sufficient clarity and distinctness to carve with rigorous representational precision the realities of the emotional brain at, as it were, its real joints. This is the exact juncture at which a proper Hegelian gesture with respect to Pansepp's neuroscience of affects is both possible and productive, a gesture mobilizing the interrelated life-scientific facts and notions of neuroplasticity and epigenetics.[63] (It's no accident that Malabou's philosophically fruitful turn to the neurosciences was initially motivated by her sophisticated appreciation of the role of plasticity in Hegel's anthropology.)[64] The Hegel-style move to be made in this context is to assert that the difficulty of naming affective phenomena is not external to the thing itself. Worded differently, the ambiguities, vagueness, equivocations, and imprecision of the intermingled affect-languages of both *lalangue* and *les langues* don't remain neatly confined to a separate representational outside (say, scientific discourses supposedly apart from their objects of investigation) without effects on neurologically grounded emotional being. Or, put in yet other terms, the uncertainties Pansepp highlights that raise doubts about any taxonomy in affective neuroscience aren't just indicative of purely epistemological-representational inadequacies internal to scientific discourses; these uncertainties reflect the uncertainties of affective life in and of itself, a life in which felt feelings circulate among a much vaster range of unfelt and misfelt feelings.

This Hegelian gesture vis-à-vis Pansepp is justified for a number of reasons, many of which I have formulated already. To begin with, neuroplasticity is now a well-established, undisputed matter of scientific fact. Part of what the side of plasticity involving flexibility and malleability entails is the brain's genetically dictated openness to epigenetic or nongenetic dictates.[65] In Lacanian eyes, symbolic orders constitute one of the most significant sources (if not the most significant source) of more-than-genetic factors influential in the vicissitudes of ontogenetic subject formation. The physiologically and psychologically momentous period of language acquisition is a time during which (in Lacanese) *lalangue* is affected by *la langue* (an affecting for which neuroplasticity is one of the crucial material conditions of its very possibility that is contingent yet *a priori*).[66] This transition into linguistically mediated subjectivity, the time of becoming a speaking subject qua $, is a passage through which the exogenous imposition of language as *la langue* becomes metabolized by the living being undergoing this, digested, and thereby appropriated as endogenous (i.e., subjectified insofar as subjectification arises from introjections of others and internalizations of symbolic orders as big Others). Obviously, one sizable sector of the language or languages thus identified with consists of vocabularies for affective phenomena. Once created on these bases and in these ways, the *parlêtre*, the speaking subject who speaks to him-/herself and others about, among other things, affective phenomena using arguably hazy and inexact affect-vocabularies, is autoaffecting, an autoaffection that both (re)acts on the neural foundations participating in its generation and is routed through the heteroaffective mediation of others and Others.

Furthermore, it's worth remembering at this point that the contemporary sciences of the brain emphasize the co-penetrating entanglements of the cognitive and emotional systems of the massively interconnected human central nervous system (or, translated into Lacan's terminology, signifiers and affects aren't, in actuality if not in theory, cleanly partitioned and independent in relation to each other). This means that the cognitive dimension of affect-language gets woven into the emotional dimension of affects themselves, setting in motion an oscillating, back-and-forth dialectic of mutual, two-way modulation between affects and signifiers. (LeDoux draws attention to this in less technical terms.)[67] Consequently, the reflexive autoaffective dynamics of the *parlêtre* qua $, dynamics in which the confusing muddiness of the emotional lexicons of overlapping *lalangue* and *la langue* swirls about, result in fuzzy and imprecise affect-vocabularies literally bedding down in the brain itself, sculpting and rewiring this groundless neural ground. Hence, Panksepp's lack of Hegelian sensibilities when considering the linguistic naming and representation of emotions and feelings is an instructive example of what Pommier might mean when he accuses neuroscientists of "forgetting" the issue of language (particularly language as understood in Lacanian psychoanalytic theory).[68] This also lends illustrative support to Pommier's contention that "more and more of the numerous results of the neurosciences are illegible without psychoanalysis."[69]

A similar absence of Hegelian finesse afflicts the non-Lacanian neuro-psychoanalysis advocated by Solms. Alluding to both Spinoza and the American analytic philosopher of mind Donald Davidson, he and his collaborators proclaim "dual-aspect monism" to be the ontological framework through which their particular version of the synthesis of the neurosciences and psychoanalysis approaches the central matter of the mind-body relationship.[70] In either its Spinozist or Davidsonian incarnations, this framework risks maintaining too sharp a demarcating line of nondialectical distinction between mental and physical dimensions (the presupposed monistic ontological underbelly posited by dual-aspect or anomalous monism remains epistemologically inaccessible, a noumenal substratum *an sich*).[71] A philosophical paradigm sharply partitioning mind and body as separate and autonomous "aspects" (à la Spinoza's "attributes") is in danger of theoretically blinding its adherents to, among other things, precisely the phenomena brought out in stark relief through the immediately preceding Hegelian critique of Panksepp: theoretically postulating the mental-subjective and the physical-objective as independent angles of stratified refraction appears not to allow for taking into account the full extent of the consequences of linguistic mediation (including the mediations of affect-languages) on subjects emerging out of plastic neural systems sustaining both auto- and heteroaffections.

These dangers and difficulties aside, Solms and Turnbull helpfully highlight a number of interesting sites of overlap between psychoanalysis and the neurosciences. In particular, they emphasize, in a resonation with earlier discussions, the various important roles of neurologically hardwired "blanks" in the human brain, namely, hardwired absences of hardwiring. Such preprogrammed openings, openings for reprogramming, are, in their view, crucial conditions for the potential eventual genesis of the forms of subjectivity familiar to quotidian experience generally and psychoanalytic clinical practice specifically. Appropriating Panksepp's taxonomy of the evolutionarily primary basic emotion systems shared between humans and other mammals, Solms and Turnbull associate the SEEKING system with the Freudian notion of the id-level seat of the drives, that is, the motivational foundations of the libidinal economy. In so doing, they claim that Freud's crucial thesis regarding the "objectless" status of the drives[72] is vindicated by the neuroscientific discovery that the SEEKING system acquires its orienting coordinates (i.e., what exactly, in terms of objects and states of affairs, is craved, desired, wanted, and so on) exclusively over time through experience, learning, and so on.[73]

Apart from the SEEKING system, Solms and Turnbull, when addressing as a whole Panksepp's overall taxonomic schema for the evolutionary foundations of the emotional brain, are anxious to underscore that adopting this schema isn't tantamount to capitulating to a reductive naturalism or mechanistic materialism eliminating much of what a psychoanalytic approach would wish to conserve. (In relation to this, one could maintain that Freud never repudiated without reservations the neurosciences *tout court*, only the reductive or mechanistic versions of them prevalent at the time, versions centered on establishing neuroanatomical localizations of mental processes rather than appreciating these processes as involving dynamics distributed across multiple neural networks and subsystems.)[74] While admitting that the genetically shaped brain is hardly a tabula rasa to be overwritten by epigenetic or nongenetic variables— this empiricist-style (à la Locke and Hume) image of the brain is empirically quite false[75]—Solms and Turnbull nonetheless repeatedly stress (much more so than Panksepp) that the human brain's various blanks are the plastic openings through which the unique complexities of a human subject's life sculpt the idiosyncratic contours of a person's absolutely singular brain and corresponding psyche.[76] As Damasio puts it, "Each brain is unique."[77] One can't help but hear echoes of the original French title of the Lacanian neuro-psychoanalytic book by Ansermet and Magistretti: "To each his own brain" (*À chacun son cerveau*).

In what seems to be a strangely neglected book, *La causalité psychique: Entre nature et culture* (1995), the ex-Lacanian André Green directly confronts some of the challenging, vexing issues haunting any effort to bring together psychoanalysis and the neurosciences. (Borrowing David Chalmers's phrase,[78] one could credit Green with tackling head-on the neuro-psychoanalytic version of the "hard problem" around which mind-body debates in Anglo-American analytic philosophy orbit.) Green touches on a number of claims and topics dealt with earlier here: the significant influence of language as a higher-order cognitive function on the embodied psyche;[79] the contextual mediation of the brain as dependent for its structures and dynamics on its particular physical and cultural-symbolic environs;[80] the inseparable entanglement of nature and nurture in human subjects, to the point of the difference often being indiscernible for all intents and purposes;[81] the biologically inborn incompleteness of human beings as naturally destining humans to sociosexual denaturalization;[82] the drive-level intersections at which soma and psyche are soldered to each other while nonetheless remaining relatively distinct from one another.[83] For anyone acquainted with Lacan's writings, the title of Green's book is likely to call to mind the *écrit* "Presentation on Psychical Causality" (1946). Therein, Lacan speaks of "the intersection of the biological and the social."[84] He proceeds to remark that "man is far more than his body, even though he can know [*savoir*] nothing more about his being."[85] Lest this remark be mistaken for marking an abrupt break with anything biological, Lacan, consonant with contemporaneous lines of his thought expressed elsewhere,[86] hints a page later at the relevance of psychoanalytic insights and concepts for the life sciences.[87] These indications from 1946 audibly reverberate in Green's book published in 1995.

When it comes to what "causes" human subjects to be what they are, Green insists again and again that the psychical causality isolated and explained exclusively by psychoanalysis is neither natural nor cultural.[88] He identifies the Freudian id as "the genuine intercessor between the brain and the psyche."[89] Emergentism also is alluded to by Green:[90] "psychical causality is that which *emerges* from the relations between nature and culture."[91] Such thus constituted, ontogenetically emergent subjects, as loci of convergence for a vast multitude of overdetermining vectors of "natural" and "cultural" influences, are therefore, in part, incredibly dense condensations of "hypercomplexity."[92] Both the theory and practice of analysis allegedly address themselves to this hypercomplexity, attending, through free association, to the irrational reason and illogical logics arising out of beings situated at the multifaceted intersections of so many converging (and frequently conflicting) forces and factors.[93]

Despite displaying the gesture of reaching out a little bit to the natural sciences, Green ends up unfortunately perpetuating the inaccurate image of these disciplines as essentially hostile to any nonscientific (read "antireductive") explanatory discourse (such as psychoanalysis).[94] Situating psychoanalysis with respect to the Enlightenment and post-Enlightenment tension between science and religion, Green depicts analysis as sharing religions' ostensibly warranted worries regarding the reductive tendencies of the natural sciences and their institutional and ideological offshoots. However, in supposed solidarity with the sciences, the Freudian field is said to be adamantly materialist. And yet, Green's analytic "materialism" refuses to ground the psyche in the brain.[95] Instead, with a nod to certain religious notions, he "pleads for a 'laicized' soul that we designate as such in order to oppose it to cerebral machinery, which is nothing but a pale caricature of that which is the psyche."[96] He immediately warns one not to "confound this psyche with the religious soul of a divine essence."[97] And yet, he subsequently resumes flirting with religiosity, laying out a vision of psychoanalysis as raising the truth of religious antireductionism (as opposed to the purportedly reductive mechanistic materialism of the sciences, including the neurosciences) to the dignity of its secular, demystified Notion.[98]

However, in contrast with Green's compromise position between religion and science, what if, reenacting the uncompromising Leninist stance of *Materialism and Empirio-Criticism* (1908), one objects that this psyche qua secularized soul really isn't all that secular except for a scientific explanation of how this entity escaping the jurisdiction of scientific explanation emerges from the lone immanent material ground(s) of concern to the physical sciences? (Similarly, one could treat the choice between religion and science as a Badiouian "point," that is, a fundamental, unavoidable choice between two mutually exclusive alternatives in which no honest third way is truly possible.)[99] This isn't to plead, against Green, in favor of a science-fetishizing reductivism. Rather, this is to insist that any materialism worthy of the title must perform, in order to be truly materialist yet simultaneously nonreductive, a sort of theoretical jujitsu trick, namely, a vaguely Gödelian-style in- or decompletion of the natural sciences. A materialism entirely divorced from the natural sciences (i.e., a staunchly antinaturalist materialism) is materialist in name only; a materialist (as opposed to idealist) antinaturalism requires a natural-scientific account of the material possibility conditions for the emergence of the antinatural (as more than natural or material).[100] Playing off an irreducible nonnatural subject, portrayed as a mystery utterly inexplicable in scientific terms, against the fictional straw man caricature of a natural neuronal machine governed exclusively by the blind mechanisms of the efficient causalities of evolution and genetics merely reinstates a version of those dualisms that rightly are so anathema to the tradition of authentic (dialectical) materialism.[101]

When it comes to the subjects of concern to psychoanalysis (i.e., human beings as speaking subjects), the real challenge is to pinpoint and link up two parallel, complementary nodes of explanatory incompleteness within scientific and psychoanalytic discourses. A properly formulated neuro-psychoanalysis does precisely this. It engages in the double move of (1) complementing Freudian-Lacanian psychoanalysis with a naturalist or biological account of the material underpinnings of denaturalized or more-than-biological subjectivity and (2) complementing the neurosciences with a sophisticated, systematic metapsychological theory of subjects whose geneses, although tied to brains, involve much more than bare organic anatomy. (These emergent subjects also come to have significant repercussions for the biomaterial bases that are the necessary-but-not-sufficient aleatory conditions of possibility for their very existences.) One can and should strive to develop a scientifically shaped (although not purely and strictly scientific) account of how humans defying and escaping explanatory encapsulation by the sciences become what they are.[102] Correlatively, a materialist psychoanalysis must be, as Lacan would put it, not without its scientific reasons, while maintaining itself as a specific discipline whose objects of inquiry cannot be absorbed unreservedly into subjectless material being(s).[103] I believe that psychoanalysis nowadays can make a convincing case, on natural-scientific grounds, for its irreducible autonomy and specificity vis-à-vis the sciences of nature (especially the life sciences). The brittle, doomed strategy of unconvincing recourse to dogmatic foot stamping and fist banging about irreducibility in the face of advancing scientific knowledge is no longer necessary or appropriate.

As regards Green specifically, of even greater interest in connection with outlining a neuro-psychoanalytic metapsychology of affect is an early essay by him, "The Logic of Lacan's *objet (a)* and Freudian Theory: Convergences and Questions," written under the influence of Lacan and published in 1966 in the third issue of the journal *Cahiers pour l'Analyse*. Therein, in a subsection of his essay on "The Problem of the Distinction Between the Representative of Drive and the Affect," he addresses the relations between, on the one hand, Freud's *Vorstellung* and Lacan's signifier and, on the other hand, affective phenomena as distinct from such ideational representations and their logics or structures. Speaking of the later Freud, Green enigmatically proposes that *"the affect takes on the status of signifier."*[104] (He reiterates this a few years later in *Le discours vivant*.)[105] To Lacanian ears, this sounds odd, to the point of perhaps sounding paradoxical or self-contradictory insofar as Lacan tirelessly insists on the difference in kind separating affects and signifiers. A few paragraphs later, Green seems to reinstate Lacan's distinction between signifier and affect by claiming that the latter, unlike the former, is noncombinatory: *"The specificity of affect is that it cannot enter into combination."*[106] Unlike Lacan, the early Green, in line with Freud, allows for the possibility of affects succumbing to repression.[107] But, in Green's view, whereas repressed signifiers qua *Vorstellungen* come to light only through indirect, winding webs of associative combinations involving multiple ideational representations of the same type, repressed affects "can be expressed directly— that is, without passing through the connecting links of the preconscious"[108] (i.e., the matrix of word-presentations [*Wortvorstellungen*], as per Freud's schema according to which unconscious thing-presentations [*Sachvorstellungen*], in order to gain the potential of possibly entering into consciousness, must be matched up with word-presentations in the preconscious).[109] One of the guiding assumptions apparently steering Green's proposals in 1966 (an assumption he appears to abandon by 1973) is the notion that affective phenomena, in contrast with linguistic-symbolic signifiers as structured ideational representations, enjoy a nonrelational self-sufficiency, an immediate identity-to-self as sameness, in contrast with the mediated non-self-identity of signifiers as (to quote Saussure) "differences *without positive terms*."[110]

The final move I want to make, the explication of which will occupy me in the remainder of what follows, can be introduced through reference to Green's text from 1966. In terms of this reference, this move consists of rejecting his manners of maintaining a clear contrast between affects and signifiers as a consequence of putting a new twist on his suggestion that *"the affect takes on the status of signifier."* This proposition can be twisted into the ultimate infinite judgment (as per the Hegelian infinite judgment) of a Lacan-inflected neuropsychoanalysis: affects are signifiers. Interestingly, both Lacanian psychoanalysis and affective neuroscience seem to concur that this equation is problematic, if not nonsensically impossible. Empirical studies of the brain have uncovered evidence supporting the Freudian-Lacanian thesis regarding the distinction between emotional affects and cognitive representations.[111] However, one should bear in mind that the neurosciences also often simultaneously maintain that, in most real-time brain dynamics, emotions and cognitions, although distinguishable through neuroanatomical analysis, are de facto indistinguishable through neurodynamic synthesis insofar as they are inextricably intertwined in lived reality. Apropos Lacan, one of the best ways to secure a grip on the nature of and justifications for his fashion of differentiating between signifiers and affects is to return to the topic of deception.

For Lacan, both signifiers and affects are deceptive. But, they each deceive, according to him, in ways that are fundamentally different in kind. Going through Lacan's corpus and cataloguing the numerous forms of deception engendered by signifiers detailed therein would be a daunting, protracted task (one not to be undertaken here). Žižek, for instance, often draws attention to the title of Lacan's twenty-first seminar of 1973–1974: *Les non-dupes errant* ("the non-dupes err," roughly homophonous with *le Nom-du-Père* [the Name-of-the-Father]). Succinctly summarized, the Name-of-the-Father, as a master signifier (S1) underpinning the symbolic order as the universe of other signifiers (S2), is a bluff, fake, fiction, illusion, myth, semblance, and so on.[112] The entire Symbolic big Other constitutes a fantasmatic "virtual reality" not entirely governed by what is presumed to be actual concrete being.[113] The late Lacan, in the twenty-fourth seminar, goes so far as to declare that "the symbolic tells nothing but lies."[114] And yet, as Žižek, following Lacan, is fond of reminding his readers, he/she who refuses to be "taken in" by the trickery of the signifier-mediated virtual reality of the symbolic order—such a cynical nominalist, empiricist, or positivist "non-dupe" stubbornly sticks to beliefs in absolutely singular and unique entities, conceptually unprocessed raw perceptual experience, and brute facts-in-themselves wholly independent of sociosymbolic mediation—errs most, losing contact with those abstractions that, in the topsy-turvy inverted world of human existence, arguably are more concrete than the (imagined) concrete itself.[115] Near the end of his life, Lacan counts himself among the dupes (who presumably don't err).[116] One contextually appropriate manner of fleshing out what is meant here involves referring back to the preceding Hegelian critique of Panksepp's handling of the issue of linguistic labeling in constructing a taxonomy of emotion systems in the brain: those who cling to the conviction that clear-cut affective distinctions dwell in the posited extrarepresentational concrete real of the central nervous system entirely apart from the hazy, murky representational fuzziness of abstract affect-languages are the ones who err, both theoretically and empirically; the vagaries of affect-languages are not without their impacts on the emotional brain itself. That is to say, the "lies" of "inaccurate" emotional terminology in natural languages become the (partial) truths of affective life *an sich*, right down to its material bases.

In the sixteenth seminar, Lacan distinguishes between "dupery" (*duperie*) and "deception" (*tromperie*). The latter implies a standard of representational accuracy or faithfulness vis-à-vis an extrarepresentational point of reference. Degrees of deception, in Lacan's specific sense, are measured according to the criteria of a correspondence theory of truth. As he rightly observes, psychoanalysis is not in the least bit invested in a correspondence theory of truth, at least as it's commonly construed. Analysts aren't (or, at least, shouldn't be) preoccupied with speculations about the representational veracity of, say, childhood memories or depictions of recent events transpiring off the couch outside the analytic consulting room. One could say that analysis concerns itself more with a coherence theory of truth, with the consistencies and inconsistencies of the networks of associative connections internal to the webs of analysands' monologues. Whether the nodes in these verbal networks are realistic renditions or fictitious fantasies is both unknowable within the framework of an analysis and ultimately unimportant to its long-term progress. For example, an analysand who consistently lies to his/her analyst, fabricating all of his/her reported dreams, fantasies, and so on, still discloses to the analyst the truths of his/her unconscious, telling "true lies" despite him-/herself insofar as the very selection of the fabricated verbal material cannot help but be itself revealing; such an inadvertent "telling the truth in the guise of lying" would be the mirror-image correlate of the Lacanian notion of "lying in the guise of truth." This is one very Freudian reverberation of Lacan's opening line from his television appearance: "I always speak the truth" ("*Je dis toujours la vérité*"),[117] the "I" ("*je*") in question here being the (subject of the) unconscious. But, although not preoccupied by deception, psychoanalysis indeed is very interested in dupery, specifically, "the dupery of consciousness." Lacan defines a dupe as "someone who someone else exploits." Consciousness is duped to the extent that it's "exploited" (i.e., pushed around, manipulated, and so on) by those signifiers forming symptomatic formations of the unconscious generating perturbations within the narrow, restricted field of self-awareness.[118]

As regards the topic of affect in psychoanalysis, Lacan appears to maintain that affects deceive whereas signifiers dupe. Generally speaking, he reduces affects to felt feelings (*Empfindungen*) and characterizes such consciously registered sentiments (or *senti-ments*) as either opaque signals confusedly gesturing at a reality of a different order than their own (i.e., the unconscious "other scene" composed of signifiers as nonaffective ideational representations [*Vorstellungen*]) or the red herrings of *affectuations* disguising and concealing repressed signifying structures. In a sense, Lacan judges affects according to a correspondence theory of truth, albeit one internal to the (in)coherent "psychical reality" of the *parlêtre* talking on the couch: the relative truth or falsity, honesty or dishonesty, of affects (as felt feelings) is measured against the standards of signifiers (as purportedly different in kind from feelings).

Another angle of approach to these issues is to observe that, from Lacan's perspective, signifiers and affects both can be misleading, although they mislead in utterly distinct modes. In this view, affects tend to mislead at the level of why they are, but not what they are. When one feels angry, sad, and so on, what's misleading is not the qualitative phenomenal feel of the feeling per se, but rather the true (unfeeling) causes, logics, objects, and reasons (all situated within nonaffective representational registers) responsible for the emergence in conscious experience of this feeling state—and this insofar as Lacan, as already noted (in chapter 11), regularly argues that affects, limited to the status of felt feelings and nothing more, are only ever displaced within consciousness along unfurling chains of signifiers, some of which are repressed or unconscious in ways that affects, according to him, cannot be repressed or unconscious. Lacan's psychoanalytic appropriation of Saussurian linguistics combines, among other things, Saussure's definition of the signifier as a purely differential (non)entity determined by its relations with other such (non)entities and Freud's psychoanalytic thesis that representational contents and associative connections in mental life—for Lacan, these contents are signifiers and these connections are their relations—can be (and often are) unconscious. One implication of this, in terms of the modes in which signifiers and affects can be misleading, is that, unlike affects, signifiers can and do mislead even as to what they are. If a signifier is what it is by virtue of the sum total of its differential relations with other signifiers, and if repression and other defense mechanisms delineated by psychoanalysis are able to render one or more of these other signifiers unconscious, then consciousness can be misled (or duped) about what a given signifier really is if some of this signifier's co-determining relations with repressed other signifiers are unknown to this same consciousness.

The entire preceding project, especially through its return to the textual details of Freud's discussions of affective phenomena and explorations of current affective neuroscience, undermines this Lacanian fashion of differentiating between affects and signifiers. In the combined lights of Freud and the neurosciences, if the term *affect* refers to much more than just consciously felt feelings (i.e., Freudian *Empfindungen*, as distinct from *Affekte* and *Gefühle*), then a very disturbing, unsettling truth reveals itself: affects can and do mislead at the level of not only why they are, but what they are, that is, how they feel.

In a Hegelian-style formulation, perhaps it could be said that the distinction between affects and signifiers is a distinction internal to the category of the signifier itself. With respect to Lacan, this formulation isn't as objectionable as it might seem at first glance. To cut a long story short, Lacan's signifier isn't necessarily a unit of language as per linguistics. Rather, anything can be a signifier if its status and function rely upon its positions in constellations of synchronic systems and diachronic dynamics in which spatial and temporal differences are decisive. Other materials besides the phonetic and graphic materials of natural languages can and do operate as signifiers as defined by both Lacan and various versions of a post-Saussurian general semiotics.[119]

But, one lingering, nagging question remains: if affects can be signifiers insofar as the category of signifier is a formal rather than a substantial category, then what are affects? During his television appearance, Lacan, in response to Miller drawing attention to the word *unconscious*, says regarding this master word for psychoanalysis: "Freud didn't find a better one, and there's no need to go back on it. The disadvantage of this word is that it is negative, which allows one to assume anything at all in the world about it, plus everything else as well. Why not? To that which goes unnoticed, the word *everywhere* applies just as well as *nowhere*."[120] If, as these observations indicate, the problem with the word *unconscious* is that it's a negative term (*un-*) for a positive *x*—Lacan immediately adds, "It is nonetheless a very precise thing"[121]—the problem with the word *affect* might be the exact opposite: it's a positive term for a negative *x*, namely, the absence of a coherent concept referring, in a precise one-to-one correspondence, to a clearly identifiable set of phenomena. Even drawing boundary lines circumscribing a general domain that would be the realm of the affects proper (as manifestly distinct from other things) is incredibly tricky and uncertain. And yet, just as Lacan chooses not to jettison the word *unconscious* despite its noted drawbacks, maybe the fuzzy word *affect* ought to be retained precisely because the realities it designates are themselves fuzzy. If *affect* is indeed a positive term for a negative x, this negativity isn't merely epistemological-representational (i.e., a deficiency or lack at the level of the concept alone).

Redeploying the distinctions between emotions and various shades and sorts of feelings uncovered by recent affective neuroscience, one should perhaps retain the term *affect* precisely to designate the uniquely human desynchronizations between emotions and feelings as well as among feelings themselves, that is, the actual, palpable absences of in-synch harmonies afflicting the bodies, brains, and psyches of partially denaturalized subjects of signifiers. For such subjects, affective life must be lived under the permanent shadow of doubts about passions and sentiments as self-evident, self-transparent, and self-sufficient experiences. Reflexive self-consciousness, thanks to the reflexivity of feeling itself, never will seize upon solid guarantees vouching for the ultimate, final truths of why it feels, how it feels, or even what it feels. A lot can happen in the gaps between emotions, feelings, and the feelings of feelings. With the combined resources of Lacan's Freudian foundations and the rapidly accumulating findings of the neurosciences, the time is ripe for Lacanian explorations in both psychoanalysis and neurobiology of this terrain that no longer justifiably can be neglected.

POSTFACE

THE PARADOXES OF
THE PRINCIPLE OF CONSTANCY

I believe it possible to affirm more than ever that a confrontation between psychoanalysis, neurobiology, and Continental philosophy has not been attempted before. It is this confrontation that our work undertakes here, a work insisting on the importance of the new libidinal economy currently emerging at the intersection of these disciplines and revealing new definitions of affects.

The most striking affirmations of contemporary neurobiologists like Damasio or LeDoux concern the importance of the emotional brain. All the cognitive operations closely depend on it. Affects function initially at a primitive biological and cerebral level that does not involve consciousness. There therefore exists nonconscious affects, and the brain is their place of origin. This is why it is important, for the neurobiologists, to redefine the psyche according to this primordial emotionality. What challenges do such affirmations throw at psychoanalysis and philosophy?

Psychoanalysis: Are There Unconscious Feelings?

During the course of a meticulous and passionate investigation, Adrian Johnston explores, in Freud and Lacan, the fate of the feelings of guilt and anxiety first, and then those of shame and modesty. Why this exploration? Johnston recalls, with a great deal of pertinence, that the question of affects seems in many respects to have been neglected by psychoanalysis. For one thing, this is because, for Freud as for Lacan, emotions and feelings cannot but be conscious. This is why emotions and feelings can be displaced or inhibited, but never repressed. In other words, and paradoxically, the unconscious, where the pleasure principle is located, is little concerned with affects as such.

In his metapsychological writings, Freud declares, in 1915, that it is incoherent to assume the existence of unconscious affects. How could one feel something without being conscious of it? In response to this question appears Johnston's very beautiful formulation: How can there be seen to be something like *misfelt feelings*? How can it be supposed that "one can feel without feeling that one feels, namely, that there can be, so to speak, unfelt (or, more accurately, misfelt) feelings?" Lacan will return to this Freudian position in affirming that feelings, if they merit their name, cannot but be experienced in consciousness and that neither unconscious nor, thus, "misfelt" feelings exist. As is well known, Lacan takes care to distinguish between, on the one hand, affects, which always are conscious, and, on the other hand, signifiers, which truly and totally constitute the register of the unconscious. An "affective" unconscious therefore is nonsense.

All the same, from 1907 on, Freud circles around the possibility of admitting the existence of "an unconscious feeling of guilt," an idea picked back up in "The Unconscious" of 1915. We should remember that the third section of that metapsychological essay is entitled "Unconscious Emotions." Nevertheless, after having envisaged this hypothesis, Freud pushes it aside. He employs some very interesting terms that he never takes the trouble to define and distinguish, such as *affective structures* (*Affektbildungen*), *affects* (*Affekte*), *emotions* (*Gefühle*), and *feelings* (*Empfindungen*).

In much later texts, like *The Ego and the Id* (1923), Freud speaks again of an "unconscious sense of guilt." He seems at this point to recognize, in the second topography, a structural relationship of the unconscious with affects via the feeling of guilt. He already had opened the possibility of such a feeling in texts such as "Some Character-Types Met with in Psycho-Analytic Work" of 1916 (in the section entitled "Criminals from a Sense of Guilt"), where there appears a feeling of guilt certainly conscious but where that consciousness does not know what this guilt is about: an obscure guilt that is unaware of itself.

This unconscious feeling of guilt is able to manifest itself also in the form of a diffuse anxiety originating from the superego. Guilt even is assimilated to a "topographical variety of anxiety." Freud thus considers that guilt perhaps can be a "misfelt feeling" which gives itself to be felt as an uneasiness, a dissatisfaction—once again, as an anxiety that is vague and without apparent object.

Lacan seems more radical still than the Freud of the first topography in terms of negating the existence of unconscious feelings or affects. In the seminar *The Ethics of Psychoanalysis*, he denounces the confused nature of the recourse to affects and the mixing together of representations and affects. The latter play only a secondary role in relation to the unconscious. It is not a question of confusing affects and the ideational representations they can merely accompany. There is no representational rapport between affect and signifier.

In reality, Lacan's position is more nuanced. In the tenth seminar, *Anxiety*, he correctly states that anxiety is an affect, an affect that it really is necessary to call unconscious. And, perhaps it is possible to reconcile here what Lacan calls a *senti-ment*, playing with the two verbs *sentir* (to feel) and *mentir* (to lie), with what Johnston names a "misfelt feeling." Anxiety does not know in the face of what it is anxious. For this reason, like guilt, it manifests itself as an uneasiness, as a dissatisfaction more than as an affect that is clear and perfectly certain of its object. Consequently, anxiety is well defined as "the central affect, the one around which everything is organized," the "fundamental affect."

‰ ‰ ‰

If psychoanalysis ends with recognizing the importance of affects, can one now envision possible points of passage between psychoanalysis and contemporary neurobiology? The problem is that psychoanalysis has never admitted the central importance of cerebral activity in psychical functioning.

Freud never contested the appropriateness of the metaphor of the brain as an "electrical center" developed by Breuer in the *Studies on Hysteria*. According to this metaphor, the brain is a pure and simple place where the transmission of energy occurs, a simple mechanism. Breuer declares:

> We ought not to think of a cerebral path of conduction as resembling a telephone wire which is only excited electrically at the moment at which it has to function (that is, in the present context, when it has to transmit a signal). We ought to liken it to a telephone line through which there is a constant flow of galvanic current and which can no longer be excited if that current ceases. Or better, let us imagine a widely-ramified electrical system for lighting and the transmission of motor power; what is expected of this system is that simple

establishment of a contact shall be able to set any lamp or machine in operation. To make this possible, so that everything shall be ready to work, there
must be a certain tension present throughout the entire network of lines of
conduction, and the dynamo engine must expend a given quantity of energy
for this purpose. In just the same way there is a certain amount of excitation
present in the conductive paths of the brain when it is at rest but awake and
prepared to work.[1]

Now, there exists "an optimum for the height of the intracerebral tonic excitation."[2] When this is exceeded, it produces in the system the equivalent of a
"short circuit": "I shall venture once more to recur to my comparison with an
electrical lighting system. The tension in the network of lines of conduction in
such a system has an optimum too. If this is exceeded its functioning may easily
be impaired; for instance, the electric light filaments may be quickly burned
through. I shall speak later of the damage done to the system itself through a
break-down of its insulation or through 'short-circuiting.'"[3]

The brain therefore has no other possibility for coping with energetic excess
than malfunctioning. It is not equipped with any structure of fluidification via
detour—that is to say, via differentiation (*différenciation*)—of energy. In other
words, it does not enjoy *any mechanism of representation*. Lacan will affirm
exactly the same thing: the brain, a purely biological and organic entity, is not
endowed with representations.

Thus, for Freud as for Lacan, the drive (*Trieb, pulsion*) is never a cerebral
given. The "thrust" (*poussée*) of the drive, despite the urgency of the pressure
it exerts, does not effectively manifest itself, as Johnston recalls, except by *representation* or *delegation*. At its temporal origins, it splits itself into a commis-
sioning power (*mandateur*) and its commissioned proxy (*mandataire*). The
drive then sends representatives in order to say that it cannot wait. It is this
representative structure that qualifies and characterizes the particular rapport
between the somatic and the psychical which is at work in the drive's structure.

Freud develops on this point two conceptions that are contradictory only in
appearance. According to Laplanche and Pontalis, "Sometimes the instinct [*la
pulsion*] itself is presented as 'the psychical representative of the stimuli originating from within the organism and reaching the mind.' At other times the
instinct becomes part of the process of somatic excitation, in which case it is
represented in the psyche by 'instinctual representatives' [*les représentants de la
pulsion*] which comprise two elements—the ideational representative [*Vorstellungsrepräsentanz, représentant-représentation*] and the quota of affect."[4]

It should be noted that the drive representative itself is split, in an additional splitting, into a representation or group of representations and a quota of affect. The extreme pressure exercised by the drive on the nervous system therefore is not only quantitative but also qualitative: that which pushes is simultaneously the quantity of force *and* the division of instances put in relation in the force, namely, representative and quota. The cut or separation between the two, obtained by repression, is hence the sole possible solution to the excess of stressful endogenous urgings: division, procrastinating, and delaying permit deferring (*différer*) the pressure of the inside without provoking "short circuits."

From the perspective of Freudian-Lacanian psychoanalysis, this separation provoked by repression certainly cannot be the result of a biological operation.[5] In effect, for the cut to take place, it is necessary that psychical energy detach itself from neural (*nerveuse*) energy. The vicissitudes of the drives—"reversal into its opposite, turning round upon the subject's own self, repression, sublimation"[6]—assume a place other than the cerebral topography. Psychical energy is, in a way, the rhetorical detour of neural energy. Unable to discharge itself in the nervous system, endogenous excitation makes detours comparable to the tropes or figures of discourse.

Because, for Freud, symbolic activity does not exist in the nervous system, psychical energy represents this very absence in a style that is foreign to the brain. This brain does not have any initiative in the treatment of an energy it can only transmit and maintain at a constant level to the extent that this is possible.[7]

"Psychical" energy therefore comes to reveal the absence of a representational and symbolic power in cerebral organization. The nervous system, of which the first task is to master excitations, does not represent the relation of representation that originally unites and divides the psyche and the body. It does not develop representations of the "sources of internal excitation of the organism." Insofar as it cannot affect itself, it also is not a *psyche*.

※ ※ ※

In Freud's thinking, as is known, sexuality does not designate primarily the sexual drives or sexual life, but actually a certain regime of events governed by a specific causality. Now, this causality finds its source in the possibility of the cut—this cut is at work in every drive, sexual or not (the drives are all similar qualitatively, writes Freud)—between representation and affect.

The sexual drive is, in a sense, reducible to an upsurge of energy that pushes and knocks at the door in demanding to be liquidated. But, this liquidation is never simple or immediate: the energy there undergoes circumnavigations, splittings, and divisions so as to transform itself into the coded message of a "representative." Sexuality is the hermeneutic adventure of psychical energy. The exogenous event, when it happens, necessarily finds itself separated from its very exteriority in enlisting itself in the endogenous adventure of meaning (*sens*).

Thus, one will not be surprised that what "libido" (qua affect related initially to the sexual drive *stricto sensu*) ends up designating, in Freud, is the mobility or the "rhetoric" of the quota of affect in general. In the same manner that there exists an "enlarged" meaning of sexuality (as a type of causality and specific regime of events), there also exists, by way of consequence, an "enlarged" sense of the word *libido*. The mobile character of the libido, which renders it susceptible to detours, becomes the dominant trait of psychical energy as a whole. The treatment of the sexual drive becomes paradigmatic for every drive vicissitude.

Lacan shows that the libido, far from being only a dynamic manifestation of the sexual drive, designates, in fact, "an undifferentiated quantitative unit susceptible of entering into relations of equivalence."[8] Even if, as one will see later on here, it is far from being the only psychical energy at work in the psyche, the libido gives its name to every energetic transaction. "Hence one would talk," Lacan continues, "of transformations, regressions, fixations, sublimations of the libido, a single term which is conceived of quantitatively."[9] The libido therefore truly has for its function the unification of a *field* (*champ*)—not simply that of different phases and structures of sexual development, but also, and precisely, that of the "field of psychoanalytic effects" (*champ des effets psychanalytiques*) in general, the energetic tropes or tropisms that go beyond the organization of the nervous system.[10]

※ ※ ※

Contemporary neurobiological discoveries put into question these analytic notions. The Freudian conception of a brain foreign to symbolic activity, a brain that is a purely material base without autonomy in the treatment of its own energetic urgings, is in the process of totally disappearing today. Contrary to what the psychoanalysts affirm, the "emotional brain" is apt to support endogenous excitations or drives. In light of this fact, the frontiers between, on the one side, the brain and the cerebral organization and, on the other side, the psychical apparatus and the unconscious find themselves reelaborated.

What is an emotion from a neurobiological point of view, what we are calling here affects? The word is old, thus seeming to drive us back well behind what is designated by the word *drive*. Emotion, according to its literal sense, designates a relational dynamic between brain and body, the very movement of the psycho-somatic totality, comprises an individual body and a nervous system. It is this totality in movement that, as I have shown in my text, Damasio interprets in terms of conatus. Between the nervous system and the body a constant exchange of information takes place (which draws these "maps" of which we spoke much earlier). In fact, only one word is needed in order to designate the two entities: *organism*, which refers as much to cerebral organization as to bodily structure.

The dynamic of emotion has its origin precisely in this elementary activity of exchange of information and autoregulation of the organism. In the beginning, emotion does not designate this or that passion, but actually is a process at work in vital regulation. There is consequently a sort of pure emotion of vitality, without any object other than the "self," namely, the cerebral "self," which Damasio calls the "protoself."

Far from being a mechanical energetic process, comparable to the functioning of an electrical switchboard or telephone exchange, homeostasis, the self's information about itself and the maintenance of life, is an affective and emotional economy—something psychoanalysis has never envisaged.

The maintenance of excitation at its lowest level, necessary for the survival and elementary activity of the system, is the producer of affects: the brain affects itself in regulating life. There is therefore no "principle of inertia"—this is the name Freud gives to the principle of constancy—without emotion, that is to say, without the autoaffection of the mechanism that produces the maintenance of the system. "Curiously enough," writes Damasio, "emotions are part and parcel of the regulation we call homeostasis."[11] We thus arrive at this astonishing paradox: maintenance, constancy, inertia, and homeostasis are the products of an autoexcitation. The "emotional brain" must be understood precisely starting from this paradox.

The emotions organize and coordinate cerebral activity. Whether concerning primary emotions (sadness, joy, fear, surprise, disgust), secondary or "social" emotions (embarrassment, jealousy, guilt, pride), or even emotions said to be "in the background" (well-being, uneasiness, calm, despondency), the emotions are all elaborate ensuing continuations of affective processes at work in homeostatic regulation. Therefore, in the brain, there are no regulatory mechanisms of adaptation to the external world and the environment without emotional adaptation to the inside of the brain by the brain itself.

Now, it seems that psychoanalysis remains blind to this cerebral autoexcitation. However, does Freud not say that homeostasis, or the "principle of inertia," is regulated precisely by the pleasure principle? We recall here the celebrated remark that "the most highly developed mental apparatus is subject to the pleasure principle, i.e. is automatically regulated by feelings belonging to the pleasure-unpleasure series. . . . [U]npleasurable feelings are connected with an increase and pleasurable feelings with a decrease of stimulus."[12]

Nevertheless, in Freud, the pleasure principle does not produce any pleasure to the extent that it doesn't affect itself. The mechanism of the pleasure principle remains impassive, insensitive to that of which it is the principle. Even Damasio insists that pleasure is not exactly an emotion, although, unlike Freud, he ties the pleasure-pain spectrum quite closely to affective phenomena.[13] Moreover, Damasio affirms that emotion is a reflexive structure through which vital regulation affects itself: "the status of life regulation is expressed in the form of affects."[14]

The cerebral sites that produce emotion occupy a zone which starts at the level of the brain stem and goes up to the cortex. Outside of a part of the frontal lobe called the prefrontal ventromedial cortex, the majority of these sites are subcortical—sites that Freud had considered as being without relation to the unconscious. The principle subcortical sites are located in regions of the brain stem, the hypothalamus, and the basal telencephalon. The amygdala, or the amygdala complex—this is the almond-shaped group of neurons situated in the temporal lobe in front of the hippocampus—is equally a determinant subcortical site in the triggering of emotions. It forms that part of the limbic system implicated notably in fear and aggression.

What the anatomy of the relation between the triggering and execution of emotions shows is that the distribution of emotional processes over many sites permits the brain to discipline and treat the internal sources of excitation without being overwhelmed by them, without producing, contrary to what Breuer affirms, "short circuits." These sites are not rigid and fixed, but instead constitute functional systems. Damasio emphasizes that "none of these triggering sites produces an emotion by itself. For an emotion to occur the site must cause subsequent activity in other sites. . . . As with any other form of complex behavior, emotion results from the concerted participation of several sites within a brain's system."[15] It is hence clear that the intensity of internal sources of excitation is treated from within the nervous system in a functional and interactive manner that assumes the collaboration of many sites. The psychical detour of neural or nervous energy is no longer necessary. Thus, there are no longer two types of energy.

Hence, the brain takes the drives and energetic tensions upon itself alone. This supposes that there exists a cerebral activity of representation different from that put forward by Freud under the name of representation (*représentance*), which was examined earlier. This change of conception has considerable consequences, since it has to do with nothing less than a change in the very meaning of the unconscious.

※ ※ ※

We do not seek here to situate biologically this unconscious in opposing emotion and drive. Researchers such as Mark Solms, for example, categorically refuse to localize the unconscious. In any case, writes Solms, it is not a question of saying that "the unconscious is located in the right hemisphere" nor that it merges with the inductive sites for emotions. If a cerebral unconscious exists, related to the emotional brain, then it necessarily is, like the emotional brain, also a distributed functional system and, consequently, cannot be situated in this or that anatomical "region."

All the same, anatomy plays a major role here. To insist on the biological spatiality of the sites for emotion permits establishing that the cerebral unconscious is first of all related both to the brain's treatment of internal excitations as well as to the autorepresentative activity that is tied to this treatment there. This unconscious is constituted by the "core" (*noyau*) that corresponds to the neuronal elaboration of a representation, constant and changing, of the psychosomatic rapport and that determines the original, primitive attachment of the attachment to life.

The representative activity internal to the brain and the unconscious corresponds to a certain type of image-making (*mise en image*). Damasio writes: "*core consciousness occurs when the brain's representation devices generate an imaged, nonverbal account of how the organism's own state is affected by the organism's processing of an object.*"[16] This cartography of the relationship between the inside and the outside reveals the biological history of the organism "*caught in the act of representing its own changing state as it goes about representing something else.*"[17]

The core "protoself," the primitive form of identity, is therefore a constant interaction between the internal milieu and the external world. The state of the internal milieu, the viscera and the musculo-skeletal framework (the elementary homeostatic indices), produces a continuous, dynamic representation by which life maintains itself in producing constant loops of information. Second after second, the brain represents the interaction between internal state and external stimuli. The sources of internal excitation are thus always identified: "*The proto-self is a coherent collection of neural patterns which map, moment by moment, the state of the physical structure of the organism in its many dimensions.* This ceaselessly maintained first-order collection of neural patterns occurs not in one brain place but in many, at a multiplicity of levels, from the brain stem to the cerebral cortex, in structures that are interconnected by neural pathways. These structures are intimately involved in the process of regulating the state of the organism. The operation of acting on the organism and of sensing the state of the organism are closely tied."[18]

The devices described here form part of a set of structures that simultaneously regulate and represent bodily states. Therefore, in the brain, there is no regulation without representation. This double economy precisely defines cerebral identity as a constant synthesis of different states of relation between body and psyche, as an equilibrium, in a word, of the organism.

⁜ ⁜ ⁜

A question poses itself at this moment of the analysis: Is not defining the unconscious as a nonconscious activity to fall back into the famous trap, denounced by Freud, that consists in conflating the unconscious (*Unbewußt*) and the nonconscious (*Bewußtlos*)? Would this not be to remain outside the significance of the psychical unconscious?

It is certain that if one simply characterizes the cerebral unconscious as the nonconscious place where homeostatic processes are afoot, one risks, in effect, falling into this trap and clinging to an insufficient and uncritically pre-Freudian definition of the unconscious. Things proceed entirely otherwise if one calls "cerebral unconscious" the "*cerebralization*" *of affects,*[19] that is to say, an active and sui generis process of regulation. All the data that the brain gives (itself) on the internal state of the organism and on the relations of the organism with objects is accompanied by the production of affects. The autorepresentative activity of the brain, which ceaselessly maps psychosomatic states, hence scrutinizes its own inside, putting it into images and affecting itself by this activity of which it is, as seen, the receiver and addressee. The "cerebral unconscious" consequently designates less the ensemble of nonconscious processes than the autoaffection of the brain in its entirety.

From the start, *homeostatic processes, the birth of the self,* and *the birth of the object* intertwine themselves in the brain as a single and the same phenomenon. The logic of cerebral autoaffection does not presume the intervention of an extra supplementary energy that is endowed with the status of the libido. The distinction between the self (*moi*) and the object appears before any and every narcissism and sexual investment. The psychical apparatus appears hence as the core that gathers together, in the same energetic economy, the constant exigency of survival, the relation to self, and the desire of the other.

How can one comprehend more exactly the concept of the brain's autoaffection? Traditionally, as I have shown in my analysis of wonder, the notion of autoaffection designates, in philosophy, the original and paradoxical manner in which the subject feels itself to be identical to itself in addressing itself to itself as to another in the strange space of its inner depths. It has to do with a sort of primordial touching of self—the subject senses itself, speaks itself, hears itself speaking, experiences the succession of states of consciousness. This contact produces the difference of self to self without which, paradoxically, there would be neither identity nor permanence. Autoaffection is the original power of the subject to interpellate itself, to autosolicit itself and constitute itself as a subject in this double movement of identity and alterity to self.

Homeostatic regulation is, in a certain sense, a mirroring structure of specularity within which the brain informs itself of itself.[20] Emotion plays a fundamental role in the constitution of this cerebral psyche: the brain affects itself, that is to say, modifies itself in the constant course of vital regulation. The stakes of neurobiological research consist in drawing out from the elementary rapport of the brain with itself and with the other the idea of a cerebral identity that is the unconscious part of subjectivity.

This is the paradox that I have sought to illuminate in my essay: autoaffection is not opposed to the idea of the unconscious; instead, the former constitutes the latter. In this resides one of the most important teachings of contemporary neurobiology. Cerebral autoaffection is not of the same nature as the autoaffection of a subject such as philosophers define it. Cerebral autoaffection does not redouble its specularity up to the point of giving itself the form of consciousness. Nobody feels his/her brain—nobody any longer speaks to him-/herself of it, hears him-/herself speak of it, or hears him-/herself in it. Cerebral autoaffection is paradoxically and necessarily accompanied by an impassibility and neutrality of the conscious subject as regards it. If the subject can affect itself, it is really thanks to the brain: the first contact with the self that is homeostasis renders this contact possible. But, at the same time, this original solicitation dissimulates itself in the very thing that it makes possible. My brain never appears in my inner depths. The brain is not visible except in an objective manner through the snapshots produced by brain-imaging techniques. Hence, original emotions remain forever lost for consciousness. But, this does not signify that the cerebral unconscious limits itself solely to the nonconscious. In effect, an entire history hides itself in primitive emotions, and it is evident that events lived by the subject play a role in cerebral autoaffection in the manner in which the conatus informs and maintains itself.

The neurobiologists seem in other places sometimes to recognize a certain proximity between the functioning of the protoself and the ego (*moi*) of the Freudian second topography.[21] The ego, like core consciousness, effectively appears as a perceptive surface where internal excitations and external demands meet each other coming from opposite directions. Jaak Panksepp elsewhere defines the protoself as a "Simple Ego-like Life Form" (SELF). Solms comments that "this primal SELF forms the foundational 'ego' upon which all our more complex representations of our selves are built."[22] The "ego" of Freud and the "self" (*soi*) of the neurobiologists have the common characteristic of being frontier or limit concepts between the perception of internal states and the perception of external events, interfaces between inner sensations, sensibility, and mobility.

But, the analogy brings itself to a halt abruptly. Damasio point-blank compares the self to a "homunculus," this "little man" that many psychologists and neurologists—Freud included—have conceived of as "inhabiting" the interior of the ego. In *The Ego and the Id*, Freud declares that, as regards the ego, "If we wish to find an anatomical analogy for it we can best identify it with the 'cortical homunculus' of the anatomists, which stands on its head in the cortex, sticks up its heels, faces backwards and, as we know, has its speech-area on the left-hand side."[23] The homunculus corresponds to a figural representation of a part of the nervous system. There is, in a sense, a sort of subject in the subject, devoted to interpreting the images and representations formed in the brain.[24]

Damasio affirms that "the protoself" is not "to be confused with the rigid homunculus of old neurology."[25] It is necessary to avoid this confusion to the extent that "the proto-self does not occur in one place only, and it emerges dynamically and continuously out of multifarious interacting signals that span varied orders of the nervous system. Besides, the proto-self is not an interpreter of anything. It is a reference point at each point in which it is."[26] Certainly, we know and can localize the cerebral structures necessary to the constitution of the protoself. But, the latter remains paradoxically unlocalizable, dynamic, and distributed.

In the brain, affect does not cut itself off from its own energy, does not delegate or metaphorize itself. But, it is not, for all that, an expression of a unity. In effect, the "self" is not substantial. Its manifestation is fundamentally temporal. The self is not what it is except inasmuch as it endures and fabricates itself at each instant: "The story contained in the images of core consciousness is not told by some clever homunculus. Nor is the story really told by *you* as a self because the core *you* is only born as the story is told, *within the story itself.* You exist as a mental being when primordial stories are being told, and only then; as long as primordial stories are being told, and only then. You are the music while the music lasts."[27]

Cerebral autoaffection is the biological process, both logical and affective, by which finitude is constituted in the core of subjectivity without ever being able to become, at the same time, the knowledge (*savoir*) of the subject. The cerebral self has no presence-to-self. In this sense, it is always anonymous; it is no one in wholly being the most elementary form of identity.

It is thus possible to measure the entire distance that separates the neuronal unconscious from the unconscious as traditionally defined. The former merges in a certain fashion with the passage of time, whereas the latter ignores time. Freud writes, "The processes of the system *Ucs.* are *timeless*; i.e. they are not ordered temporally, are not altered by the passage of time; they have no reference to time at all. Reference to time is bound up . . . with the work of the system *Cs.*"[28] To these assertions are related those according to which the unconscious does not know death: "Our unconscious, then, does not believe in its own death; it behaves as if it were immortal."[29] By contrast, cerebral autoaffection is the announcement and the incessant internal reminder of mortality. Damasio declares, "We do not have a self sculpted in stone and, like stone, resistant to the ravages of time. Our sense of self is a state of the organism, the result of certain components operating in a certain manner and interacting in a certain way, within certain parameters. It is another construction, a vulnerable pattern of integrated operations whose consequence is to generate the mental representation of a living individual being. The entire biological edifice, from cells, tissues, and organs to systems and images, is held alive by the constant execution of construction plans, always on the brink of partial or complete collapse."[30]

The brain never conducts itself as if it were immortal. The cerebral unconscious, in diametrical opposition to the Freudian unconscious, is therefore fundamentally a destructible unconscious. This is why emotions and affects are exposed to their potential disappearance. Faced with a menacing event, the self, as we have seen, can detach itself from its own affects.

※ ※ ※

I have perhaps been more negative than Adrian in my critique of psychoanalysis here. He departs from a recognition, by Freud and by Lacan, of misfelt feelings and concludes from this that there is a point of common passage between analysis and neurobiology. I certainly also think this, but I believe that it is necessary to insist all the same that the contempt of psychoanalysis vis-à-vis the brain and neurobiology in general has been erroneous. This lack of regard is also shared with contemporary philosophy, something that I have, for my part, tried to show.

Despite everything, the recent teachings of the neurobiological approach to emotions permit us, Adrian as well as me, to revisit the two traditions of psychoanalysis and philosophy with a new gaze and to discover there theses or positions on the subject of affects that had not necessarily been discovered previously.

The cutting edge of the cerebral unconscious passes through anxiety to wonder, an unconscious via which, as we teach, one can become a stranger to oneself at any moment, as well as a stranger to every kind of tradition that one believes to be immortal. Today, a new subject arrives in the world, a subject potentially denuded of the feeling of guilt, of wonder, of the capacity for surprise, of moral sentiments. Is it only the sick subject that presents itself thus? Where is the new face of the unconscious? Contemporary neurobiology is caught up in this paradox: insisting on the fundamental importance of affects, it describes their possible loss. Hence, at the very heart of biological life and homeostasis, a new chapter in the history of the death drive (*Todestrieb, pulsion de mort*) writes itself.

Catherine Malabou
Paris, August 2011

NOTES

INTRODUCTION: FROM THE PASSIONATE SOUL
TO THE EMOTIONAL BRAIN

1. Gilles Deleuze, *Lectures on Spinoza at Vincennes*, BDSweb: University Courses, 1978.
2. In the French translation of the *Ethics*, "affects" appears as "emotions."
3. Deleuze, *Lectures on Spinoza at Vincennes*, January 24, 1978; Baruch Spinoza, *Ethics*, trans. Samuel Shirley (Indianapolis: Hackett, 1992), bk. 3, def. 3.
4. Immanuel Kant, *Critique of Pure Reason*, trans. by J.M.D. Meiklejohn (Amherst: Prometheus Books, 1990), 106.
5. Ibid., 108.
6. Martin Heidegger, *Kant and the Problems of Metaphysics*, trans. Richard Taft, (Bloomington: Indiana University Press, 1990), §34, "Time as Pure Self-Affection and the Temporal Character of the Self," p. 132.
7. René Descartes, *The Passions of the Soul*, in *The Philosophical Writings of Descartes*, trans. John Cottingham, Robert Stoothof, and Dugald Murdoch, vol. 1 (Cambridge: Cambridge University Press, 1985), §27, pp. 338–339.
8. Antonio Damasio, *Descartes' Error: Emotions, Reason, and the Human Brain* (New York: HarperCollins, 1995), xvi.
9. Ibid.
10. Wonder is also a state in which one wants to learn more about something (curiosity), the desire to know that motivates investigation and study.
11. Descartes, *Passions of the Soul*, §53, p. 350.
12. Spinoza, *Ethics*, bk. 3, prop. 52, proof, p. 134.

13. Aristotle, *Metaphysics*, trans. W. D. Ross, in *The Basic Works of Aristotle*, ed. Richard McKeon (New York: Random House, 1941), 1.2.982b10.

14. Descartes, *Passions of the Soul*, §25, p. 337.

15. Spinoza, *Ethics*, bk. 3, prop. 53, p. 135.

16. Ibid.

1. WHAT DOES "OF" MEAN IN DESCARTES'S EXPRESSION, "THE PASSIONS *OF* THE SOUL"?

1. René Descartes, *The Passions of the Soul*, in *The Philosophical Writings of Descartes*, trans. John Cottingham, Robert Stoothof, and Dugald Murdoch, vol. 1 (Cambridge: Cambridge University Press, 1985), part 2, "The Number and Order of the Passions," §§51–148.

2. Ibid., §§53, 70–78, 150.

3. Ibid., §2, p. 328.

4. Ibid., §7, p. 330.

5. Ibid., §10, pp. 331–332.

6. Ibid., §12.

7. We also find an explanation of muscular movements in §11, "How the Movements of the Muscles Take Place," and §13, "[The] Action of External Objects May Direct the Spirits Into the muscles in Various Different Ways."

8. Ibid., 342–343.

9. Ibid., 335.

10. Ibid.

11. Ibid., §19, p. 335.

12. Ibid., §25, pp. 337–338.

13. Ibid., §27, p. 339.

14. Ibid., §28.

15. Luce Irigaray finds a connection between Descartes's account of the passions and psychoanalysis: "Situating the passions at the junction of the physical and the psychological, he [Descartes] constructs a theory of the ego's affects which is close to Freud's theory of the drives" Irigaray, *The Ethics of Sexual Difference* (Ithaca: Cornell University Press, 1993), 80.

16. Descartes, *Passions Of The Soul*, §40.

17. Ibid., §§31–32, p. 340.

18. Cf. ibid., §75.

19. Ibid.

20. Ibid., 103, 121–122.

21. Ibid., 105.

22. Ibid., 103.
23. Ibid., 104.
24. Ibid.
25. Ibid., 105.
26. Ibid., 109.
27. Ibid., 105.

2. A "SELF-TOUCHING YOU": DERRIDA AND DESCARTES

1. Jacques Derrida, *On Touching—Jean-Luc Nancy*, trans. Christine Irizarry (Stanford: Stanford University Press, 2005), 180.
2. Jacques Derrida, "To Speculate—on 'Freud,'" in *The Postcard: From Socrates to Freud and Beyond*, trans. Alan Bass (Chicago: University of Chicago Press, 1987), 359.
3. Jacques Derrida, *Of Grammatology*, trans. Gayatri Chakravorty Spivak (Baltimore: Johns Hopkins University Press, 1976), 165.
4. Derrida, *On Touching—Jean-Luc Nancy*, 34.
5. Ibid., 35.
6. Ibid., 273.
7. Ibid.
8. René Descartes, *The Passions of the Soul*, in *The Philosophical Writings of Descartes*, trans. John Cottingham, Robert Stoothof, and Dugald Murdoch, vol. 1 (Cambridge: Cambridge University Press, 1985), §30.
9. Ibid.
10. Ibid., §31, p. 340.
11. Derrida, *On Touching—Jean-Luc Nancy*, 155.
12. Ibid.
13. Jean-Luc Nancy, *Corpus*, trans. Richard Rand (New York: Fordham University Press, 2008).
14. Derrida, *On Touching—Jean-Luc Nancy*, 156.
15. Nancy, *Corpus*, 2–121 ("Corpus"), 161–170 ("The Intruder").
16. Derrida, *On Touching—Jean-Luc Nancy*, 34.
17. See ibid., 273, 282.
18. Ibid., 21. In *Experience of Freedom*, Nancy declares: "The generosity of being offers nothing other than existence, and the offering, as such, is *kept* in freedom. All this means: a space is offered whose spacing, each time, only takes place by the way of a decision. But there is not 'the' decision. There is, each time, my own, yours, his or hers, ours. And this is the generosity of being." Jean-Luc Nancy, *Experience of Freedom*, trans. Bridget McDonald (Stanford: Stanford University Press, 1993), 146–147.
19. Derrida, *On Touching—Jean-Luc Nancy*, 282.

3. THE NEURAL SELF: DEMASIO MEETS DESCARTES

1. Antonio Damasio, *Descartes' Error: Emotions, Reason, and the Human Brain* (New York: HarperCollins, 1995), 236.

2. Oliver Sacks, foreword to *The Brain and The Inner World: An Introduction to the Neuroscience of Subjective Experience*, by Mark Solms and Oliver Turnbull (New York: Other Press, 2002), viii.

3. Cf. Alexander Luria, *Higher Cortical Functions in Man*, trans. Basil Haigh (New York: Basic Books, 1982).

4. V. S. Ramachandran and Sandra Blakeslee, *Phantoms in the Brain: Probing the Mysteries of the Human Mind* (New York: Quills Edition, 1999), 56.

5. Solms and Turnbull, *The Brain and the Inner World*, 4.

6. International Neuropsychoanalysis Society's website, www.neuropsa.org.uk. Let's recall that Mark Solms is a neurologist and a psychoanalyst at the same time. His two main books are *Neuropsychology of Dreams* and *Clinical Studies in Neuropsychology*. Damasio is also a member of The International Neuropsychoanalysis Society.

7. Solms and Turnbull, *The Brain and the Inner World*, 307.

8. Damasio, *Descartes' Error*, 251.

9. Ibid.

10. Antonio Damasio, *The Feeling of What Happens: Body and Emotion in the Making of Consciousness* (London: Heinemann, 1999), 174–175.

11. Damasio, *Descartes' Error*, 243.

12. Ibid., 238.

13. For a view of this chain (primary emotions, social emotions, feelings), see Antonio Damasio, *Looking for Spinoza: Joy, Sorrow, and the Feeling Brain* (New York: Harcourt, 2003), 45–46.

14. Damasio, *Descartes' Error*, 237.

4. AFFECTS ARE ALWAYS AFFECTS OF ESSENCE: BOOK 3 OF SPINOZA'S *ETHICS*

1. Baruch Spinoza, *Ethics*, trans. Samuel Shirley (Indianapolis: Hackett, 1992), bk. 3, preface, p. 102.

2. Ibid.

3. Ibid., 102–103.

4. See ibid., bk. 1, prop. 14: "There can be, or be conceived, no other substance but God." On Necessity, see ibid., bk. 1, prop. 17: "God acts solely from the laws of his own nature, constrained by none." On attributes and modes, see ibid., bk. 1, defs. 4 and 5, p. 31.

5. Deleuze, *Lectures on Spinoza at Vincennes*, BDSweb: University Courses, March 24, 1981.

6. Spinoza, *Ethics*, bk. 3, props. 1–59. The fifty-nine propositions can be divided into four parts: (a) 1–5; (b) 6–10; (c) 11–51; and (d) 52–59.

7. Ibid., 103.

8. Ibid., bk. 2, props. 6–7, p. 108.

9. Ibid., prop. 11, p. 110.

10. "When this conatus is related to the mind alone," Spinoza says, "it is called Will [*voluntas*]; when it is related to mind and body together, it is called Appetite [*appetites*]," which is also "desire [*cupiditas*]" when it is conscious. Ibid., prop. 9, scholium, p. 109.

11. The translation says "Pleasure and Pain." Following Deleuze's translations, we use "Joy" and "Sorrow."

12. Gilles Deleuze, *Expressionism in Philosophy: Spinoza*, trans. Martin Joughin (New York: Zone Books, 1992), 222.

13. Spinoza, *Ethics*, bk. 3, p. 141.

14. Deleuze, *Lectures on Spinoza at Vincennes*, January 24, 1978.

15. See the discussion of the central role played by imagination in Spinoza, *Ethics*, bk. 3, prop. 40.

16. Ibid., bk. 3, prop. 9, scholium.

17. Ibid., prop. 52, p. 134.

18. Ibid.

19. Deleuze, *Expressionism in Philosophy*, 222–223.

5. THE FACE AND THE CLOSE-UP: DELEUZE'S SPINOZIST APPROACH TO DESCARTES

1. Gilles Deleuze, *Cinema 1: The Movement-Image*, trans. Hugh Tomlinson and Barbara Habberjam (Minneapolis: University of Minnesota Press, 1986). Deleuze's reading of Descartes was first presented at Vincennes in a series of lectures given in February of 1982. Gilles Deleuze and Felix Guattari, *What Is Philosophy?*, trans. Hugh Tomlinson and Grahman Burchell (New York: Columbia University Press, 1994), 24–32.

2. Deleuze, *Lectures on Spinoza at Vincennes*, BDSweb: University Courses, January 24, 1978.

3. Baruch Spinoza, *Ethics*, trans. Samuel Shirley (Indianapolis: Hackett, 1992), bk. 2, props. 40–45.

4. Ibid., bk. 2, prop. 40, scholium 2, p. 90.

5. Ibid.

6. Ibid.

7. Deleuze, *Lectures on Spinoza at Vincennes*, January 24, 1978.

8. Gilles Deleuze and Felix Guattari, *A Thousand Plateaus: Capitalism and Schizophrenia 2*, trans. Brian Massumi (Minneapolis: University of Minnesota Press, 1987), 13.

9. René Descartes, *The Passions of the Soul*, in *The Philosophical Writings of Descartes*, trans. John Cottingham, Robert Stoothof, and Dugald Murdoch, vol. 1 (Cambridge: Cambridge University Press, 1985), §122.

10. See Deleuze, *Cinema 1*, chap. 6, "Affection-Image: The Face and the Close-Up."

11. Deleuze, *Lectures on Spinoza at Vincennes*, February 2, 1982.

12. Deleuze, *Cinema 1*, 87–88.

13. Deleuze, *Lectures on Spinoza at Vincennes*, February 2, 1982. See Deleuze, *Cinema 1*, 88.

14. Deleuze, *Cinema 1*, 88.

15. Ibid., 99.

16. Ibid.

17. Deleuze, *What Is Philosophy?*, 36.

18. Ibid., 64.

6. DAMASIO AS A READER OF SPINOZA

1. Antonio Damasio, *Looking for Spinoza: Joy, Sorrow, and the Feeling Brain* (New York: Harcourt, 2003).

2. Antonio Damasio, *The Feeling of What Happens: Body and Emotion in the Making of Consciousness* (London: Heinemann, 1999), 284.

3. Damasio, *Looking for Spinoza*, 8.

4. Ibid., 12.

5. See ibid., 156.

6. Ibid., 13.

7. Ibid., 15.

8. Ibid., 36.

9. Damasio, *Looking For Spinoza*, 13.

10. Ibid., 217.

11. The quotations are from Baruch Spinoza, *Ethics*, trans. Samuel Shirley (Indianapolis: Hackett, 1992), bk. 2, props. 13, 19, 23, 15.

12. Damasio, *Looking For Spinoza*, 212–213.

13. Ibid., 213.

14. Ibid., 137–138.

7. ON NEURAL PLASTICITY, TRAUMA, AND THE LOSS OF AFFECTS

1. Antonio Damasio, *Descartes' Error: Emotions, Reason, and the Human Brain* (New York: HarperCollins, 1995), 112–113.

2. Joseph LeDoux , *Synaptic Self: How Our Brain Becomes Who We Are* (New York: Penguin, 2002), 377–378.

230 •   6. DAMASIO AS A READER OF SPINOZA

3. Mark Solms and Oliver Turnbull, *The Brain and The Inner World: An Introduction to the Neuroscience of Subjective Experience* (New York: Other Press, 2002), 2–3.

4. Ibid., 4.

5. Antonio Damasio, *The Feeling of What Happens: Body and Emotion in the Making of Consciousness* (London: Heinemann, 1999), 53.

6. Ibid., 41.

7. Damasio, *Descartes' Error*, 16.

8. Ibid., 36.

9. Ibid., 45.

10. Ibid., 38.

11. Damasio, *Feeling of What Happens*, 102–103.

12. Damasio, *Descartes' Error*, 64.

13. Sigmund Freud, *Civilization and Its Discontents*, in *The Standard Edition of the Complete Psychological Works of Sigmund Freud*, ed. and trans. James Strachey, in collaboration with Anna Freud, assisted by Alix Strachey and Alan Tyson (London: Hogarth Press and the Institute of Psycho-Analysis, 1953–1974), 21:70.

14. Sigmund Freud, "Thoughts for the Times on War and Death," in *The Standard Edition*, 24:285–286.

15. Solms and Turnbull, *The Brain And The Inner World*, 208.

16. Ibid., 210.

CONCLUSION

1. Baruch Spinoza, *Ethics*, trans. Samuel Shirley (Indianapolis: Hackett, 1992), bk. 3, p. 135.

2. Jacques Derrida, *On Touching—Jean-Luc Nancy*, trans. Christine Irizarry (Stanford: Stanford University Press, 2005), 112–113.

3. Gilles Deleuze and Felix Guattari, *What Is Philosophy?*, trans. Hugh Tomlinson and Grahman Burchell (New York: Columbia University Press, 1994), 173.

4. Antonio Damasio, *The Feeling of What Happens: Body and Emotion in the Making of Consciousness* (London: Heinemann, 1999), 74–75.

5. Maurice Merleau-Ponty, *Phenomenology of Perception*, trans. Colin Smith (London: Routledge and Kegan Paul, 1962), 92.

6. Derrida, *On Touching—Jean-Luc Nancy*, 156.

7. Deleuze and Guattari, *What is Philosophy?*, 178–179.

8. Antonio Damasio, *Descartes' Error: Emotions, Reason, and the Human Brain* (New York: HarperCollins, 1995), 16.

9. Jacques Derrida, "Maddening the Subjectile," trans. Mary Ann Caws, in *Yale French Studies* 84, Boundaries: Writing & Drawing (New Haven: Yale University Press, 1994), 122.

10. Derrida, *On Touching—Jean-Luc Nancy*, 156.

11. Sigmund Freud, note left on August 22, 1938, in *Schriften aus dem Nachlass*, in *Gesammelte Werke*, ed. E. Bibring, W. Hoffer, E. Kris, and O. Isakower, vol. 17 (Frankfurt: S. Fischer, 1952). The English translation is found in *The Standard Edition of the Complete Psychological Works of Sigmund Freud*, ed. and trans. James Strachey, in collaboration with Anna Freud, assisted by Alix Strachey and Alan Tyson, vol. 24 (London: Hogarth Press and the Institute of Psycho-Analysis, 1953–1974).

12. See Sigmund Freud, *Beyond the Pleasure Principle*, trans. James Strachey (New York: W. W. Norton, 1961).

13. Sigmund Freud, *The Ego And The Id* (London: Hogarth Press, 1949), 72.

14. Derrida, *On Touching—Jean-Luc Nancy*, 16.

15. Jacques Lacan, *Le Séminaire de Jacques Lacan*, book 19, trans. Cormac Gallagher from unedited French typescripts, 114–126.

16. Oliver Sacks, *The Man Who Mistook His Wife for a Hat, and Other Clinical Tales* (London: Picador, 1985), 36.

17. Thomas Metzinger, *Being No One: The Self-Model Theory of Subjectivity* (Cambridge, Mass.: MIT Press, 2003), 1.

8. GUILT AND THE FEEL OF FEELING: TOWARD A NEW CONCEPTION OF AFFECTS

All citations of works by Sigmund Freud are references to his *Gesammelte Werke* (German) or *Standard Edition* (English). These are abbreviated as *GW* or *SE*, followed by the volume number and the page number (*GW/SE #:#*). See Sigmund Freud, *Gesammelte Werke*, ed. E. Bibring, W. Hoffer, E. Kris, and O. Isakower (Frankfurt: S. Fischer, 1952); and Sigmund Freud, *The Standard Edition of the Complete Psychological Works of Sigmund Freud*, ed. and trans. James Strachey, in collaboration with Anna Freud, assisted by Alix Strachey and Alan Tyson, 24 vols. (London: Hogarth Press and the Institute of Psycho-Analysis, 1953–1974).

1. Aristotle, *Metaphysics*, trans. W. D. Ross, in *The Basic Works of Aristotle*, ed. Richard McKeon (New York: Random House, 1941), 1.2.982b12–22.

2. *SE* 14:95.

3. *SE* 22:69–70.

4. *SE* 19:52.

5. *SE* 14:332–333.

6. *SE* 9:123.

7. *SE* 14:178.

8. *GW* 10:277; *SE* 14:178.

9. *GW* 10:276; *SE* 14:177.

10. Adrian Johnston, "Repeating Engels: Renewing the Cause of the Materialist Wager for the Twenty-First Century," *Theory @ Buffalo* 15 (2011): 141–182; Adrian Johnston, *A Weak Nature Alone: Prolegomena to Any Future Materialism*, vol. 2 (unpublished manuscript).

11. Adrian Johnston, *Žižek's Ontology: A Transcendental Materialist Theory of Subjectivity* (Evanston: Northwestern University Press, 2008), 270–272; Adrian Johnston, "What Matter(s) in Ontology: Alain Badiou, the Hebb-Event, and Materialism Split from Within," *Angelaki: Journal of the Theoretical Humanities* 13, no. 3 (April 2008): 27–49; Adrian Johnston, "The Weakness of Nature: Hegel, Freud, Lacan, and Negativity Materialized," in *Hegel and the Infinite: Into the Twenty-First Century*, ed. Clayton Crockett, Creston Davis, and Slavoj Žižek (New York: Columbia University Press, 2011), 159–179; Adrian Johnston, "Second Natures in Dappled Worlds: John McDowell, Nancy Cartwright, and Hegelian-Lacanian Materialism," *Umbr(a): A Journal of the Unconscious—The Worst*, ed. Matthew Rigilano and Kyle Fetter (Buffalo: Center for the Study of Psychoanalysis and Culture, State University of New York at Buffalo, 2011), 71–91; Adrian Johnston, "Turning the Sciences Inside Out: Revisiting Lacan's 'Science and Truth,'" in *Concept and Form: The Cahiers pour l'Analyse and Contemporary French Thought*, ed. Peter Hallward, Knox Peden, and Christian Kerslake (London: Verso, 2012); Adrian Johnston, "On Deep History and Lacan," in "Lacan and Philosophy: The New Generation," ed. Lorenzo Chiesa, special issue, *Journal of European Psychoanalysis* (2012); Adrian Johnston, "'Naturalism or anti-naturalism? No, thanks—both are worse!': Science, Materialism, and Slavoj Žižek," in "On Slavoj Žižek," special issue, *La Revue Internationale de Philosophie* (2012); Adrian Johnston, *Alain Badiou and the Outcome of Contemporary French Philosophy: Prolegomena to Any Future Materialism*, vol. 1 (Evanston: Northwestern University Press, 2013).

12. André Green, *Le discours vivant: La conception psychanalytique de l'affect* (Paris: Presses Universitaires de France, 1973), 6, 237.

13. Colette Soler, *Les affects lacaniens* (Paris: Presses Universitaires de France, 2011), viii, x, 3–5, 11.

14. Adrian Johnston, "Sigmund Freud," in *The History of Continental Philosophy*, vol. 3, *The New Century*, ed. Keith Ansell Pearson (Chesham: Acumen Press, 2010), 322–324, 328–330.

15. *SE* 16:284–285.

16. Jacques Lacan, "The Subversion of the Subject and the Dialectic of Desire in the Freudian Unconscious," in *Écrits: The First Complete Edition in English*, trans. Bruce Fink (New York: W. W. Norton, 2006), 674.

17. Blaise Pascal, *Pensées*, ed. Léon Brunschvicg (Paris: Flammarion, 1976), 158; translation: Blaise Pascal, *Pensées*, trans. A. J. Krailsheimer (New York: Penguin, 1966), 59.

18. Pascal, *Pensées*, 59; translation: Pascal, *Pensées*, 158.

19. Jacques Lacan, *The Seminar of Jacques Lacan*, book 7, *The Ethics of Psychoanalysis, 1959–1960*, ed. Jacques-Alain Miller, trans. Dennis Porter (New York: W. W. Norton, 1992), 14.

20. René Descartes, "Meditations: Objections et réponses," in *Oeuvres de Descartes*, vol. 9, *Meditations et principes*, ed. Charles Adam and Paul Tannery (Paris: Vrin, 1996), 180, 190.

21. René Descartes, *The Passions of the Soul*, trans. Robert Stoothoff, in *The Philosophical Writings of Descartes*, trans. John Cottingham, Robert Stoothoff, and Dugald Murdoch, vol. 1 (Cambridge: Cambridge University Press, 1985), §26, p. 338.

22. Wilfrid Sellars, *Empiricism and the Philosophy of Mind* (Cambridge, Mass.: Harvard University Press, 1997), 14, 45.

23. John McDowell, *Mind and World* (Cambridge, Mass.: Harvard University Press, 1994), ix, 9–13, 18, 24, 41, 46, 64, 66–67, 69–70, 87, 98; John McDowell, "Preface," in *Having the World in View: Essays on Kant, Hegel, and Sellars* (Cambridge, Mass.: Harvard University Press, 2009), viii; John McDowell, "Sellars on Perceptual Experience," in *Having the World in View*, 5–6; John McDowell, "The Logical Form of an Intuition," in *Having the World in View*, 23–43; John McDowell, "Sensory Consciousness in Kant and Sellars," in *Having the World in View*, 124; John McDowell, "On Pippin's Postscript," in *Having the World in View*, 198; Johnston, "Second Natures in Dappled Worlds," 73–77, 80–81, 85–86.

24. Georg Lukács, "Class Consciousness," in *History and Class Consciousness*, trans. Rodney Livingstone (Cambridge, Mass.: MIT Press, 1971), 52, 73–74.

25. Jacques Lacan, "Remarque sur le rapport de Daniel Lagache: 'Psychanalyse et structure de la personnalité,'" in *Écrits* (Paris: Éditions du Seuil, 1966), 683.

9. FEELING WITHOUT FEELING: FREUD AND THE UNRESOLVED PROBLEM OF UNCONSCIOUS GUILT

1. *GW* 13:254–255, 263; *SE* 19:26–27, 35.

2. *GW* 7:135; *SE* 9:123.

3. *GW* 10:276; *SE* 14:177.

4. *SE* 9:123.

5. Ibid.

6. *SE* 21:142.

7. *GW* 10:390; *SE* 14:332.

8. *GW* 13:282; *SE* 19:52.

9. *SE* 19:28, 39, 48–49.

10. Ibid., 17–19, 23.

11. Ibid., 28.

12. Ibid.

13. *SE* 19:26.

14. *GW* 13:254–255; *SE* 19:26–27.

15. *SE* 19:35.

16. *GW* 14:254; *SE* 20:224.

17. *SE* 22:109–110.

18. *SE* 19:49.

19. *GW* 13:279; *SE* 19:49–50.

20. *SE* 14:95–96.

21. *SE* 19:54, 167.

22. *GW* 13:373; *SE* 19:161.

23. *SE* 19:161.

24. Ibid., 166.

25. *GW* 13:379; *SE* 19:166.

26. *SE* 19:168–169.

27. *GW* 14:493.

28. *SE* 21:134.

29. *GW* 14:499; *SE* 21:139.

30. *SE* 21:125.

31. Ibid., 112.

32. *SE* 21:125–126.

33. *GW* 14:494; *SE* 21:134.

34. *GW* 14:494–495; *SE* 21:134–135.

35. *GW* 14:497; *SE* 21:137.

36. *SE* 19:51.

37. *SE* 22:109.

38. *GW* 14:495; *SE* 21:135–136.

39. *SE* 21:139.

40. *SE* 20:132.

41. *GW* 13:282; *SE* 19:53.

42. *GW* 13:281; *SE* 19:52.

43. *GW* 15:116; *SE* 22:109.

10. AFFECTS, EMOTIONS, AND FEELINGS: FREUD'S METAPSYCHOLOGIES OF AFFECTIVE LIFE

1. *SE* 1:327.

2. Jean Laplanche and Jean-Bertrand Pontalis, *The Language of Psycho-Analysis*, trans. Donald Nicholson-Smith (New York: W. W. Norton, 1973), 13–14.

3. *SE* 1:295, 298–300.

4. *GW* 1:65–66; *SE* 3:51–52.

5. *SE* 3:49.

6. Ibid., 48–50.

7. Jacques Lacan, *The Seminar of Jacques Lacan*, book 11, *The Four Fundamental Concepts of Psycho-Analysis, 1964*, ed. Jacques-Alain Miller, trans. Alan Sheridan (New York: W. W. Norton, 1977), 217.

8. *SE* 3:53.

9. *SE* 18:60.

10. *GW* 10:275; *SE* 14:177.

11. *SE* 14:148, 152–153.

12. Ibid., 122–123.

13. Ibid., 177.

14. *GW* 10:276; *SE* 14:177.

15. *GW* 10:276; *SE* 14:177.

16. *GW* 10:276; *SE* 14:177.

17. Jacques Lacan, *The Seminar of Jacques Lacan*, book 17, *The Other Side of Psychoanalysis, 1969–1970*, ed. Jacques-Alain Miller, trans. Russell Grigg (New York: W. W. Norton, 2007), 144.

18. André Green, *Le discours vivant: La conception psychanalytique de l'affect* (Paris: Presses Universitaires de France, 1973), 61–62.

19. *GW* 10:276; *SE* 14:177–178.

20. *GW* 10:278; *SE* 14:179.

21. *GW* 10:276–277; *SE* 14:178.

22. *SE* 1:321–322.

23. Laplanche and Pontalis, *The Language of Psycho-Analysis*, 14.

24. *SE* 14:179.

25. *GW* 10:277; *SE* 14:178.

26. Green, *Le discours vivant*, 63, 100.

27. Ibid., 17.

28. *GW* 13:250; *SE* 19:22–23.

29. Sydney E. Pulver, "Can Affects Be Unconscious?," *International Journal of Psycho-Analysis* 52 (1971): 350, 353.

30. Ibid., 348.

31. Sydney E. Pulver, "Unconscious Versus Potential Affects," *Psychoanalytic Quarterly* 43 (1974): 78.

32. Ibid., 83–84.

33. Pulver, "Can Affects be Unconscious?," 349–350; Pulver, "Unconscious Versus Potential Affects," 80.

34. Pulver, "Can Affects be Unconscious?," 351.

35. Pulver, "Unconscious Versus Potential Affects," 80–81.

36. Pulver, "Can Affects be Unconscious?," 348, 353.

37. Ibid., 347.

11. FROM SIGNIFIERS TO *JOUIS-SENS*: LACAN'S *SENTI-MENTS* AND *AFFECTUATIONS*

1. Bruce Fink, *Lacan to the Letter: Reading Écrits Closely* (Minneapolis: University of Minnesota Press, 2004), 142.

2. *GW* 10:278–279; *SE* 14:179.

3. Jacques Lacan, *Le Séminaire de Jacques Lacan*, book 19, *Le savoir du psychanalyste, 1971–1972* (unpublished typescript), session of November 4, 1971.

4. Bruce Fink, *Fundamentals of Psychoanalytic Technique: A Lacanian Approach for Practitioners* (New York: W. W. Norton, 2007), 130.

5. Fink, *Lacan to the Letter*, 142.

6. Fink, *Fundamentals of Psychoanalytic Technique*, 130.

7. Jacques Lacan, *The Seminar of Jacques Lacan*, book 1, *Freud's Papers on Technique, 1953–1954*, ed. Jacques-Alain Miller, trans. John Forrester (New York: W. W. Norton, 1988), 57.

8. Fink, *Lacan to the Letter*, 51–52.

9. Green, *Le discours vivant: La conception psychanalytique de l'affect* (Paris: Presses Universitaires de France, 1973), 99–100.

10. Lacan, *The Seminar of Jacques Lacan*, book 1, 57.

11. Jacques Lacan, "The Function and Field of Speech and Language in Psychoanalysis," in *Écrits: The First Complete Edition in English*, trans. Bruce Fink (New York: W. W. Norton, 2006), 254.

12. Fink, *Lacan to the Letter*, 51.

13. *SE* 14:152.

14. Jacques Lacan, *Le Séminaire de Jacques Lacan*, book 6, *Le désir et son interprétation, 1958–1959* (unpublished typescript), session of November 26, 1958.

15. Roberto Harari, *Lacan's Seminar on "Anxiety": An Introduction*, ed. Rico Franses, trans. Jane C. Lamb-Ruiz (New York: Other Press, 2001), 22.

16. Harari, *Lacan's Seminar on "Anxiety,"* 12–13; Roberto Harari, *Lacan's Four Fundamental Concepts of Psychoanalysis: An Introduction*, trans. Judith Filc (New York: Other Press, 2004), 268; Bruce Fink, *A Clinical Introduction to Lacanian Psychoanalysis: Theory and Technique* (Cambridge, Mass.: Harvard University Press, 1997), 113–114.

17. Lacan, *Le Séminaire de Jacques Lacan*, book 6, session of November 26, 1958.

18. Jacques Lacan, *The Seminar of Jacques Lacan*, book 7, *The Ethics of Psychoanalysis, 1959–1960*, ed. Jacques-Alain Miller, trans. Dennis Porter (New York: W. W. Norton, 1992), 102.

19. Jacques Lacan, *Le Séminaire de Jacques Lacan*, book 9, *L'identification, 1961–1962* (unpublished typescript), session of May 2, 1962.

20. Harari, *Lacan's Seminar on "Anxiety,"* 27.

21. Colette Soler, *Les affects lacaniens* (Paris: Presses Universitaires de France, 2011), 11.

22. Jacques Lacan, "Television," trans. Denis Hollier, Rosalind Krauss, and Annette Michelson, in *Television/A Challenge to the Psychoanalytic Establishment*, ed. Joan Copjec (New York: W. W. Norton, 1990), 20.

23. Ibid., 20.

24. Jacques Lacan, *Le Séminaire de Jacques Lacan*, book 23, *Le sinthome, 1975–1976*, Jacques-Alain Miller (Paris: Éditions du Seuil, 2005), 149.

25. Jacques Lacan, *Le Séminaire de Jacques Lacan*, book 27, *Dissolution, 1979–1980* (unpublished typescript), session of March 18, 1980.

26. Bruce Fink, *The Lacanian Subject: Between Language and Jouissance* (Princeton: Princeton University Press, 1995), 8, 73–74; Fink, *A Clinical Introduction to Lacanian Psychoanalysis*, 167–168.

27. *SE* 14:121–122.

28. Ibid., 148.

29. *GW* 10:276; *SE* 14:177–178.

30. Fink, *The Lacanian Subject*, 74; Bruce Fink, "The Real Cause of Repetition," in *Reading Seminar XI: Lacan's Four Fundamental Concepts of Psychoanalysis*, ed. Richard Feldstein, Bruce Fink, and Maire Jaanus (Albany: SUNY Press, 1995), 227–228.

31. *GW* 10:250–251; *SE* 14:148.

32. Elisabeth Roudinesco, *Jacques Lacan & Co.: A History of Psychoanalysis in France, 1925–1985*, trans. Jeffrey Mehlman (Chicago: University of Chicago Press, 1990), 312.

33. Green, *Le discours vivant*, 58–59, 125, 128, 212, 230, 233–234, 253, 287, 333.

34. Jacques Lacan, "In Memory of Ernest Jones: On His Theory of Symbolism," in *Écrits*, 598.

35. Lacan, *The Seminar of Jacques Lacan*, book 7, 103.

36. Ibid., 102–103.

37. Lacan, *Le Séminaire de Jacques Lacan*, book 6, session of November 26, 1958.

38. Lacan, *The Seminar of Jacques Lacan*, book 7, 61.

39. Lacan, *Le Séminaire de Jacques Lacan*, book 19, session of February 3, 1972; Jacques Lacan, *Le Séminaire de Jacques Lacan*, book 25, *Le moment de conclure, 1977–1978* (unpublished typescript), session of November 15, 1977; Jean-Claude Milner, *Le périple structural: Figures et paradigms* (Paris: Éditions du Seuil, 2002), 144–146.

40. Lacan, *The Seminar of Jacques Lacan*, book 7, 61.

41. Ibid., 102, 118.

42. Jacques Lacan, "Discours aux catholiques," in *Le triomphe de la religion, précédé de Discours aux catholiques*, ed. Jacques-Alain Miller (Paris: Éditions du Seuil, 2005), 50–51.

43. Jacques Lacan, *The Seminar of Jacques Lacan*, book 11, 216.

44. Ibid., 216–217.

45. Ibid, 60.

46. Ibid., 217.

47. Ibid.

48. Jacques Lacan, *Le Séminaire de Jacques Lacan*, book 13, *L'objet de la psychanalyse, 1965–1966* (unpublished typescript), session of June 1, 1966.

49. Harari, *Lacan's Four Fundamental Concepts of Psychoanalysis*, 267–268.

50. Lacan, *The Seminar of Jacques Lacan*, book 11, 218.

51. Ibid., 236.

52. Jacques Lacan, *Le Séminaire de Jacques Lacan*, book 15, *L'acte psychanalytique, 1967–1968* (unpublished typescript), session of November 15, 1967.

53. Jacques Lacan, *Le Séminaire de Jacques Lacan*, book 16, *D'un Autre à l'autre, 1968–1969*, ed. Jacques-Alain Miller (Paris: Éditions du Seuil, 2006), 261.

54. Lacan, *The Seminar of Jacques Lacan*, book 7, 102.

55. Lacan, *The Seminar of Jacques Lacan*, book 11, 218.

56. Jacques Lacan, *Le Séminaire de Jacques Lacan*, book 14, *La logique du fantasme, 1966–1967* (unpublished typescript), session of December 14, 1966; Jacques Lacan, *Le Séminaire de Jacques Lacan*, book 18, *D'un discours qui ne serait pas du semblant, 1971*, ed. Jacques-Alain Miller (Paris: Éditions du Seuil, 2006), 14.

57. Lacan, *The Seminar of Jacques Lacan*, book 1, 191.

58. Lacan, *Le Séminaire de Jacques Lacan*, book 14, session of December 14, 1966; Jacques Lacan, *The Seminar of Jacques Lacan*, book 17, *The Other Side of Psychoanalysis, 1969–1970*, ed. Jacques-Alain Miller, trans. Russell Grigg (New York: W. W. Norton, 2007), 144.

59. Lacan, *The Seminar of Jacques Lacan*, book 11, 220.

60. Ibid., 220.

61. *SE* 14:278–279, 287–288.

62. Ibid., 287–288.

63. Green, *Le discours vivant*, 54.

64. Fink, *The Lacanian Subject*, 73–74, 188.

65. Jacques Lacan, *Le Séminaire de Jacques Lacan*, book 10, *L'angoisse, 1962–1963*, ed. Jacques-Alain Miller (Paris: Éditions du Seuil, 2004), 23, 28.

66. Ibid., 23.

67. Ibid.

68. Lacan, *The Seminar of Jacques Lacan*, book 17, 144; Lacan, "Television," 21.

69. Lacan, *Le Séminaire de Jacques Lacan*, book 10, 24.

70. *SE* 16:395, 405; *SE* 20:140–141, 166–167, 202; *SE* 22:84, 93–95; *SE* 23:146, 199.

71. Harari, *Lacan's Seminar on "Anxiety,"* 4–5.

72. Lacan, *The Seminar of Jacques Lacan*, book 17, 144.

73. Ibid.

74. *GW* 10:250–251; *SE* 14:148.

75. Jean Laplanche and Serge Leclaire, "L'inconscient: Une étude psychanalytique," in Jean Laplanche, *Problématiques IV: L'inconscient et le ça* (Paris: Presses Universitaires de Frances, 1981), 289.

76. Jean Laplanche and Serge Leclaire, "The Unconscious: A Psychoanalytic Study," trans. Patrick Coleman, in "French Freud—Structural Studies in Psychoanalysis," *Yale French Studies* 48 (1972): 144.

77. Jean Laplanche and Jean-Bertrand Pontalis, *The Language of Psycho-Analysis*, trans. Donald Nicholson-Smith (New York: W. W. Norton, 1973), 203–204.

78. Ibid., 203–204.

79. Green, *Le discours vivant*, 289.

80. Lacan, *The Seminar of Jacques Lacan*, book 17, 144.

81. Ibid.

82. Ibid., 150.

83. Ibid., 150–151.

84. Ibid., 151.

85. Ibid.

86. Ibid.

87. Joan Copjec, "May '68, The Emotional Month," in *Lacan: The Silent Partners*, ed. Slavoj Žižek (London: Verso, 2006), 92.

88. Lacan, *The Seminar of Jacques Lacan*, book 17, 151.

89. Ibid., 34.

90. Slavoj Žižek, "The Undergrowth of Enjoyment: How Popular Culture Can Serve as an Introduction to Lacan," in *The Žižek Reader*, ed. Elizabeth Wright and Edmond Wright (Oxford: Blackwell, 1999), 28–29; Slavoj Žižek, *Iraq: The Borrowed Kettle* (London: Verso, 2004), 133–134, 144; Adrian Johnston, *Žižek's Ontology: A Transcendental Materialist Theory of Subjectivity* (Evanston: Northwestern University Press, 2008), 251–253, 259–260.

91. Johnston, *Žižek's Ontology*, 251–252; Paul Verhaeghe, "From Impossibility to Inability: Lacan's Theory on the Four Discourses," in *Beyond Gender: From Subject to Drive* (New York: Other Press, 2001), 22.

92. Mladen Dolar, "Hegel as the Other Side of Psychoanalysis," in *Jacques Lacan and the Other Side of Psychoanalysis: Reflections on Seminar XVII*, ed. Justin Clemens and Russell Grigg (Durham: Duke University Press, 2006), 143–144.

93. Green, *Le discours vivant*, 224–225.

94. Soler, *Les affects lacaniens*, 6.

95. Lacan, *Le Séminaire de Jacques Lacan*, book 23, 66.

96. Jacques Lacan, "*La mort est du domaine de la foi*," October 13, 1972, www.ecole-lacanienne.net/pastoutlacan70.php.

97. Slavoj Žižek, *The Parallax View* (Cambridge, Mass.: MIT Press, 2006), 229.

98. Lacan, *Le Séminaire de Jacques Lacan*, book 19, sessions of November 4, 1971, December 2, 1971.

99. Jacques Lacan, *The Seminar of Jacques Lacan*, book 20, *Encore, 1972–1973*, ed. Jacques-Alain Miller, trans. Bruce Fink (New York: W. W. Norton, 1998), 138; Jacques Lacan, "Alla Scuola Freudiana: Conférence à Milan," March 30, 1974, www.ecole-lacanienne.

net/pastoutlacan70.php; Jacques Lacan, "Conférence à Genève sur 'Le symptôme,'" October 4, 1975, www.ecole-lacanienne.net/pastoutlacan70.php; Jacques Lacan, "Conférences et entretiens dans des universités nord-américaines: Columbia University Auditorium School of International Affairs" (delivered December 1, 1975), *Scilicet* 6/7 (1976): 47.

100. Lacan, *Le Séminaire de Jacques Lacan*, book 25, session of November 15, 1977.

101. Jacques Lacan, *Le Séminaire de Jacques Lacan*, book 21, *Les non-dupes errent, 1973–1974* (unpublished typescript), session of June 11, 1974; Lacan, *Le Séminaire de Jacques Lacan*, book 23, 117.

102. Lacan, *Le Séminaire de Jacques Lacan*, book 25, session of November 15, 1977.

103. Jacques Lacan, *Le Séminaire de Jacques Lacan*, book 24, *L'insu que sait de l'une-bévue, s'aile à mourre, 1976–1977* (unpublished typescript), session of April 19, 1977; Lacan, *Le Séminaire de Jacques Lacan*, book 25, sessions of November 15, 1977, April 11, 1978.

104. Colette Soler, *Lacan, l'inconscient réinventé* (Paris: Presses Universitaires de France, 2009), 34.

105. Laplanche and Pontalis, *The Language of Psycho-Analysis*, 339–341.

106. Lacan, *Le Séminaire de Jacques Lacan*, book 21, session of January 8, 1974; Lacan, "Television," 9–10.

107. Jacques Lacan, " . . . ou pire: Compte rendu du Séminaire 1971–1972," in *Autres écrits*, ed. Jacques-Alain Miller (Paris: Éditions du Seuil, 2001), 551.

108. Slavoj Žižek, *Looking Awry: An Introduction to Jacques Lacan through Popular Culture* (Cambridge, Mass.: MIT Press, 1991), 128–129.

109. Lacan, "Television," 10.

110. Ibid.

111. Lacan, "The Function and Field of Speech and Language in Psychoanalysis," 248; Jacques Lacan, "Discours de Rome," in *Autres écrits*, 137–138; Jacques Lacan, "Problèmes cruciaux pour la psychanalyse: Compte rendu du Séminaire 1964–1965," in *Autres écrits*, 199; Lacan, *Le Séminaire de Jacques Lacan*, book 14, sessions of February 1, 1967, May 10, 1967; Johnston, *Žižek's Ontology*, 87–88; Adrian Johnston, "Slavoj Žižek's Hegelian Reformation: Giving a Hearing to *The Parallax View*," *Diacritics: A Review of Contemporary Criticism* 37, no. 1 (Spring 2007): 9.

112. Lacan, *The Seminar of Jacques Lacan*, book 20, 139.

113. Ibid.

114. Ibid.

115. Soler, *Lacan, l'inconscient réinventé*, 29–32; Soler, *Les affects lacaniens*, 84, 103, 106–107.

116. Lacan, *Le Séminaire de Jacques Lacan*, book 10, 91–92, 252–253; Jacques Lacan, "Introduction to the Names-of-the-Father Seminar," ed. Jacques-Alain Miller, trans. Jeffrey Mehlman, in Copjec, *Television/A Challenge to the Psychoanalytic Establishment*, 82; Žižek, *The Parallax View*, 229.

117. Lacan, *Le Séminaire de Jacques Lacan*, book 18, 104.

118. Lacan, *The Seminar of Jacques Lacan*, book 17 151.

119. Lacan, *Le Séminaire de Jacques Lacan*, book 10, 24.

120. Lacan, *The Seminar of Jacques Lacan*, book 17, 144.

121. Lacan, *Le Séminaire de Jacques Lacan*, book 10, 91–92; Jacques-Alain Miller, "Introduction to Reading Jacques Lacan's Seminar on *Anxiety*," trans. Barbara P. Fulks, *Lacanian Ink* 26 (Fall 2005): 63–64; Jacques-Alain Miller, "Introduction to Reading Jacques Lacan's Seminar on *Anxiety* II," trans. Barbara P. Fulks, *Lacanian Ink* 27 (Spring 2006): 22.

12. EMOTIONAL LIFE AFTER LACAN: FROM PSYCHOANALYSIS TO THE NEUROSCIENCES

1. Jacques Lacan, *Le Séminaire de Jacques Lacan*, book 10, *L'angoisse, 1962–1963*, ed. Jacques-Alain Miller (Paris: Éditions du Seuil, 2004), 93; Adrian Johnston, *Badiou, Žižek, and Political Transformations: The Cadence of Change* (Evanston: Northwestern University Press, 2009), 144–156.

2. Lacan, *Le Séminaire de Jacques Lacan*, book 10, 92.

3. Ibid.

4. Ibid.

5. Jacques Lacan, *The Seminar of Jacques Lacan*, book 11, *The Four Fundamental Concepts of Psycho-Analysis, 1964*, ed. Jacques-Alain Miller, trans. Alan Sheridan (New York: W. W. Norton, 1977), 35, 44; Jacques Lacan, *Le Séminaire de Jacques Lacan*, book 12, *Problèmes cruciaux pour la psychanalyse, 1964–1965* (unpublished typescript), session of June 9, 1965; Adrian Johnston, *Time Driven: Metapsychology and the Splitting of the Drive* (Evanston: Northwestern University Press, 2005), 62, 64–65, 70, 279–280.

6. Jacques Lacan, *The Seminar of Jacques Lacan*, book 17, *The Other Side of Psychoanalysis, 1969–1970*, ed. Jacques-Alain Miller, trans. Russell Grigg (New York: W. W. Norton, 2007), 180–183, 192–193.

7. Jacques-Alain Miller, "On Shame," ed. Catherine Bonningue, trans. Russell Grigg, in *Jacques Lacan and the Other Side of Psychoanalysis: Reflections on Seminar XVII*, ed. Justin Clemens and Russell Grigg (Durham: Duke University Press, 2006), 13, 15, 23–24, 26–27; Paul Verhaeghe, "Enjoyment and Impossibility: Lacan's Revision of the Oedipus Complex," in Clemens and Grigg, *Jacques Lacan and the Other Side of Psychoanalysis*, 47; Dominiek Hoens, "Toward a New Perversion: Psychoanalysis," in Clemens and Grigg, *Jacques Lacan and the Other Side of Psychoanalysis*, 96–97; Éric Laurent, "Symptom and Discourse," in Clemens and Grigg, *Jacques Lacan and the Other Side of Psychoanalysis*, 234.

8. Jacques Lacan, "Impromptu at Vincennes," trans. Jeffrey Mehlman, in Copjec, *Television/A Challenge to the Psychoanalytic Establishment*, ed. Joan Copjec (New York: W. W. Norton, 1990), 117–128; Lacan, *The Seminar of Jacques Lacan*, book 17, 181.

9. Adrian Johnston, "Lacanian Theory Has Legs: Structures Marching in the Streets," *South Atlantic Review* 72, no. 2 (Spring 2007): 100–105.

10. Jacques Lacan, *The Seminar of Jacques Lacan*, book 20, *Encore, 1972–1973*, ed. Jacques-Alain Miller, trans. Bruce Fink (New York: W. W. Norton, 1998), 3, 7–8; Adrian Johnston, *Time Driven: Metapsychology and the Splitting of the Drive* (Evanston: Northwestern University Press, 2005), xxxvii–xxxviii, 295–299, 331, 335–337.

11. Joan Copjec, "May '68, The Emotional Month," in *Lacan: The Silent Partners*, ed. Slavoj Žižek (London: Verso, 2006), 91.

12. Johnston, "Lacanian Theory Has Legs," 100–102.

13. Copjec, "May '68, The Emotional Month," 92–93, 96.

14. Ibid., 93.

15. Alenka Zupančič, "When Surplus Enjoyment Meets Surplus Value," in Clemens and Grigg, *Jacques Lacan and the Other Side of Psychoanalysis*, 155, 158.

16. Copjec, "May '68, The Emotional Month," 92–93.

17. Ibid., 91–92.

18. Jacques Lacan, *Le Séminaire de Jacques Lacan*, book 17, *L'envers de la psychanalyse, 1969–1970*, ed. Jacques-Alain Miller (Paris: Éditions du Seuil, 1991), 209–210, 223.

19. Jacques Lacan, *Le Séminaire de Jacques Lacan*, book 8, *Le transfert, 1960–1961*, ed. Jacques-Alain Miller (Paris: Éditions du Seuil, 2001), 213–214; Jacques Lacan, *Le Séminaire de Jacques Lacan*, book 11, *Les quatre concepts fondamentaux de la psychanalyse, 1964*, ed. Jacques-Alain Miller (Paris: Éditions du Seuil, 1973), 166.

20. Johnston, "Lacanian Theory Has Legs," 103.

21. Copjec, "May '68, The Emotional Month," 91–92, 111; Joan Copjec, *Imagine There's No Woman: Ethics and Sublimation* (Cambridge, Mass.: MIT Press, 2004), 216–217.

22. Jacques Lacan, *Le Séminaire de Jacques Lacan*, book 6, session of December 10, 1958.

23. Lacan, *Le Séminaire de Jacques Lacan*, book 8, 213–214.

24. Jacques Lacan, "*Le signification du phallus*," in *Écrits* (Paris: Éditions du Seuil, 1966), 692; Jacques Lacan, "The Signification of the Phallus," in *Écrits: The First Complete Edition in English*, trans. Bruce Fink (New York: W. W. Norton, 2006), 581; Jacques Lacan, *Le Séminaire de Jacques Lacan*, book 5, *Les formations de l'inconscient, 1957–1958*, ed. Jacques-Alain Miller (Paris: Éditions du Seuil, 1998), 384; Lacan, *Le Séminaire de Jacques Lacan*, book 8, 213–214.

25. Lacan, "The Signification of the Phallus," 581; Jacques Lacan, *Le Séminaire de Jacques Lacan*, book 21, *Les non-dupes errent, 1973–1974* (unpublished typescript), session of March 12, 1974.

26. Lacan, "The Signification of the Phallus," 581.

27. Ibid.

28. Jacques Lacan, *Le Séminaire de Jacques Lacan*, book 4, *La relation d'objet, 1956–1957*, ed. Jacques-Alain Miller (Paris: Éditions du Seuil, 1994), 155–157, 165–166, 194, 271–272, 357; Lacan, *Le Séminaire de Jacques Lacan*, book 5, 384; Lacan, *The Seminar of Jacques Lacan*, book 11, 103, 111–112; Adrian Johnston, *Žižek's Ontology: A Transcendental Materialist Theory of Subjectivity* (Evanston: Northwestern University Press, 2008), 34–35, 138–139.

29. Lacan, *Le Séminaire de Jacques Lacan*, book 6, session of June 3, 1959; Jacques Lacan, "*Préface à* L'Éveil du printemps," in *Autres écrits*, ed. Jacques-Alain Miller (Paris: Éditions du Seuil, 2001), 562; Colette Soler, *Les affects lacaniens* (Paris: Presses Universitaires de France, 2011), 91.

30. Johnston, *Žižek's Ontology*, 24–25.

31. Jacques Lacan, *Le Séminaire de Jacques Lacan*, book 16, *D'un Autre à l'autre, 1968–1969*, ed. Jacques-Alain Miller (Paris: Éditions du Seuil, 2006), 315.

32. Copjec, "May '68, The Emotional Month," 91.

33. Jacques Lacan, *The Seminar of Jacques Lacan*, book 7, *The Ethics of Psychoanalysis, 1959–1960*, ed. Jacques-Alain Miller, trans. Dennis Porter (New York: W. W. Norton, 1992), 216–217.

34. Ibid., 260–261.

35. Ibid., 295.

36. Ibid., 247.

37. Ibid., 298.

38. Jacques Lacan, *Le Séminaire de Jacques Lacan*, book 7, *L'éthique de la psychanalyse, 1959–1960*, ed. Jacques-Alain Miller (Paris: Éditions du Seuil, 1986), 345.

39. Lacan, *Le Séminaire de Jacques Lacan*, book 21, session of March 12, 1974.

40. Lacan, *Le Séminaire de Jacques Lacan*, book 8, 364.

41. Lacan, *The Seminar of Jacques Lacan*, book 7, 299.

42. Ibid.

43. Johnston, *Time Driven*, 234–241.

44. Lacan, *Le Séminaire de Jacques Lacan*, book 12, session of May 19, 1965; Jacques Lacan, *Le Séminaire de Jacques Lacan*, book 22, *R.S.I., 1974–1975* (unpublished typescript), session of March 11, 1975.

45. Slavoj Žižek, "Da Capo senza Fine," in Judith Butler, Ernesto Laclau, and Slavoj Žižek, *Contingency, Hegemony, Universality: Contemporary Dialogues on the Left* (London: Verso, 2000), 256.

46. Žižek, "Da Capo senza Fine," 256.

47. Antonio Damasio, *Looking for Spinoza: Joy, Sorrow, and the Feeling Brain* (New York: Harcourt, 2003), 159–160.

48. Antonio Damasio, *The Feeling of What Happens: Body and Emotion in the Making of Consciousness* (New York: Harcourt, 1999), 27, 228, 297; Damasio, *Looking for Spinoza*, 184.

49. Antonio Damasio, *Descartes' Error: Emotion, Reason, and the Human Brain* (New York: Avon Books, 1994), 185, 187–189; Damasio, *Feeling of What Happens*, 36–37, 279–281, 283–284.

50. Damasio, *Feeling of What Happens*, 37.

51. Damasio, *Descartes' Error*, 149–150, 159, 163–164; Damasio, *Feeling of What Happens*, 35, 57, 218–219, 311; Damasio, *Looking for Spinoza*, 71, 78–79.

52. Paul Thagard, "Mental Mechanisms," in *Hot Thought: Mechanisms and Applications of Emotional Cognition* (Cambridge, Mass: MIT Press, 2006), 7–8, 10; Paul Thagard and Josef Nerb, "Emotional Gestalts: Appraisal, Change, and the Dynamics of Affect," in *Hot Thought*, 55–56, 63; Paul Thagard, "How Molecules Matter to Mental Computation," in *Hot Thought*, 127.

53. Damasio, *Feeling of What Happens*, 42–43; Damasio, *Looking for Spinoza*, 27; Antonio Damasio, *Self Comes to Mind: Constructing the Conscious Brain* (New York: Pantheon Books, 2010), 109–110.

54. Damasio, *Looking for Spinoza*, 7, 28.

55. Ibid., 30, 80, 101.

56. Damasio, *Feeling of What Happens*, 37.

57. Ibid., 11, 20–22; Damasio, *Self Comes to Mind*, 63–64, 89–90, 187.

58. Damasio, *Self Comes to Mind*, 10, 72.

59. Ibid., 319.

60. Ibid., 283–284.

61. Ibid., 150.

62. Ibid., 36, 279–281.

63. Jean-Pierre Changeux, *The Physiology of Truth: Neuroscience and Human Knowledge*, trans. M. B. DeBevoise (Cambridge, Mass.: Harvard University Press, 2004), 76.

64. Johnston, *Žižek's Ontology*, 89.

65. Ibid., 256–257.

66. Damasio, *Looking for Spinoza*, 12; Baruch Spinoza, *Ethics*, ed. James Gutmann (New York: Hafner Press, 1949), 89–90, 101–102.

67. Damasio, *Looking for Spinoza*, 29.

68. Ibid., 33.

69. Ibid., 55, 60–61; Damasio, *Self Comes to Mind*, 143, 275.

70. Damasio, *Descartes' Error*, 143, 145–146, 159; Damasio, *Looking for Spinoza*, 85, 91; Damasio, *Self Comes to Mind*, 75–76, 101.

71. Damasio, *Looking for Spinoza*, 85.

72. Ibid., 85–86.

73. Ibid., 88.

74. Ibid., 109.

75. Damasio, *Descartes' Error*, 162–163.

76. Damasio, *Looking for Spinoza*, 72.

77. Johnston, *Time Driven*, xxvii, 46, 63, 140.

78. Damasio, *Feeling of What Happens*, 30–31, 282, 285, 313.

79. Ibid., 88–89, 100, 107–109, 113, 121–123, 125–127, 154, 172–173, 175, 177, 185–186, 191, 198, 200, 217–219, 222, 226–230.

80. Slavoj Žižek, "Descartes and the Post-Traumatic Subject," *Filozofski Vestnik: Radical Philosophy?*, ed. Peter Klepec, 29, no. 2 (2008): 23, 26–27, 29; Johnston, *Time Driven*, 83–84, 107; Johnston, *Žižek's Ontology*, 11–12, 21–22, 196, 210, 218–220, 231–232.

81. Slavoj Žižek, *The Parallax View* (Cambridge, Mass.: MIT Press, 2006), 226–227.

82. Johnston, *Žižek's Ontology*, xxiii–xxiv, 218–220, 284–286; Adrian Johnston, "Slavoj Žižek's Hegelian Reformation: Giving a Hearing to *The Parallax View*," *Diacritics: A Review of Contemporary Criticism* 37, no. 1 (Spring 2007): 12–13.

83. Damasio, *Feeling of What Happens*, 107–108, 185–186.

84. Ibid., 198.

85. Ibid., 218–219, 222.

86. Ibid., 200, 228–230.

87. Ibid., 22, 172, 175, 177; Damasio, *Self Comes to Mind*, 190, 202–203.

88. Žižek, *The Parallax View*, 227.

89. Ibid.

90. Slavoj Žižek, *In Defense of Lost Causes* (London: Verso, 2008), 440.

91. Adrian Johnston, "The Weakness of Nature: Hegel, Freud, Lacan, and Negativity Materialized," in *Hegel and the Infinite: Into the Twenty-First Century*, ed. Clayton Crockett, Creston Davis, and Slavoj Žižek (New York: Columbia University Press, 2011), 159–179.

92. Žižek, *In Defense of Lost Causes*, 435, 442; Johnston, *Žižek's Ontology*, 171, 174, 194, 207–208, 272, 286–287; Johnston, "Slavoj Žižek's Hegelian Reformation," 18–19; Adrian Johnston, "Conflicted Matter: Jacques Lacan and the Challenge of Secularizing Materialism," *Pli: The Warwick Journal of Philosophy* 19 (Spring 2008): 172–176, 185–188; Johnston, "The Weakness of Nature," 159–179; Adrian Johnston, "Second Natures in Dappled Worlds: John McDowell, Nancy Cartwright, and Hegelian-Lacanian Materialism," in *Umbr(a): A Journal of the Unconscious—The Worst*, ed. Matthew Rigilano and Kyle Fetter (Buffalo: Center for the Study of Psychoanalysis and Culture, State University of New York at Buffalo, 2011), 81–85.

93. Johnston, *Žižek's Ontology*, xxiii, 176, 270–273; Adrian Johnston, "What Matter(s) in Ontology: Alain Badiou, the Hebb-Event, and Materialism Split from Within," *Angelaki: Journal of the Theoretical Humanities* 13, no. 3 (April 2008): 38–39, 42.

94. Adrian Johnston, *A Weak Nature Alone: Prolegomena to Any Future Materialism*, vol. 2 (unpublished manuscript).

95. Damasio, *Looking for Spinoza*, 79–80; Damasio, *Self Comes to Mind*, 63, 93, 124, 269–271.

96. Žižek, *The Parallax View*, 226–227.

97. Ibid., 228.

98. Joseph LeDoux, *Synaptic Self: How Our Brains Become Who We Are* (New York: Penguin, 2002), 197–198.

99. Damasio, *Self Comes to Mind*, 288.

100. LeDoux, *Synaptic Self*, 203–204.

101. Francisco J. Varela, Evan Thompson, and Eleanor Rosch, *The Embodied Mind: Cognitive Science and Human Experience* (Cambridge, Mass.: MIT Press, 1991), 106–107.

102. LeDoux, *Synaptic Self*, 31.

103. Joseph LeDoux, *The Emotional Brain: The Mysterious Underpinnings of Emotional Life* (New York: Simon & Schuster, 1996), 105.

104. Ibid.

105. Damasio, *Descartes' Error*, 185.

106. Alain Badiou, *Being and Event*, trans. Oliver Feltham (London: Continuum, 2005), 140.

107. Damasio, *Feeling of What Happens*, 331; Damasio, *Self Comes to Mind*, 314.

108. Damasio, *Self Comes to Mind*, 250–251.

109. David J. Linden, *The Accidental Mind: How Brain Evolution Has Given Us Love, Memory, Dreams, and God* (Cambridge, Mass.: Harvard University Press, 2007), 6.

110. Ibid., 245.

111. Ibid., 2–3, 5–7, 21–24, 26, 245–246.

112. Ibid., 235–246.

113. Gary Marcus, *Kludge: The Haphazard Evolution of the Human Mind* (New York: Houghton Mifflin Harcourt, 2008), 6–16, 161–163.

114. François Jacob, "Evolution and Tinkering," *Science* 196, no. 4295 (June 10, 1977): 1161–1166.

115. LeDoux, *The Emotional Brain*, 16, 106, 127.

116. Jaak Panksepp, *Affective Neuroscience: The Foundations of Human and Animal Emotions* (Oxford: Oxford University Press, 1998), 353.

117. Ibid., 147.

118. Ibid., 70.

119. Ibid., 75–76.

120. LeDoux, *Synaptic Self*, 322–323.

121. Keith E. Stanovich, *The Robot's Rebellion: Finding Meaning in the Age of Darwin* (Chicago: University of Chicago Press, 2004), 12, 13, 20–21, 21–22, 67, 82–83, 247.

122. Žižek, *The Parallax View*, 229.

123. Ibid.

124. François Ansermet and Pierre Magistretti, *Biology of Freedom: Neural Plasticity, Experience, and the Unconscious*, trans. Susan Fairfield (New York: Other Press, 2007), 33–34; Gérard Pommier, *Comment les neurosciences démontrent la psychanalyse* (Paris: Flammarion, 2004), 215.

125. LeDoux, *The Emotional Brain*, 29–30.

126. Damasio, *Feeling of What Happens*, 228.

127. Ibid., 228–230.

128. Damasio, *Descartes' Error*, 130, 185, 187–188; Damasio, *Looking for Spinoza*, 72.

129. Johnston, *Time Driven*, xxvii, 140.

130. Damasio, *Descartes' Error*, 139; Damasio, *Feeling of What Happens*, 42–43; Damasio, *Looking for Spinoza*, 27–29.

131. Adrian Johnston, "'Naturalism or anti-naturalism? No, thanks—both are worse!': Science, Materialism, and Slavoj Žižek," in "On Slavoj Žižek," special issue, *La Revue Internationale de Philosophie* (2012).

132. Žižek, *The Parallax View*, 231.

133. Johnston, *Žižek's Ontology*, 105, 109, 180–194, 209–210, 222–223, 236–238.

134. Slavoj Žižek, "From *objet a* to Subtraction," *Lacanian Ink* 30 (Fall 2007): 138.

135. Žižek, "From *objet a* to Subtraction," 139.

136. Johnston, *Žižek's Ontology*, 241; Johnston, "Slavoj Žižek's Hegelian Reformation," 4.

137. Johnston, "The Weakness of Nature," 159–179.

138. *SE* 21:97, 112, 114, 122–124, 143, 145.

13. AFFECTS ARE SIGNIFIERS: THE INFINITE JUDGMENT OF A LACANIAN AFFECTIVE NEUROSCIENCE

1. Adrian Johnston, "The Weakness of Nature: Hegel, Freud, Lacan, and Negativity Materialized," in *Hegel and the Infinite: Into the Twenty-First Century*, ed. Clayton Crockett, Creston Davis, and Slavoj Žižek (New York: Columbia University Press, 2011), 159–179.

2. Jean-Pierre Changeux, *The Physiology of Truth: Neuroscience and Human Knowledge*, trans. M. B. DeBevoise (Cambridge, Mass.: Harvard University Press, 2004), 81–82; Benjamin Libet, *Mind Time: The Temporal Factor in Consciousness* (Cambridge, Mass.: Harvard University Press, 2004), 28, 56, 66–67, 70–72, 107–109, 120–122, 208; Francisco J. Varela, Evan Thompson, and Eleanor Rosch, *The Embodied Mind: Cognitive Science and Human Experience* (Cambridge, Mass.: MIT Press, 1991), 48–51.

3. Adrian Johnston, "What Matter(s) in Ontology: Alain Badiou, the Hebb-Event, and Materialism Split from Within," *Angelaki: Journal of the Theoretical Humanities* 13, no. 3 (April 2008): 28–44; Adrian Johnston, "Conflicted Matter: Jacques Lacan and the Challenge of Secularizing Materialism," *Pli: The Warwick Journal of Philosophy* 19 (Spring 2008): 177–182; Adrian Johnston, "Slavoj Žižek's Hegelian Reformation: Giving a Hearing to *The Parallax View*," *Diacritics: A Review of Contemporary Criticism* 37, no. 1 (Spring 2007): 4–14, 16–17; Johnston, "The Weakness of Nature," 159–179; Changeux, *The Physiology of Truth*, 33, 207–208; Antonio Damasio, *Looking for Spinoza: Joy, Sorrow, and the Feeling Brain* (New York: Harcourt, 2003), 162–164, 173–174; Douglas Hofstadter, *I Am a Strange Loop* (New York: Basic Books, 2007),

31; Eric R. Kandel, "Psychotherapy and the Single Synapse: The Impact of Psychiatric Thought on Neurobiologic Research," in *Psychiatry, Psychoanalysis, and the New Biology of Mind* (Washington, D.C.: American Psychiatric Publishing, 2005), 21; Eric R. Kandel, "A New Intellectual Framework for Psychiatry," in *Psychiatry, Psychoanalysis, and the New Biology of Mind*, 42–43, 47; Eric R. Kandel, "Biology and the Future of Psychoanalysis: A New Intellectual Framework for Psychiatry Revisited," in *Psychiatry, Psychoanalysis, and the New Biology of Mind*, 94, 97–98; Joseph LeDoux, *Synaptic Self: How Our Brains Become Who We Are* (New York: Penguin, 2002), 2–3, 5, 12, 20, 66–67; Libet, *Mind Time*, 5; Catherine Malabou, *Que faire de notre cerveau?* (Paris: Bayard, 2004), 27–28, 30–31, 84–85, 156, 161–163; Catherine Malabou, *La plasticité au soir de l'écriture: Dialectique, destruction, déconstruction* (Paris: Éditions Léo Scheer, 2005), 19; Thomas Metzinger, *Being No One: The Self-Model Theory of Subjectivity* (Cambridge, Mass.: MIT Press, 2003), 115; Lesley Rogers, *Sexing the Brain* (New York: Columbia University Press, 2001), 2–3, 5, 20, 23–24, 47–48, 68, 97–98; Mark Solms and Oliver Turnbull, *The Brain and the Inner World: An Introduction to the Neuroscience of Subjective Experience* (New York: Other Press, 2002), 64, 218, 244, 271–272.

4. Jaak Panksepp, *Affective Neuroscience: The Foundations of Human and Animal Emotions* (Oxford: Oxford University Press, 1998), 4, 10, 43, 47, 50–51, 56, 77, 79, 122–123, 325–330.

5. Ibid., 52.

6. Ibid., 52–54.

7. Ibid., 54.

8. Ibid., 47.

9. Solms and Turnbull, *The Brain and the Inner World*, 112–133, 277–278.

10. Antonio Damasio, *Descartes' Error: Emotion, Reason, and the Human Brain* (New York: Avon Books, 1994), 267.

11. *SE* 5:600–604.

12. Joseph LeDoux, *The Emotional Brain: The Mysterious Underpinnings of Emotional Life* (New York: Simon & Schuster, 1996), 123.

13. LeDoux, *The Emotional Brain*, 17–18, 20, 33–34, 40–41, 64–66, 71, 161, 203.

14. Panksepp, *Affective Neuroscience*, 34.

15. Ibid., 28.

16. LeDoux, *The Emotional Brain*, 137.

17. Eva Jablonka and Marion J. Lamb, *Evolution in Four Dimensions: Genetic, Epigenetic, Behavioral, and Symbolic Variation in the History of Life* (Cambridge, Mass.: MIT Press, 2005), 1–2, 5–7, 58–60, 62–65, 67, 72–75, 77–78, 109–111, 144–145, 160–161, 166, 176, 189, 191, 193, 204–205, 220–223, 238, 285–286, 319, 344, 378–380.

18. Ibid., 226.

19. Ibid., 372.

20. LeDoux, *The Emotional Brain*, 302.

21. Ibid.

22. Damasio, *Descartes' Error*, 134, 149–150.

23. Antonio Damasio, *Self Comes to Mind: Constructing the Conscious Brain* (New York: Pantheon Books, 2010), 294.

24. Adrian Johnston, *Žižek's Ontology: A Transcendental Materialist Theory of Subjectivity* (Evanston: Northwestern University Press, 2008), 61, 108, 118, 186, 237, 245.

25. Panksepp, *Affective Neuroscience*, 16–17, 27.

26. Ibid., 21, 72.

27. Ibid., 26–27, 31, 33–34, 37.

28. Ibid., 26.

29. Ibid., 122.

30. Ibid., 39, 301, 334, 352; Catherine Malabou, *The Future of Hegel: Plasticity, Temporality and Dialectic*, trans. Lisabeth During (New York: Routledge, 2005), 8–9; Malabou, *Que faire de notre cerveau?*, 15–17, 29–30, 40, 65–66, 145–146; Malabou, *La plasticité au soir de l'écriture*, 21, 25–26, 110–111.

31. Gérard Pommier, *Comment les neurosciences démontrent la psychanalyse* (Paris: Flammarion, 2004), 142.

32. Ibid.

33. Giorgio Agamben, *Homo Sacer: Sovereign Power and Bare Life*, trans. Daniel Heller-Roazen (Stanford: Stanford University Press, 1998), 1.

34. Michel Foucault, *"Society must be defended": Lectures at the Collège de France, 1975–1976*, ed. Mauro Bertani and Alessandro Fontana, trans. David Macey (New York: Picador, 2003), 240–247, 249–250, 253; Agamben, *Homo Sacer*, 4–5, 148, 165, 179.

35. Agamben, *Homo Sacer*, 83.

36. Giorgio Agamben, *State of Exception*, trans. Kevin Attell (Chicago: University of Chicago Press, 2005), 87–88.

37. Agamben, *Homo Sacer*, 35, 37, 105–106, 109.

38. Ibid., 17–19, 24–25, 37, 83, 105; Agamben, *State of Exception*, 1, 4–6, 14, 24, 26, 31, 35, 38–39, 50–51, 69–70.

39. Panksepp, *Affective Neuroscience*, 39, 69.

40. Ibid., 42–43, 301.

41. Ibid., 166.

42. Ibid., 51.

43. Damasio, *Descartes' Error*, 128.

44. Pommier, *Comment les neurosciences démontrent la psychanalyse*, 18.

45. Johnston, *Žižek's Ontology*, 87–90; Johnston, "Slavoj Žižek's Hegelian Reformation," 9; Adrian Johnston, *Badiou, Žižek, and Political Transformations: The Cadence of Change* (Evanston: Northwestern University Press, 2009), 119–124; Jacques Lacan, "The Function and Field of Speech and Language in Psychoanalysis," in *Écrits: The First Complete Edition in English*, trans. Bruce Fink (New York: W. W. Norton,

2006), 248; Jacques Lacan, "The Direction of the Treatment and the Principles of Its Power," in *Écrits*, 496; Jacques Lacan, "Discours de Rome," in *Autres écrits*, ed. Jacques-Alain Miller (Paris: Éditions du Seuil, 2001), 137–138; Jacques Lacan, "Problèmes cruciaux pour la psychanalyse," in *Autres écrits*, 199; Jacques Lacan, "Petit discours à l'ORTF," in *Autres écrits*, 224; Jacques Lacan, "Of Structure as an Inmixing of an Otherness Prerequisite to Any Subject Whatever," in *The Structuralist Controversy: The Languages of Criticism and the Sciences of Man*, ed. Richard Macksey and Eugenio Donato (Baltimore: Johns Hopkins University Press, 1970), 187; Jacques Lacan, *The Seminar of Jacques Lacan*, book 1, *Freud's Papers on Technique, 1953–1954*, ed. Jacques-Alain Miller, trans. John Forrester (New York: W. W. Norton, 1988), 244; Jacques Lacan, *The Seminar of Jacques Lacan*, book 2, *The Ego in Freud's Theory and in the Technique of Psychoanalysis, 1954–1955*, ed. Jacques-Alain Miller, trans. Sylvana Tomaselli (New York: W. W. Norton, 1988), 82; Jacques Lacan, *The Seminar of Jacques Lacan*, book 3, *The Psychoses, 1955–1956*, ed. Jacques-Alain Miller, trans. Russell Grigg (New York: W. W. Norton, 1993), 32; Jacques Lacan, *Le Séminaire de Jacques Lacan*, book 9, *L'identification, 1961–1962* (unpublished typescript), session of January 10, 1962; Jacques Lacan, *Le Séminaire de Jacques Lacan*, book 14, *La logique du fantasme, 1966–1967* (unpublished typescript), session of February 1, 1967; Jacques Lacan, *Le Séminaire de Jacques Lacan*, book 16, *D'un Autre à l'autre, 1968–1969*, ed. Jacques-Alain Miller (Paris: Éditions du Seuil, 2006), 88–90; Jacques Lacan, *Le Séminaire de Jacques Lacan*, book 24, *L'insu que sait de l'une-bévue, s'aile à mourre, 1976–1977* (unpublished typescript), session of April 19, 1977.

46. Pommier, *Comment les neurosciences démontrent la psychanalyse*, 23–24.

47. Changeux, *The Physiology of Truth*, 201–202; Jean-Pierre Changeux, *Du vrai, du beau, du bien: Une nouvelle approche neuronale* (Paris: Odile Jacob, 2008), 293–294, 296–297.

48. Jean-Pierre Changeux, *Neuronal Man: The Biology of Mind*, trans. Laurence Garey (Princeton: Princeton University Press, 1997), 246–249; Changeux, *The Physiology of Truth*, 61–62.

49. Changeux, *The Physiology of Truth*, 58, 60–62, 64.

50. Ibid., 113–114, 118.

51. Immanuel Kant, *Anthropology from a Pragmatic Point of View*, trans. Victor Lyle Dowdell (Carbondale: Southern Illinois University Press, 1978), 175–176; Slavoj Žižek, *The Plague of Fantasies* (London: Verso, 1997), 237; Johnston, *Žižek's Ontology*, 180–181.

52. LeDoux, *Synaptic Self*, 72–74.

53. Changeux, *The Physiology of Truth*, 114.

54. Ibid., 113, 129, 132, 140–141, 201–202.

55. Pommier, *Comment les neurosciences démontrent la psychanalyse*, 24–28, 45–47.

56. Ibid., 27.

57. Johnston, *Žižek's Ontology*, 106–111, 114–115, 172–173, 200, 204–205, 208, 277–278; Johnston, "What Matter(s) in Ontology," 33–34; Johnston, "Slavoj Žižek's Hegelian Reformation," 16; Johnston, "Conflicted Matter," 177–181; Johnston, "The Weakness of Nature," 159–179; François Ansermet, "*Des neurosciences aux logosciences*," in *Qui sont vos psychanalystes?*, ed. Nathalie Georges, Jacques-Alain Miller, and Nathalie Marchaison (Paris: Éditions du Seuil, 2002), 377–378, 383; François Ansermet and Pierre Magistretti, *Biology of Freedom: Neural Plasticity, Experience, and the Unconscious*, trans. Susan Fairfield (New York: Other Press, 2007), xvi, 8, 10, 239; Changeux, *The Physiology of Truth*, 152–153; Changeux, *Du vrai, du beau, du bien*, 39–40, 104–105; Daniel Dennett, *Freedom Evolves* (New York: Viking, 2003), 90–91, 93; LeDoux, *Synaptic Self*, 8–9, 20, 91, 296; Malabou, *Que faire de notre cerveau?*, 7–8, 14–17, 20–23, 31–32, 84–85; Malabou, *La plasticité au soir de l'écriture*, 112; Catherine Malabou, "Préface," in *La chambre du milieu: De Hegel aux neurosciences* (Paris: Hermann, 2009), 9–10; Solms and Turnbull, *The Brain and the Inner World*, 220; Slavoj Žižek, *The Parallax View* (Cambridge, Mass.: MIT Press, 2006), 213–214.

58. Pommier, *Comment les neurosciences démontrent la psychanalyse*, 27.

59. Ansermet and Magistretti, *Biology of Freedom*, 8.

60. *SE* 14:187.

61. *SE* 21:69–71.

62. Panksepp, *Affective Neuroscience*, 47, 52, 149, 302, 318–319.

63. Changeux, *The Physiology of Truth*, 37, 39.

64. Malabou, *The Future of Hegel*, 8–9, 73–74, 192–193.

65. Changeux, *The Physiology of Truth*, 184–185; Lesley Rogers, *Sexing the Brain* (New York: Columbia University Press, 2001), 21–22; Keith E. Stanovich, *The Robot's Rebellion: Finding Meaning in the Age of Darwin* (Chicago: University of Chicago Press, 2004), 82, 201–202.

66. Changeux, *The Physiology of Truth*, 62.

67. LeDoux, *Synaptic Self*, 203–204.

68. Pommier, *Comment les neurosciences démontrent la psychanalyse*, 18.

69. Ibid., 17.

70. Karen Kaplan-Solms and Mark Solms, *Clinical Studies in Neuro-Psychoanalysis: Introduction to a Depth Neuropsychology* (New York: Other Press, 2002), 250–251, 255; Solms and Turnbull, *The Brain and the Inner World*, 54–56, 72, 78.

71. Johnston, *Žižek's Ontology*, 275–280.

72. *SE* 7:147–148; *SE* 14:122–123; Adrian Johnston, *Time Driven: Metapsychology and the Splitting of the Drive* (Evanston: Northwestern University Press, 2005), 20–21, 168.

73. Solms and Turnbull, *The Brain and the Inner World*, 118–119, 122–123.

74. Kaplan-Solms and Solms, *Clinical Studies in Neuro-Psychoanalysis*, 18–23, 43, 55; Ansermet and Magistretti, *The Biology of Freedom*, 216.

75. Changeux, *The Physiology of Truth*, 8–9, 23, 25, 28, 32–33, 36, 246, 247; Metzinger, *Being No One*, 51; Johnston, "What Matter(s) in Ontology," 35.

76. Solms and Turnbull, *The Brain and the Inner World*, 120, 133–134, 277–278.

77. Damasio, *Self Comes to Mind*, 299.

78. David J. Chalmers, *The Conscious Mind: In Search of a Fundamental Theory* (Oxford: Oxford University Press, 1997), xii–xiii.

79. André Green, *La causalité psychique: Entre nature et culture* (Paris: Éditions Odile Jacob, 1995), 43.

80. Ibid., 45.

81. Ibid., 118, 252, 290–291.

82. Ibid., 279.

83. Ibid., 289–290.

84. Jacques Lacan, "Presentation on Psychical Causality," in *Écrits*, 150.

85. Ibid. 153.

86. Jacques Lacan, "Les complexes familiaux dans la formation de l'individu: Essai d'analyse d'une fonction en psychologie," in *Autres écrits*, 33–34; Jacques Lacan, "The Mirror Stage as Formative of the *I* Function as Revealed in Psychoanalytic Experience," in *Écrits*, 77–78; Jacques Lacan, "Aggressiveness in Psychoanalysis," in *Écrits*, 92; Jacques Lacan, "Some Reflections on the Ego," *International Journal of Psycho-Analysis* 34 (1953): 13; Johnston, "The Weakness of Nature," 159–179.

87. Lacan, "Presentation on Psychical Causality," 154.

88. Green, *La causalité psychique*, 14, 252, 292, 298.

89. Ibid., 21.

90. Ibid., 124–125, 239–240.

91. Ibid., 124.

92. Ibid., 126, 292.

93. Ibid., 87–89, 104, 303.

94. Ibid., 252.

95. Ibid., 85.

96. Ibid., 223.

97. Ibid.

98. Ibid., 254.

99. Alain Badiou, *Logiques des mondes: L'être et l'événement, 2* (Paris: Éditions du Seuil, 2006), 96, 426–427, 438–439, 442–443, 459, 461, 601, 612, 614.

100. Adrian Johnston, "'Naturalism or anti-naturalism? No, thanks—both are worse!': Science, Materialism, and Slavoj Žižek," in "On Slavoj Žižek," special issue, *La Revue Internationale de Philosophie* (2012); Adrian Johnston, "Second Natures in Dappled Worlds: John McDowell, Nancy Cartwright, and Hegelian-Lacanian Materialism," in *Umbr(a): The Worst*, ed. Matthew Rigilano and Kyle Fetter (Buffalo: Center for the Study of Psychoanalysis and Culture, State University of New York at Buffalo, 2011), 71–91.

101. Adrian Johnston, *The Outcome of Contemporary French Philosophy: Prolegomena to Any Future Materialism*, vol. 1 (Evanston: Northwestern University Press, 2013); Adrian Johnston, *A Weak Nature Alone: Prolegomena to Any Future Materialism*, vol. 2 (unpublished manuscript).

102. Johnston, *The Outcome of Contemporary French Philosophy*; Johnston, *A Weak Nature Alone*.

103. Johnston, "Conflicted Matter," 167–168, 174–176, 178–182, 187–188; Johnston, "What Matter(s) in Ontology," 38–42, 44.

104. André Green, "The Logic of Lacan's *objet (a)* and Freudian Theory: Convergences and Questions," trans. Kimberly Kleinert and Beryl Schlossman, in *Interpreting Lacan*, ed. Joseph H. Smith and William Kerrigan (New Haven: Yale University Press, 1983), 180.

105. André Green, *Le discours vivant: Le conception psychanalytique de l'affect* (Paris: Presses Universitaires de France, 1973), 139–141, 223, 239, 330.

106. Green, "The Logic of Lacan's *objet (a)* and Freudian Theory," 181.

107. Ibid., 180–181.

108. Ibid., 181.

109. *SE* 14:202–203; Johnston, *Time Driven*, 301–302.

110. Ferdinand de Saussure, *Course in General Linguistics*, ed. Charles Bally and Albert Sechehaye, in collaboration with Albert Riedlinger, trans. Wade Baskin (New York: McGraw-Hill, 1966), 120.

111. LeDoux, *The Emotional Brain*, 299; Solms and Turnbull, *The Brain and the Inner World*, 34.

112. Jacques Lacan, *The Seminar of Jacques Lacan*, book 7, *The Ethics of Psychoanalysis, 1959–1960*, ed. Jacques-Alain Miller, trans. Dennis Porter (New York: W. W. Norton, 1992), 181; Jacques Lacan, *Le Séminaire de Jacques Lacan*, book 18, *D'un discours qui ne serait pas du semblant, 1971*, ed. Jacques-Alain Miller (Paris: Éditions du Seuil, 2006), 15; Jacques Lacan, *Le Séminaire de Jacques Lacan*, book 23, *Le sinthome, 1975–1976*, ed. Jacques-Alain Miller (Paris: Éditions du Seuil, 2005), 121.

113. Jacques Lacan, *Le Séminaire de Jacques Lacan*, book 10, *L'angoisse, 1962–1963*, ed. Jacques-Alain Miller (Paris: Éditions du Seuil, 2004), 91–95; Lacan, *Le Séminaire de Jacques Lacan*, book 23, 164–165.

114. Lacan, *Le Séminaire de Jacques Lacan*, book 24, session of February 15, 1977.

115. Jacques Lacan, *Le Séminaire de Jacques Lacan*, book 21, *Les non-dupes errent, 1973–1974* (unpublished typescript), sessions of November 13, 1973, December 11, 1973, January 8, 1974, January 15, 1974; Jacques Lacan, *Le Séminaire de Jacques Lacan*, book 22, *R.S.I., 1974–1975* (unpublished typescript), sessions of November 19, 1974, December 17, 1974; Slavoj Žižek, *The Indivisible Remainder: An Essay on Schelling and Related Matters* (London: Verso, 1996), 206; Slavoj Žižek, *The Ticklish Subject: The Absent Centre of Political Ontology* (London: Verso, 1999), 323; Slavoj Žižek,

The Fragile Absolute; Or, Why Is the Christian Legacy Worth Fighting for? (London: Verso, 2000), 127–128; Slavoj Žižek, "Neighbors and Other Monsters: A Plea for Ethical Violence," in Slavoj Žižek, Eric L. Santner, and Kenneth Reinhard, *The Neighbor: Three Inquiries in Political Theology* (Chicago: University of Chicago Press, 2005), 179; Slavoj Žižek, "Author's Afterword: Where Do We Stand Today?," in *The Universal Exception: Selected Writings*, ed. Rex Butler and Scott Stephens (London: Continuum, 2006), 2:304–305.

116. Jacques Lacan, *Le Séminaire de Jacques Lacan*, book 27, *Dissolution, 1979–1980* (unpublished typescript), session of January 15, 1980.

117. Jacques Lacan, *Télévision* (Paris: Éditions du Seuil, 1973), 9; Jacques Lacan, "Television," trans. Denis Hollier, Rosalind Krauss, and Annette Michelson, in *Television/A Challenge to the Psychoanalytic Establishment*, ed. Joan Copjec (New York: W. W. Norton, 1990), 3.

118. Lacan, *Le Séminaire de Jacques Lacan*, book 16, 208.

119. Johnston, *Time Driven*, 300–315.

120. Lacan, "Television," 5.

121. Ibid.

POSTFACE: THE PARADOXES
OF THE PRINCIPLE OF CONSTANCY

This chapter was translated by Adrian Johnston.

1. *SE* 2:193–194.

2. Ibid., 198.

3. Ibid., 198–199.

4. Jean Laplanche and Jean-Bertrand Pontalis, *La vocabulaire de la psychanalyse* (Paris: Presses Universitaires de France, 1967), 413; Jean Laplanche and Jean-Bertrand Pontalis, *The Language of Psycho-Analysis*, trans. Donald Nicholson-Smith (New York: W. W. Norton, 1973), 364.

5. *SE* 14:121–123.

6. Ibid., 126.

7. Freud's affirmations hence clarify themselves, according to which "research has given irrefutable proof that mental activity is bound up with the function of the brain as it is with no other organ. We are taken a step further—we do not know how much—by the discovery of the unequal importance of the different parts of the brain and their special relations to particular parts of the body and to particular mental activities. But every attempt to go on from there to discover a localization of mental processes, every endeavour to think of ideas as stored up in nerve-cells and of excitations as travelling along nerve-fibres, has miscarried completely. The same fate would await any

theory which attempted to recognize, let us say, the anatomical position of the system *Cs.*—conscious mental activity—as being in the cortex, and to localize the unconscious processes in the sub-cortical parts of the brain. There is a hiatus here which at present cannot be filled, nor is it one of the tasks of psychology to fill it. Our psychical topography has *for the present* nothing to do with anatomy; it has reference not to anatomical localities, but to regions in the mental apparatus, wherever they may be situated in the body" (*SE* 14:174–175).

8. Jacques Lacan, *The Seminar of Jacques Lacan*, book 2, *The Ego in Freud's Theory and in the Technique of Psychoanalysis, 1954–1955*, ed. Jacques-Alain Miller, trans. Sylvana Tomaselli (New York: W. W. Norton, 1988), 222. We quote also the following: "So the notion of libido is a form of unification for the domain of psychoanalytical effects" (ibid.).

9. Ibid.

10. Jacques Lacan, *Le Séminaire de Jacques Lacan*, book 2, *Le moi dans la théorie de Freud et dans la technique de la psychanalyse, 1954–1955*, ed. Jacques-Alain Miller (Paris: Éditions du Seuil, 1978), 260.

11. Antonio Damasio, *The Feeling of What Happens: Body and Emotion in the Making of Consciousness* (New York: Harcourt, 1999), 40.

12. *SE* 14:120–121.

13. Damasio, *Feeling of What Happens*, 76.

14. Antonio Damasio, *Looking for Spinoza: Joy, Sorrow, and the Feeling Brain* (New York: Harcourt, 2003), 174.

15. Ibid, 59.

16. Damasio, *Feeling of What Happens*, 169.

17. Ibid., 170.

18. Ibid., 154.

19. Marcel Gauchet, *L'inconscient cérébral* (Paris: Éditions du Seuil, 1992), 37.

20. It is necessary to signal here the existence of those remarkable neurons called "mirror neurons," which activate in perceiving activity engaged in by another, coding the movement in the same manner as if it had been executed by the observing subject itself. See Marc Jeannerod, *Le cerveau intime* (Paris: Éditions Odile Jacob, 2002), 189.

21. And this contra the statements of Freud himself which affirm that "we know two kinds of things about what we call our psyche (or mental life): firstly, its bodily organ and scene of action, the brain (or nervous system) and, on the other hand, our acts of consciousness, which are immediate data and cannot be further explained by any sort of description. Everything that lies between is unknown to us, and the data do not include any direct relation between these two terminal points of our knowledge. If it existed, it would at the most afford an exact localization of the processes of consciousness and would give us no help towards understanding them" (*SE* 23:144–145).

22. Mark Solms and Oliver Turnbull, *The Brain and the Inner World: An Introduction to the Neuroscience of Subjective Experience* (New York: Other Press, 2002), 110.

23. *SE* 19:26.

24. Damasio, *Feeling of What Happens*, 189.

25. Ibid., 154.

26. Ibid.

27. Ibid., 191.

28. *SE* 14:187.

29. Ibid., 296.

30. Damasio, *Feeling of What Happens*, 144–145.

INDEX

affects (*continued*)

and signifiers, 200; unconscious
(*see* affects, unconscious); and warfare,
132; without subjects, 6–7. *See also*
anxiety; emotions; feelings; Freudian-
Lacanian psychoanalysis; Freudian
metapsychology of affects; generosity;
guilt; hatred; joy; Lacan-inspired
metapsychology of affects; love;
passions; sadness; shame; wonder;
*specific philosophers, psychoanalysts, and
neuroscientists*

affects, detachment from/absence of, 7–8;
and brain damage, 58–60; Damasio
and, 33–34, 58–60, 64; Elliot case, 11,
59–60; impaired capacity for wonder,
10–11; and lack of concern, 59–60, 71;
"L" case, 60; Phineas Gage case, xii–xiv,
57–58; Sacks and, 71

affects, unconscious, xvii, xviii; Copjec's
denial of, 155; Damasio and, 163–65;
distinguished from potential affects,
114–16; and false connections, 107,
122; Fink and, 122; and Freud's *Affekte/
Gefühle/Emfindungen* terminology,
112–13; Freud's vacillations over, xvii,
75–80, 88–101, 105–13, 118, 119, 155,
212; Harari and, 122; Lacan's denial
of, 76, 84, 111, 119, 122, 129, 134, 149,
212–13; as misfelt feelings, 94–95; and
neurobiology, 87; and pleasure and
pain, 166–67; as potential-to-feel,
108–9; Pulver and, 113–17; and
resistance to attempts to reconcile
psychoanalytic theory with
neuroscience, 81–82; and shame, 162.
See also feelings, misfelt; guilt

Les affects lacaniens (Soler), 82

affectuation (Lacan's neologism), 141,
146–47, 208

Affektbildungen, 110–13, 157–58, 212

Affekte, 111–14, 119, 212

agalma, 70–71

Agamben, Giorgio, 192–93

All About Eve (film), 11

alterity, xvi, 6, 9, 10, 17, 24, 64, 221

Alzheimer's disease, xiii, xiv

amygdala, 218

anger, 13, 186

animals, 151, 170, 182, 186, 187, 189, 192

animal spirits, Descartes and, 13–14, 17, 46

anosognosia, 33, 60, 71. *See also* brain damage

*Anthropology from a Pragmatic Point of
View* (Kant), 196

antinaturalism, xi, 172, 180–84, 187–88,
190, 193, 197, 204

Anton's Syndrome, 60

anxiety: and bodily movements, 13; Freud
and, 89–90, 99–100, 110; and gap
between cognitive and emotional
abilities, 174; guilt felt as, 89–91,
99–101, 110, 212–13; Harari and, 134–35;
and hysteria, 87; Lacan and, 82, 133,
139–40, 151–52; and obsessive disorders,
89–90; relationship to doubt, 151–52;
and repression, 110; as a signal, not
representing itself, 134–35; as sole or
central affect, 147–48, 151, 213; Žižek
and, 172, 174

autoaffection, xvi; autoaffection as
temporality as the origin of all other
affects (Heidegger's concept), 6; cerebral
autoaffection, 221–23; Damasio and,
31, 33–34, 51, 64; deconstruction of, 7;
defined, 5–6, 21, 221; Deleuze and, 45,
48–49; Deleuze's reading of Descartes
and, 46; Deleuze's reading of Spinoza
and, 36, 45; Derrida and, 19–25, 63; and
feeling of existence, 6, 20; Heidegger
and, 5–6; and homeostasis, 31, 64;
impaired mechanism for, 34 (*see also*
brain damage); and imprecise vocabulary

for affects, 199; and the "inner voice," 20, 21; and mapping between affects and concepts, 42; as mutual mirroring of mind and body, 55; and neurobiology, 26; nonsubjective autoaffection, 55; and plane of immanence, 45–46; and self-touching, 19–21, 63; and spatiality, 46; term origin, 5–6; and types of knowledge, 45; and the unconscious, 221–23; and wonder, 9–11, 63–64

autobiographical self, 31–33, 169–70

auto-heteroaffection, 55

Badiou, Alain, 175

beauty, 160–61

Beyond the Pleasure Principle (Freud), 77–78

big Other, 173–75, 188, 200, 206

bios, 192–93

blood circulation, 13–14

body: bodily movements, 13–15, 37–38, 40, 46–48; delocalization of, 68–69. *See also* organism

body-mind connection: and conatus, 38; Damasio and, 29–30, 164–66; Derrida and, 21–23; Descartes and, 12–15, 18, 21–22, 30; emotions and physiological processes, 164–67; and generosity, 18; Green and, 202–3; and inadequacy of brain events, 29–30; and linguistic mediation, 201; mind and body as expressions of the same substance, 36, 51; mind as the idea of the body, 51, 53, 166; and "organism" term, 55; and passions "in" the soul, 12–15; and pineal gland, 14–16, 21–23; and spatiality of the soul, 21–23; Spinoza and, 36, 38, 51, 53; substance of Descartes' error, 30

brain: and autoexcitation, 216–19; and bodily movements, 13–14; cerebral autoaffection, 221–23; Changeux

and, 195–98; computer model of, 27; Damasio and, 26–34, 163–70, 187, 217; Descartes and, 16, 30; and drives, 213–16; as "electrical center" (Breuer's conception), 213–14; and evolution, 175–76, 180–83, 187–89, 201; Freud and, 60–62, 214–16, 255–56nn7,21; hardwired absences of hardwiring, 201–2; as hodgepodge of modules without overall coherent function, 175–77; interconnectedness of, 177, 194, 200; and language, 177, 195–201; and language acquisition, 195–96, 199–200; and learning, 195–98; LeDoux and, 175–79, 187–88; Linden and, 176; location of cerebral sites producing emotion, 218–19; mirror neurons, xi, 256n20; and mortality, 223–24; neural plasticity, xi, 26–28, 56–58, 190–91, 194, 202; Panksepp and, 176–77, 190–91; and perception, 27, 166–67; Pommier and, 197; self-mapping, 164–67; and subjectivity, 28; substance of Descartes' error, 30; and symbolic activity, 213–14, 216, 219–23; trinity of cognition, emotion, and motivation, 163, 176, 177; and the unconscious, 71, 219–21

The Brain and the Inner World (Solms and Turnbull), 27–28, 57, 186

brain damage, xii–xiv, 56–62, 71; and damaged subjectivity, 28, 33–34; and detachment from one's own affects, 7–8, 33, 58–60; and dreaming, 62; Elliot case, 11, 59–60; "L" case, 60; and loss of wonder, 11, 33, 60; and neuropsychoanalysis, 29; Phineas Gage case, xii–xiv, 57–58; and plasticity of the brain, 56–58; and role of emotions in reason, 8; and transformation of personality, xiii–xiv, 57–61

Breuer, Josef, 213–14, 218

care for self and others: CARE emotional system, 186; relationship between feelings, emotions, and care for self and others, 51

cathexes, 110, 125, 131

La causalité psychique: Entre nature et culture (Green), 202–3

causes. *See* adequate and inadequate causes

Chalmers, David, 202

Changeux, Jean-Pierre, 165, 195–97

Cinema I (Deleuze), 46

civilization, 132, 184

Civilization and Its Discontents (Freud), 95–98, 100–101, 184

class consciousness, 86

cognition: differences between cognition and emotion, 194; entanglement of emotional and nonemotional dimensions, 177–78, 190–91, 194, 200; trinity of cognition, emotion, and motivation, 163, 176, 177. *See also* rationality; thought

cognitive games, 195–96

conatus, 6, 217; affects and variability of conatus, 37–41, 54; defined, 38; and definition of emotions, 41–42; feelings, emotions, and self-attachment, 51; and joy and sorrow, 39–40; and origin of personal identity, 52; and self-preservation, 52; and wonder, 40–41

conscience, 77–79, 91–92, 95. *See also* guilt

consciousness: as awareness of a disturbance caused by an external object, 30; and dupery, 208; LeDoux on, 188–89; link between consciousness and emotion, 30–31; as outgrowth of self-mapping dynamics, 164–67; as two-sided instance (speaker/listener etc.), 20. *See also* mind; psyche; self; soul; subjectivity; *specific philosophers, psychoanalysts, and neuroscientists*

conscious-preconscious-unconscious triad, 69–70, 78, 92

conversion, conversion symptoms, 103–4

Copernicus, Nicolaus, 83, 148

Copjec, Joan, 154–55

core self, 31–32, 169–72

Corpus (Nancy), 23–24

criminality, 72, 78, 92–93

Critique of Judgment (Kant), 53

Critique of Pure Reason (Kant), 5–6

Damasio, Antonio, xvi, xviii; and autoaffection, 31, 33–34, 51, 64; and brain damage, 33–34, 58–60, 71–72; and debate between naturalism and antinaturalism, 180–84; definition of emotion, 51; Descartes and (*see* Damasio's reading of Descartes); distinction between pain and emotion caused by pain, 65–66; distinction between public emotions and private feelings, 163–64, 166, 179–80; and Elliot case, 11, 59–60; and evolution of the brain, 187; feelings-had and feelings-known, 165, 167–69; and Freudian-Lacanian psychoanalysis, 165–66; and heteroaffection, 34, 65–66; importance of emotions and feelings for survival, 50–53; importance of emotions in neural regulation, 7, 217; and "L" case, 60; and loss of wonder, 11, 33, 64; and mental images/ideas, 54; and nonconscious affects, 163–65; and Phineas Gage case, xii–xiv, 57–58; Spinoza and (*see* Damasio's reading of Spinoza); structure of the self, 31–33, 169–74, 217, 219–20, 222–23; three stages of processing in affective life, 164–66; and the unconscious, 163–68, 179–80; and wonder, 11, 32–33, 64; Žižek's critique of, 162–63, 165, 169–74, 179–84, 190

Damasio's reading of Descartes, 7; and body-mind connection, 29–30; Cartesian mind as a "disembodied" mind, 22; and inadequacy of brain events, 29–30; and link between consciousness and emotion, 30–31; and neural plasticity, 26–28; substance of Descartes' error, 30

Damasio's reading of Spinoza, 7, 50–55; and body-mind connection, 53; differing readings of Damasio and Deleuze, 36; emotions, feelings, and conatus, 50–53; and mapping, 51–55; and self-preservation, 52–53

Darwin, Charles, 83

Davidson, Donald, 200–201

death, 159–61; death drive, 172, 181–82; and the unconscious, 223

deceptive nature of affects and signifiers, 206–9

decision making, 7, 30

defense mechanisms, xviii, 76, 87, 127, 155; Damasio and, 168–69; and doubt and anxiety, 152; Freud and, 103–10, 115, 131; and shame, 162. *See also* repression

In Defense of Lost Causes (Žižek), 172

Deleuze, Gilles, xvi; *affect* term definition, 4–5; and conceptual personae, 48; and delocalization of the natural body, 68–69; Descartes and (*see* Deleuze's reading of Descartes); and different concepts of affects and autoaffection, 48–49; and heteroaffection, 65, 68–69; and nonmetaphysical concept of philosophy, 48–49; and perception, 67; and plane of immanence, 45–46, 48, 64, 67; privileged metaphor of the face, 64; Spinoza and (*see* Deleuze's reading of Spinoza); and touch, 66–67; and wonder, 47–48, 64, 71

Deleuze's reading of Descartes, 7, 45–48, 229n1; and facial expressions, 46–48;

two possible readings of Descartes, 48–49; and wonder, 47–48

Deleuze's reading of Spinoza: and affects as affects of essence, 36, 43–44; and *affect* term definition, 4–5; and autoaffection, 45; differing readings of Damasio and Deleuze, 36; and God/Nature, 41–42; and heteroaffection, 65; and joyful and sorrowful affects, 39–40; and nonsubjective autoaffection, 36; and touch, 66–67; and types of knowledge/ideas, 44–45, 66–67; and variability of conatus and the power of acting, 41–42

denaturalized subjectivity, 172–74, 178, 180–84, 187–88, 202. *See also* antinaturalism

Derrida, Jacques, xvi, xvii; and autoaffection, 19–25, 63; and delocalization of the natural body, 68–69; Descartes and, 19–25; and generosity, 24–25, 64; and heteroaffection, 7, 19, 20–21, 24, 25, 58, 64–65, 68–69; and pineal gland, 21–23; privileged metaphor of the graft, 64; and sense of touch, 21–24, 64, 69; and spatiality of the psyche, 69; tribute to Jean-Luc Nancy, 23; "two lovers" text, 64–65; and wonder, 11, 23–25, 64, 71

Descartes, René, xvi; and body-mind connection, 12–15, 18, 21–22, 30; definition of passions of the soul, 6, 13; Derrida's interpretation of, 19–25; Descartes-Spinoza conflict, 7, 37–38; external signs of the passions (facial expressions etc.), 45–48; and functions of the soul, 15; and generosity, 13, 17–18, 25; and immediacy, 85; Irigaray and, 226n15; and nonmetaphysical concept of philosophy, 48–49; passions "in" the soul as consequences of bodily movements, 13–15; passions "of"

167–69; and *honte* (shame as a felt feeling), 157–58; relation to *Affekte* and *Gefühle*, 111–14

epigenetics, xi, 188, 191, 194, 196–97, 199

Ethics (Spinoza), 4–5, 35–42

evolution, xi, 175–76, 180–83, 186–87, 201

existence, 5, 6, 20, 32, 39–40. *See also* self-preservation

experience, 27–28, 44, 56, 57

face and facial expressions, 46–48, 64

false connections, 103–4, 107, 122, 128, 145

fear: and bodily movements, 13, 14; FEAR emotional system, 186, 189; and wonder, 9

The Feeling of What Happens (Damasio), 58, 162–63, 169, 170

feelings, xvii–xviii; and deception, 208; distinction between affects and emotions/feelings (Lacan's conception), 151; distinction between public emotions and private feelings (Damasio's conception), 163–64, 179–80; feelings-had and feelings-known, 165, 167–69; as feelings of feelings, xviii, 85; and Lacan's distinction between *honte* and *pudeur*, 157–62; misfelt (*see* feelings, misfelt); and neural maps, 52, 165; relationship amongst affects, emotions, and feelings (Freud's conception), 110–14, 164–65; relationship amongst feelings, emotions, and care for self and others (Damasio's conception), 51. *See also* affects; emotions; *Empfindungen*; passions; *specific philosophers, psychoanalysts, and neuroscientists*

feelings, misfelt, xviii, 86, 212; Damasio and, 165; and doubts raised about feelings during analysis, 140–41; and

enigmatic nature of affects, 146–47; and false connections, 107; Freud's statements on, 106–7 (*see also* Freudian metapsychology of affects); Green and, 106–7; and guilt, 90–91, 99–101, 107, 162, 212–13; and hysteria, 87, 103; Lacan and, 106–7, 141, 146–47, 152–53, 162; and shame, 162; and three destinies of quotas of affect (felt, misfelt, unfelt), 109–10; unconscious affects as, 94–95; Žižek and, 141. *See also* defense mechanisms

Fink, Bruce, 118, 119, 122, 125–26, 145

force of existing, 5, 39–40

Foucault, Michel, 192

free association, 166, 203

free will, 18

Freud, Sigmund, x, xiii, 88–101; and affects (*see* Freudian metapsychology of affects); and anxiety, 89–90, 99–101; belief in lack of symbolic activity in the nervous system, 214–15; and the brain, 60–62, 214–16, 255–56nn7,21; city of Rome analogy for psyche, 60–61, 198; and conscience, 77–78, 91–92, 95; and "criminals from a sense of guilt," 78, 92–93; dichotomy between energy and structure, 84, 102, 126; and drives, 105–6, 109, 127, 131, 213–16; on the ego, 222; focus on guilt, 78–79; Green and, 111; and hysteria, 86–87, 103–4; Kant and, 69; Lacan and, 84, 103, 119, 148–49 (*see also* Freudian-Lacanian psychoanalysis); and moral masochism, 93, 95–97; and negative therapeutic reaction, 94; and obsessive disorders, 88–89, 98–99, 103; and plasticity (capacity to preserve the past), 60–62; and pleasure principle, 95, 218; and primacy of the unconscious, 83–84; and principle of inertia, 218; and problem of

generosity, 13, 17–18, 24–25, 64
God, 36, 41–42, 44, 53
Green, André, 106–7, 111–12, 202–5
guilt, xv, xvii, 88–101, 110–13; and
    anxiety, 89–91, 99–101, 110, 212–13;
    and civilization, 97–98; feeling of
    culpability without awareness of
    transgression, 78, 91, 110, 162, 212;
    Freud's vacillations over unconscious
    sense of guilt, 78–80, 88–101, 113,
    212–13; as fundamental philosophical
    affect in relation to ethics, 77;
    guilt-in-search-of-a-crime, 78,
    92–93; and id-ego-superego triad,
    78–80, 88, 91–93, 99–101; and moral
    masochism, 93, 95–97; and need for
    punishment, 96–97, 99, 101; and
    negative therapeutic reaction, 94; and
    obsessive disorders, 88–89, 98–99;
    as penalty imposed by conscience,
    95; as potentially misfelt feeling, 107
    (see also anxiety); reasons for focus
    on, 77; and three destinies of quotas
    of affect (felt, misfelt, unfelt), 110; two
    modes of unconscious guilt (Žižek's
    conception), 162; unconscious guilt as
    instance of *Gefühl*, not *Empfindung*,
    113; unresolved questions about, 78.
    See also conscience

haptocentrism, 21
Harari, Roberto, 122, 134–35
Harvey, William, 13–14
hatred, 9, 12, 146
heart, 13–14, 21
Hegel, G. W. F., xviii, 85, 190–91
Heidegger, Martin, xi, xvi, 5–6, 20
heteroaffection, xvi, 7; auto-
    heteroaffection, 55; and biological
    basis of subjectivity, 55; and conatus,
    42; Damasio and, 34, 65–66; defined,

20–21, 63; Deleuze and, 49, 65, 68–69;
    Derrida and, 19, 20–21, 24, 25, 58,
    64–65, 68–69; and generosity, 25;
    and Nancy's nonmetaphysical sense
    of touch, 23–24; and neural maps, 55;
    and pain, 65–66; and "self-touching
    you," 24; and source of affects, 21; and
    spatiality of the psyche, 69; Spinoza
    and, 42; and wonder, 9, 11, 63–64
hetero-heteroaffection, xvi, xviii, 11
homeostasis: and autoaffection, 31,
    64; and the cerebral unconscious,
    220–21; consciousness as awareness
    of a disturbance to an organism's
    homeostasis caused by an external
    object, 30; Damasio and, 30–33,
    50–51, 64, 168–69; role of emotions
    in homeostatic regulation, 31, 50–51,
    217–18; and structure of the self, 33,
    220–23; and symbolic activity in the
    brain, 219–23
homunculus, 222–23
honte, 82, 157–62
Husserl, Edmund, xi, 20
hysteria, 86–87, 103–4
hystericization of the analysand,
    140–41, 153

icon, 47, 49
id: as intercessor between the brain and
    the psyche, 203; and SEEKING
    emotional system, 201; and spatiality
    of the psyche, 69. *See also* id-ego-
    superego triad
ideas: affects without ideas as blind/ideas
    without affects as empty, 121; ideas as
    only entities ever repressed, 155 (*see also*
    Lacan, Jacques: denial of unconscious
    affects); inextricable entanglement
    of the affective and the intellectual,
    120–22, 163; unconscious ideas, 110, 164

ideational representations, 84; affects
as aftereffects of interactions of
signifiers, 123; cross-resonating
relations between multiple
representations, 128–29; and defense
mechanisms, 103, 107–10, 125–26,
155; distinction between "affect"
(*Affekt*) and "idea" (*Vorstellung*),
102–3; and drives, 105–6; and false
connections, 107; Green and, 205;
and instincts, 214–15; Lacan and
(*see* signifiers); and misfelt feelings,
107; and obsessive disorders, 90;
priority of signifier-ideas over affects,
122–24; representation and the
confusion caused by translations of
Vorstellungsrepräsentanz, Vorstellung,
and *Repräsentanz*, 125–32. *See also*
signifiers; *Vorstellungen*
id-ego-superego triad, 101; and moral
masochism, 95–97; and possibility of
unconscious guilt, 78–80, 88, 91–93;
relation to conscious-preconscious-
unconscious triad, 78, 92; structural
dynamics between ego and superego,
92–93, 99–101; superego distinguished
from conscience, 92. *See also* ego; id;
superego
identity: conatus and origins of
personal identity, 52; personality
transformation due to brain damage,
xiii–xiv, 57–61; and the protoself,
219–20; self-model and a new
conception of materialism, 72; and the
unconscious, 92, 221
immediacy, 85–86, 134–35, 151, 192
instincts, 182, 190–91, 213
International Neuropsychoanalysis
Society, 28
intuition, 44–45, 69
Irigaray, Luce, 226n15

Jablonka, Eva, 188
Jacob, François, 176
jouis-sens (Lacan's neologism), 143–46, 165,
167, 196–98
joy: neural maps associated with, 54; as one
of six primitive passions (Descartes'
conception), 9, 12; and power of acting,
39–40, 53; Spinoza's definition, 39,
54; and states of equilibrium, 54; and
variability of conatus, 39–40; and
wonder, 40–41

Kant, Immanuel: and autoaffection, 5–6;
Freud and, 69; and intuition, 69;
Panksepp and, 190–91; and "plastic
force," 53; relationship between affects
and ideas, 121; and socialization, 196;
and subjectivity, 170
Kant and the Problem of Metaphysics
(Heidegger), 5–6
Kantbuch (Heidegger), 20
Kludge (Marcus), 176
knowledge: intuition, 44–45, 69;
knowledge from random experience,
44; knowledge from signs, 44–45;
Spinoza's conception of three kinds of
knowledge/ideas, 44–45, 66–67

Lacan, Jacques, x, 117–49, 195–200; *agalma*
and the gaze, 70–71; and alienation,
129–30; and anxiety, 82, 133, 151–52, 213;
and beauty, 160–61; contrast to Pulver,
114; Copjec and, 154–58; and deceptive
nature of signifiers and affects, 206–9;
denial of unconscious affects, 76, 84, 111,
119, 122, 129, 134, 149, 212–13; dichotomy
between the signifier and *jouissance*, 155;
distinction between "dupery" and
"deception," 207–8; and events of May '68,
154–55; formations of the unconscious,
108, 111; and free association, 166;

soul: activity and passivity of, 15, 22–23; functions of, 15; and generosity, 18; Green and, 203; passions "in" vs. passions "of," 12–18; passions "of" the soul as related to the soul alone, 15–16; and perception, 15; and pineal gland, 14–16, 21–23; and spatiality, 21–23; as two-sided instance (speaker/listener etc.), 20; and wonder, 9–11, 18. *See also* autoaffection; body-mind connection; consciousness; existence; mind; psyche; self; subjectivity; *specific philosophers*

spatiality, 21–23, 46, 64. *See also* maps, mapping; plane of immanence

Spinoza, Baruch, xvi; and active affect/ autoaffection, 45; activity and passivity, 37–41; adequate and inadequate causes, 37; affects and variability of conatus, 37–41; affects as always affects of essence, 35–36, 43–44; affects as natural ontological phenomena, 36; critique of Descartes' theory of passions, 35; definition of affects as modifications of the power of existing, 6; definition of affects related to the body's power of activity, 37, 41–42; definition of joy and sorrow, 39, 54; Descartes-Spinoza conflict, 7, 37–38; lack of knowledge of neurobiology, 54; mind and body as expressions of the same substance, 36, 37, 51; mind as the idea of the body, 51, 53; and Nature/God/Being, 36, 53; and power of acting, 38–41, 53; as protobiologist, 50, 52; Solms and, 200–201; three kinds of knowledge/ideas, 44–45, 66–67; translation of *affectio* and *affectus*, 4–5; and wonder, 8–10, 40–41. *See also* Damasio's reading of Spinoza; Deleuze's reading of Spinoza

Stanovich, Keith, 182

Studies on Hysteria (Freud and Breuer), 213–14

subject, xvi; and absence of emotions and feeling, 8, 11 (*see also* affects, detachment from/absence of); and conceptual personae, 48; and definition of autoaffection, 5–6; and heteroaffection, xvi, 7; and icons, 49; Kant on, 5–6. *See also* autoaffection

subjectivity, xvi–xvii; biological basis of, 55; and brain damage, xiii–xiv, 28, 33–34, 58; and cerebral autoaffection, 223; and denaturalization, 172–74, 178, 180–84, 187–88, 202; disembodiment of, 29–30; Kant and, 170; Lacan's barred subject ($), 151, 169–74, 187, 200; and language, 200 (*see also* language); and misfelt feelings, 86 (*see also* feelings, misfelt); neural subjectivity as a plastic structure, 26–28; and new conception of materialism, 72; and "self-touching you," 64; and time, 6; wonder and the structure of the self, 32–33; and Žižek's critique of Damasio's conception of the self, 169–72. *See also* consciousness; mind; psyche; self; soul; *specific philosophers, psychoanalysts, and neuroscientists*

superego: and civilization, 97–98; distinguished from conscience, 92; Freud's introduction of concept, 78; and moral masochism, 95–97; sadism of, 95–96, 98; and spatiality of the psyche, 69; structural dynamics between ego and superego, 92–93, 99–101; and unconscious guilt, 88, 91, 99–101, 212–13

syncope, 23–24

thought: and Deleuzian conception of autoaffection and "maps," 45; and free association, 142–43, 166; Freud's primary and secondary processes, 143–45; Lacan and, 138–39, 142–43; and perceptions, 166–67. *See also* cognition; ideational representations

Thus Spoke Zarathustra (Nietzsche), 48

time, and autoaffection, 6, 20

touch, 66–67; and activity and passivity of the soul, 22–23; Deleuze and, 66–67; Derrida and, 21–24; Nancy's nonmetaphysical sense of touch, 23–24; "touching-touched" relationship between me and myself (Merleau-Ponty's schema), 66, 67. *See also* self-touching

On Touching (Derrida), 21, 64–65, 68

Turnbull, Oliver, 27–28, 186, 201–2

unconscious: and the brain, 71, 219–21; and conscience, 78–79, 91–92; Damasio and, 163–68, 179–80; and death, 223; and defense mechanisms, 104–10, 124 (*see also* repression); discovery as revolutionary breakthrough, 83–84, 148–49; distinction between psychoanalytic unconscious and term as used in neuroscience, 177–78; Freud and (*see* Freud, Sigmund; Freudian metapsychology of affects); and id-ego-superego triad, 78–80, 92–93, 99–101; Lacan and, 82–83, 108, 119, 124–44, 155, 179–80, 208; and *lalangue* neologism, 143–45; LeDoux and, 188; as negative term for a positive *x*, 209; Panksepp and, 188; and personal identity, 92; and potential-to-feel, 108–9; repression and the confusion caused by translations of *Vorstellungsrepräsentanz, Vorstellung,* and *Repräsentanz,* 125–32; slips of the tongue, jokes, etc., 143, 196; and

spatiality of the psyche, 69–70; unconscious sense of guilt (*see* guilt); and *Vorstellungen* as signifiers, 122. *See also* affects, unconscious

"unpleasure principle," 187

virtue, 17–18, 41

vision, 62

Vorstellungen: confusion caused by translations of *Vorstellungsrepräsentanz, Vorstellung,* and *Repräsentanz,* 125–32, 136–37; Green and, 205; and inextricable entanglement of the affective and the intellectual, 121–22; as Lacan's signifiers, 119, 122, 129; and *lalangue* neologism, 143; and obsessive disorders, 90; and the unconscious, 122. *See also* ideational representations

Vorstellungsrepräsentanz, 125–32, 136–37

warfare, 132

What Is Philosophy? (Deleuze), 43, 48, 67

wonder, xv–xvi, 225n10; and alterity, 10; as ambivalent affect, 64; and autoaffection, 9–11, 63–64; and brain damage, 11, 33, 60; Damasio and, 11, 32–33, 64; deconstruction of, 10–11; defined, 8–9, 16; Deleuze and, 64, 71; Deleuze's reading of Descartes and, 47–48; Derrida and, 11, 23–25, 64, 71; Descartes and, 8–9, 12, 16–18, 25; and facial expressions, 47–48; and fear, 9; function of, 17; and generosity, 17–18, 24–25; and heteroaffection, 9, 11, 63–64; impaired capacity for, 10–11, 17, 33, 60, 64; as intermediary between passion and thought, 47; Lacan and, 70–71; nonjudgmental nature of, 17, 18; as source driving philosophizing, 77; Spinoza and, 8–10, 40–41; and the structure of the self, 32–33; and virtue, 41

Žižek, Slavoj: critique of Damasio, 169–74, 179–84, 190; and debate between naturalism and antinaturalism, 180–84, 190; LeDoux and, 174–79, 190; life 2.0, life 1.0, 172–73, 192–94, 197–98; and misfelt feelings, 141

Žižek's Ontology: A Transcendental Materialist Theory of Subjectivity (Johnston), 170

zoē, 192–93

Printed in the USA
CPSIA information can be obtained
at www.ICGtesting.com
JSHW021436221024
72172JS00002B/16